Psychosexual Medicine

Psychosexual Medicine
An introduction

Second edition

Edited by

Ruth Skrine MA MBChB MRCGP

Member of the Institute of Psychosexual Medicine,
Former GP and SCMO Psychosexual Medicine, Bath

Heather Montford MBBS DRCOG

Member of the Institute of Psychosexual Medicine,
SCMO Psychosexual Medicine and Reproductive Healthcare,
SW London Community NHS Trust

A member of the Hodder Headline Group
LONDON • NEW YORK • NEW DELHI

First published in Great Britain in 2001 by
Arnold, a member of the Hodder Headline Group,
338 Euston Road, London NW1 3BH

http://www.arnoldpublishers.com

Distributed in the USA by
Oxford University Press Inc.,
198 Madison Avenue, New York, NY10016
Oxford is a registered trademark of Oxford University Press

© 2001 Arnold

British Library Cataloguing in Publication Data
A catalogue record for this book is available from the British Library

Library of Congress Cataloging-in-Publication Data
A catalog record for this book is available from the Library of Congress

ISBN 0 340 76142 3

1 2 3 4 5 6 7 8 9 10

Publisher: Jo Koster
Development Editor: Paula O'Connell
Production Editor: James Rabson
Production Controller: Iain McWilliams
Cover Design: Terry Griffiths

Typeset in 10/12pt Palatino by Integra Software Services Pvt Ltd, Pondicherry, India; www.integra-india.com
Printed and bound in Great Britain by The Bath Press, Bath

What do you think about this book? Or any other Arnold title?
Please send your comments to feedback.arnold@hodder.co.uk

Contents

Contributors

Jane Botell MB ChB DFFP
Member of Institute of Psychosexual Medicine
SCMO Psychosexual Medicine
Southampton and Isle of Wight

Tessa Crowley MB BS DFFP
Member of the Institute of Psychosexual
Medicine
Associate Specialist in GUM
Bristol Royal Infirmary
Bristol

Marian Davis MB ChB MRCGP
Member of Institute of Psychosexual Medicine
General Practitioner
Herefordshire
and
SCMO Psychosexual Medicine
Shropshire Community and Mental Health Trust

Margaret Denman MB ChB DRCOG
Member of Institute of Psychosexual Medicine
General Practitioner
Oxford

Sue Field MRCOG
Member of Institute of Psychosexual Medicine
Consultant Obstetrician and Gynaecologist
Queen Elizabeth Hospital
Gateshead

Margaret Gill MB BS MRCS LRCP MFFP
Member of Institute of Psychosexual Medicine
SCMO Hillingdon Primary Care Trust
Bournewood Community and Mental
Health Trust

Helen Hutchinson MB BS MFFP
Member of Institute of Psychosexual Medicine
SCMO Family Planning and Psychosexual
Medicine
Addenbrooke's NHS Trust
Cambridge

Marek Miller MD FRCS
Consultant Urological Surgeon
Northampton General Hospital
Northampton

Michael Pawson MB BS FRCOG
Consultant Gynaecologist
Chelsea and Westminster Hospital
London

Janet Perrin MB ChB MRCS LRCP
Member of the Institute of Psychosexual
Medicine
SCMO North Bristol NHS Trust,
United Bristol Hospitals Trust and
Worcestershire Community Mental
Health Trust

Roseanna Pollen MSc MB BS MRCGP
Member of the Institute of Psychosexual
Medicine
General Practitioner
London

Merryl Roberts MB ChB MFFP
Member of Institute of Psychosexual Medicine
SCMO and Clinical Lead in Reproductive
Health
East Kent Community NHS Trust

Andrew Stainer-Smith MA MB BChir MRCP
MRCGP
Member of Institute of Psychosexual Medicine
General Practitioner and Hospital Practitioner
Royal Devon and Exeter (Wonford) Hospital
Exeter

Anne Smith MB BS
Member of Institute of Psychosexual Medicine
Senior Partner in General Practice
SCMO Psychosexual Medicine
Newcastle-upon-Tyne
and
Director of Training
Institute of Psychosexual Medicine

Gillian Vanhegan MB BS DRCOG MFFP
Member of Institute of Psychosexual Medicine
Specialist in Psychosexual Medicine
Medical Director, Brook Advisory Centres
London

Gill Wakley MB ChB MFFP
Member of Institute of Psychosexual Medicine
Primary Care Development Tutor
Staffordshire University
and

SCMO Psychosexual Medicine and
Reproductive Health Care
North Stafford Hospital NHS Trust

Susan Walker MB BS MRCGP MRCS LRCP
DCH MFHOM
Member of Institute of Psychosexual Medicine
General Practitioner
Bath

Lynne Webster FRCPsych
Consultant Psychiatrist
Manchester Royal Infirmary
Manchester

Jane Whitmore MB BS MFFP
Member of Institute of Psychosexual Medicine
Consultant in Family Planning and
Reproductive Health
St Helens and Knowsley

Josephine Woolf MA BM BCh MRCGP DRCOG
Member of Institute of Psychosexual Medicine
Associate Specialist in Psychosexual Medicine
Royal Free Hospital
London

Part One
Principles of Psychosexual Medicine

Introduction

Sex is a psychosomatic activity; it involves the body and the mind. Psychosexual medicine is psychosomatic medicine applied to sexual disorders. It is a specific form of body–mind doctoring where both physical and psychological factors are considered together.

Psychosexual medicine, as practised by the authors of this book, is based on the work of the psychoanalysts Dr Michael Balint and Dr Tom Main, but remains firmly rooted in the medical tradition. The Institute of Psychosexual Medicine, which trains doctors in the use of the required skills, was founded in 1974.

Since the first edition of this book was published in 1989, there have been important changes in the treatment of sexual disorders. New physical treatments have become available and further developments in physical treatments for both men and women are likely. In the medical profession as a whole, a more holistic approach is considered good practice. There is a growing recognition that many physical symptoms may be associated with or caused by sexual difficulties. The expectation for a happy and fulfilling sex life continues to increase and with it the demands of patients for a sympathetic and informed response from the medical profession.

Although primarily written for doctors, this new edition aims also to provide other health workers with an overall introduction to the subject of psychosexual medicine. It is written particularly for those who meet patients with sexual difficulties in the course of their everyday work in a variety of different settings. It will also act as an introduction for those who wish to specialize in the subject.

In recent years most doctors will have received some training in consultation skills, including those of observation, listening and being aware of the possibility of a 'hidden agenda'. Counselling, which seeks to provide an empathetic environment to enable clients to verbalize their innermost feelings and accept their situation with less anxiety and tension, is seen as the necessary accompaniment to any situation of stress. Psychosexual medicine, while embracing both consultation and counselling skills, also uses a specific psychodynamic approach which allows the patient's unconscious feelings and fantasies behind the physical symptoms to be made known and understood. Those who present their sexual problems to doctors generally believe that their problem may have, in whole or in part, a physical cause. They usually present alone rather than together with a partner.

Doctors not only have a licence but also a duty to examine the body to exclude organic disease. It has been shown that it is at this most vulnerable moment that a patient's fears and fantasies about their sexuality or sexual parts are most often revealed. The physical examination becomes a psychosomatic event where both body and mind can be studied together. In this respect, psychosexual medicine as described here differs from other forms of sex therapy, often practised by non-doctors, where behavioural and cognitive methods usually involving the couple are employed. However, each mode of treatment is not entirely exclusive. Just as those who employ more directive methods, who give the patient and their partner sexual tasks to reduce anxiety, will also study the feelings arising in the consultation, so psychosexual doctors may sometimes find it helpful to give directive advice and may see patients together as a couple on occasion.

The book consists of three parts. The first part opens with an account of the physical aspects of the sexual response. Because of the immense amount of recent research on the subject, the complex issues regarding the male sexual response are described in some detail. These chapters are followed by the consideration of psychological factors, and the interaction between physical and psychological causes. Presentation and management are discussed, followed by a description of the skills that make up the practice of psychosexual medicine. The relevance of past history and the problems arising as a result of life events are explored.

The second part of the book is devoted to a consideration of some specific sexual difficulties, and contains a chapter on disorders of sexual preference and gender identity. In the final section, the practical considerations of working in different clinical settings are explored.

Some readers may wish to start at the beginning. Others may find it more rewarding to explore an individual symptom, or to start with one of the chapters about the setting in which they work. The chapter on presentation and management is aimed at the less experienced doctor, while some of the more complicated issues arising in general practice are explored later. Readers unfamiliar with the skills of psychosexual medicine will find them fully described in chapter 6. However, these skills are demonstrated throughout the book.

This is not a book about how to do it. Psychosexual medicine is a skill that can only be learned, not taught. Each encounter with each patient is unique, and from every new encounter we can learn something more.

> Not that many useful things might be learned by that book but...that art was not to be taught by words, but practice.
>
> Izaak Walton

The method of training with the Institute of Psychosexual Medicine is described in the Appendix.

Heather Montford
Ruth Skrine

1 Physical aspects of the female sexual response

Michael Pawson

This chapter will assume that the reader has a basic knowledge of the anatomy of the female genital tract. The female sexual response will be discussed using the Masters and Johnson (1966) paradigm of four phases of sexual response: excitement, plateau, orgasm and resolution. It was Masters and Johnson who made sexuality a subject that could be looked at clinically and scientifically. Whilst the importance of the psychological and emotional aspects of sexuality had been recognized for a long time, clinical observation of sexual behaviour and response had not been seriously studied. Sexual problems present in many different guises to the gynaecologist and general practitioner, as well as to the psychiatrist, psychosexual doctor and counsellor. A knowledge and understanding of the anatomy and physiology of the female sexual response is an essential basis for any practitioner within these areas.

ANATOMY

Figure 1.1 is to provide basic reference points only. There are certain points in relation to the anatomy which are, however, helpful to emphasize.

The clitoris

Only the glans of the clitoris is visible. The clitoris, like the penis, is composed of corpus spongiosum and corpora cavernosa and is therefore

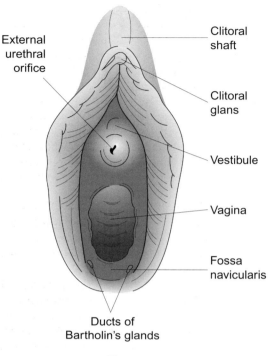

External
urethral
orifice

Clitoral
shaft

Clitoral
glans

Vestibule

Vagina

Fossa
navicularis

Ducts of
Bartholin's glands

Figure 1.1

an erectile organ. It is anchored at its base to the pubic bone. There is a rich sensory nerve supply to the clitoris. The clitoris has no other function than to act as the receptor of sexual stimuli as part of the sensory arm of the female orgasmic reflex.

The vagina

The vagina is an important structure for its role in sexual expression, but it is also essential for natural conception and birth. The upper part of the vagina is capacious; the lower one-third of the vagina is firmer and tighter because of the levator ani and perineal muscles. Histology of the anterior vaginal wall shows free nerve endings in the epithelium forming plexuses around blood vessels. The highest concentration of nerve plexuses is between the bladder and the vaginal wall. The urethra is embedded in the anterior vaginal wall and laterally and

anteriorly is surrounded by some erectile tissue. It is the response of this erectile tissue that causes the secretion of clear fluid from the urethra, which Grafenburg described as the female ejaculate.

The upper vagina is derived embryologically from the Mullerian ducts, which generally have a poor sensory supply. The lower vagina, clitoris and introitus are supplied by the pelvic plexus of nerves and are much more sensitive.

The anterior wall of the vagina, with its higher concentration of nerve plexuses and ganglia, is much more sensitive to pressure and sensory stimuli under both erotic and non-erotic conditions than the lateral and posterior walls. However, under non-erotic conditions, it remains less sensitive to electrical stimuli than the skin on the dorsum of the hand.

Zwi Hoch (1986) found the whole of the anterior vaginal wall to be erotically sensitive. Most writers remain unimpressed by the presence of a 'G' (or Grafenburg) spot, and this is not surprising as the concentration of nerve supply is widespread along the mid-line of the anterior wall.

It is reported widely that the anterior vaginal wall is sensitive to digital pressure under erotic conditions. Whilst occasionally some women report the anterior vaginal wall as being more sensitive than the clitoris, the clitoris remains more sensitive for the great majority.

THE FEMALE ORGASMIC REFLEX

The sensory arms of this reflex are the clitoris and the anterior vagina. The motor arm is a circum-vaginal muscular discharge manifested by contractions of the pubo-coccygeus muscle. Pre-coital and coital stimulation does help some women achieve intra-coital orgasm. The argument raised by Freud that vaginal orgasm is more 'mature' than clitoral orgasm, is now outdated. We now recognize the importance of both clitoris and vagina and the best term to use is 'genital orgasm'.

THE SEXUAL RESPONSE

Arousal can be mediated through a number of different pathways:

1. **Local genital areas**, the clitoris and vagina in particular, but also other sites such as the nipples.
2. **The nervous system**. Visual and olfactory stimuli are potent arousal senses. Stimulation of centres within the brain in animals can cause erection and ejaculation. The basic physiological response for sexual stimuli of widespread vasocongestion and later myotonia fits with early parasympathetic followed by sympathetic activity. The hypothalamus is the mediator of such responses and in sexual disorders is clearly affected by higher centres (e.g. anxiety).
3. **Hormones**. It is clear that hormones trigger sexual responses in many mammalian groups that only mate when fertile. In primates this activity can be reproduced in female castrates subsequently given hormones to mimic the cycle. Hormone fluctuations during the menstrual cycle, pregnancy and the peri-menopause, as well as hormonal treatment such as 'the pill', may influence sexual behaviour and responses. This may be through a direct effect on the brain and hypothalamus affecting the sexual response directly or by inducing mood changes. Hormones may act directly on the genitalia inducing a vasocongestion similar to a state of sexual arousal and may increase sexual attractiveness by a secretion of pheromones. Testosterone appears to be important in the libido of both male and female, and prenatal levels of hormone may affect later sexual behaviour. As one progresses up the evolutionary ladder, hormones are of decreasing importance, and psychological and environmental factors are of increasing importance, in sexual behaviour.

Bancroft (1983) uses the analogy of hunger and appetite in discussing the human sexual response. Hunger stimulates the search for food. As Pavlov so famously demonstrated, appetite is stimulated not only by the need for food but also by sensory perceptions associated with eating, which include smell, sight, sharing and habit or constant repetition. As there are both biological and psychological aspects to hunger and appetite, so there are to sexual arousal.

Sexual stimuli are perceived centrally through the brain and are termed psychic-stimuli. Sensory perception through the skin is a reflexive stimulus that is present even where there has been spinal cord transection.

As appetite and hunger may vary if one is ill or has just eaten, so the intrinsic ability and desire to respond sexually will vary according to libido, central arousal, peripheral arousal and genital responses.

Higher levels in the brain are important in sexual response. It was a French Prime Minister who said that the most exciting and intense moment in a sexual relationship was when she had said 'Yes' and they were going up the stairs. Continuing the appetite analogy, Winnie-the-Pooh likewise said that the best moment with a pot of honey was when the lid was off and the pot was full.

- The clitoris and, to a lesser extent, the anterior vaginal wall form the sensory arm of the orgasmic reflex.
- Sexual stimuli are perceived locally and centrally.
- Sexual perception involves all senses, including visual and olfactory.
- Hormones are less important in human sexual behaviour than psychological and environmental factors.

PHASES OF SEXUAL RESPONSE

Masters and Johnson describe four phases of sexual response. We will not be considering the emotional and psychological responses in this chapter, but of course the psyche and soma are of equal importance in sexual behaviour.

1. **Excitement phase.** This earliest phase of response can be initiated by psychological or physical stimuli, or both.
2. **Plateau phase.** Physical stimulus is now more important and must continue if orgasm is to be achieved.
3. **Orgasm.** In the female this is of varying intensity.
4. **Resolution.** In this phase the female is capable of returning to orgasm but the male is not.

Excitement phase

Vasocongestion of the external genitalia occurs within 30 seconds of the initiating stimulus, whether it is a psychogenic or physical stimulus. The clitoris and labia become engorged and erect and there may be accompanying colour changes especially in the labia minora. The tumescence of the clitoris always occurs but may not always be detectable. The labia majora flatten and appear to open out.

There is a rapid transudate that develops within the vagina, even after total hysterectomy and bilateral salpingo-oophorectomy, and it is dependent upon blood flow. This transudate will develop even in those who have an artificial vagina. The cervix and Bartholin's glands are unimportant in vaginal lubrication. This transudate reduces friction during coitus and increases the partial pressure of oxygen in the vaginal epithelium, providing more energy for sperm activity. The dilatation of the venous plexuses within the vagina and vestibule narrow the lower one-third of the vagina, forming the so-called 'turgid cuff'. The uterus also begins to engorge.

Vasodilatation also leads to erection of the nipples and engorgement of the areolar breast tissue. A slight superficial pink flush may spread over the breasts, abdomen and limbs, described by Masters and Johnson as 'the sex flush'.

Plateau phase

At the end of the excitement phase and into the plateau, the vagina continues to lengthen and distend. The turgid cuff of the distal end of the vagina increases. The elevation of the uterus continues and with the expansion of the proximal end of the vagina forms the 'tenting' or 'ballooning' effect of the upper vagina.

During this phase the clitoris normally retracts. This may mislead the male partner into believing that the sexual response is waning.

Orgasm

The female orgasm has no recognizable end point and, like pain, is an ill-defined subjective experience that is impossible to assess. It is both psychophysiological and physical in the development of myotonia and the release of vasocongestion and is a total body response that varies widely. The female experiences orgasm a few seconds before it is physiologically expressed. The turgid cuff or orgasmic platform of the distal vagina contracts regularly and briefly, and varies according to the length of the orgasm. Occasionally, the anal sphincter also contracts.

The uterus contracts during orgasm and this may be cramp-like and painful. Other voluntary and involuntary muscle contractions occur in the limbs, hands, feet, face, abdomen and buttocks. Older women in particular may experience stress incontinence at orgasm, a very distressing symptom. There is a transitory rise in blood pressure, tachycardia and hyperventilation during orgasm.

The female is capable of prolonging orgasm up to 60 seconds and can return to orgasm rapidly if she is stimulated further before her state of arousal has faded too much. The intensity of orgasm for most females is greater at masturbation, but for most is not as fulfilling as coital orgasm.

The orgasm phase starts with an intense focusing of awareness on the clitoris with a sensation of what has been described as 'receptive opening'. This is followed by a feeling of warmth, suffusing first through the pelvis and then through the whole body. The final sensation of the orgasm phase is that of approximately five involuntary vaginal and pelvic contractions.

Resolution phase

There is usually a rapid return to the normal anatomical and physiological state. The vaso-congestion and myotonia resolve, the uterus descends, the cervix dropping into the seminal pool in the ballooned upper vagina. This is less obvious in the multiparous woman than the nulliparous. This resolution phase is much quicker if the female has achieved orgasm.

Studies in prostitutes who repeatedly experience excitement and plateau phases, but do not achieve orgasm, suggest that the pelvic vessels may become increasingly congested, leading to pain or discomfort. This can be relieved by masturbating to orgasm.

Resolution of the vasocongestion may take some hours if orgasm has not been reached. The experience of orgasm is very pleasurable and serves the purpose of being an experience that both male and female want to repeat. In this way it encourages reproduction and continuation of the species. But the experience of female orgasm *per se* is not related to fertility, nor is it necessary for conception.

The above description of the whole female sexual response is based on the observations that Masters and Johnson reported. Recording these details is clearly very difficult indeed, and the authors acknowledge the artificiality of the circumstances of their subjects and the inaccuracy of measuring changes in uterine size and vaginal shape by clinical examination.

Weijmar Schultz *et al.* (1999) have now reported on the first MRI scans to be taken during coitus. They have shown that in complete penetration the penis is boomerang-shaped, reaches up to the mid-sacrum or even sacral promontory and on average measures 22 cm root to tip. The penis fills up the whole of either the anterior or posterior fornix.

They were able to confirm the lengthening of the anterior vaginal wall, upward displacement of the uterus and filling of the bladder. There was no change in the position of the uterus other than upwards unless caused by the penis. Furthermore, they were unable to demonstrate any enlargement of the uterus. Masters and Johnson's assessment of the uterine size was made by manual examination and the bladder filling and elevation of the uterus may have influenced their observations.

SEXUAL RESPONSE IN ADOLESCENCE

The age of first sexual experience is getting younger throughout the western world. In the United States, one in five girls have had their first sexual experience by the age of 15 and in the United Kingdom the same number by the age of 16, which is the legal age of consent. In parts of the United States, 50 per cent of Afro-American males are sexually active by the age of 13. One in 10 American teenagers gets pregnant every year and of these pregnancies half are aborted. In those pregnancies that continue, the baby is at greater risk of the effects of social deprivation, low birth weight, maternal drug taking and so on. And so the cycle continues.

Everyone reading this will have experience of seeing adolescent girls who have conceived, not from a biological urge, but to try to do better than the mess their own parents have made of their lives. If they are not going to be loved by their parents, they will have a baby that will compensate by needing and loving them.

There are many factors that influence sexual experimentation among today's adolescents. These include peer pressure, the media and the need for love and security in a society where the nuclear family is breaking down. These issues are discussed further in chapter 8.

SEXUAL RESPONSE IN THE MENSTRUAL CYCLE

The sexual behaviour of animals is very closely related to the hormone cycle. The female is active during oestrous alone and if ovariectomized has no sexual interest at all. Hormones may inhibit sexual activity as well as stimulate it.

The evidence as to sexual activity during the human menstrual cycle is puzzling and conflicting. Retrospective questionnaires suggest an increase in coitus pre- and post-menstrually and there appears to be no increase in sexual activity at the time of ovulation, contrary to what one would expect. It is clearly very difficult to differentiate between sexual desire and responding to male demands, especially as most females prefer to abstain from coitus during menstruation. It may also be that these times are perceived to be part of the 'safe period'.

Prospective diary records indicate increased sexual activity on day 8 and 26 of the cycle, confirming the retrospective findings. However, there is a variation related to culture and peri-menstrual sex is commoner in middle-class white women. Working-class black women and single white women have coitus more frequently about the time of ovulation. Analysis of dreams shows that the sexual content of dreams is highest during menstruation. It is at this time that hormones are at their lowest, so why should this be? Could it be associated with abstinence during menstruation?

Vaginal blood flow responds less to erotic stimuli in the peri-ovulatory time than peri-menstrually. It is suggested that this may be because testosterone is highest around ovulation. But testosterone is important in libido. The evidence relating to sexual response in relation to the hormone cycle is indeed conflicting.

Menstruation

Most women prefer to abstain from coitus during menstruation, although increased libido is reported occasionally. The cervix has been observed during orgasm at menstruation and spurts of menstrual flow reported, presumably in association with uterine contractions. It has been suggested that coitus during menstruation may shorten the duration of bleeding and may increase the risk of endometriosis; the mechanism being uterine contractions expelling

blood and endometrium either through the cervix or retrogradely through the fallopian tubes (Cutler *et al.*, 1996).

SEXUAL RESPONSE ON THE CONTRACEPTIVE PILL

Women taking the combined oral contraceptive pill have a constant level of hormones, except during the withdrawal bleed. We have already stated that the sexual cycle, if it exists, appears to be peri-menstrual rather than peri-ovulatory, so suppressing ovulation might be expected to make no difference in sexual response. The evidence is again conflicting, but for the majority there is little change in sexual activity when taking oral contraception. There is a small but significant number who get depressed, which reduces their libido. Some also report reduced libido without depression; maybe removing the reproductive purpose of coitus is responsible for this. There are also some who report increased sexual activity on the pill, presumably associated with the lifting of the anxiety in relation to unwanted conception and removing the unacceptable aspects of alternative contraception.

SEXUAL RESPONSE IN PREGNANCY

There is no cycle during pregnancy, but there are dramatic hormonal and emotional changes. There are many taboos surrounding sex and pregnancy, some of which still find their way into books on pregnancy for the lay-public.

The breasts start to increase in size early in pregnancy and the additional increase in size caused by sexual stimulation can be uncomfortable. In a state of high sexual arousal, the breasts can be quite painful. This is less of a problem in the second and third trimester than the first, because the female is now accustomed to the changes in her breasts. In late pregnancy and the puerperium, occasional spurts of milk have been reported during orgasm.

The genital organs are much more congested during pregnancy and there is a very marked increase in vaginal lubrication. The uterus is more irritable in pregnancy, and many women find the uterine contractions during orgasm more painful throughout pregnancy. In the last trimester, uterine contractions during orgasm can be tonic and have been timed to last as long as 60 seconds. There may even be a brief associated foetal bradycardia. It has been postulated that the pregnant uterus may be more sensitive to seminal prostaglandins than the non-pregnant.

Masters and Johnson reported on sexual responses in pregnancy based on interviews and also on studying six pregnant women having coitus in laboratory conditions. Of the latter, all reported an increase in sexual arousal in the second trimester and a greater facility for multiple orgasm. The authors suggest this could be due to increased pelvic congestion, but one must question whether such subjects are truly representative.

In the first trimester there is a wide variation in sexuality. In general, primiparous women and those who have lost previous pregnancies report a reduced sexual activity. They are afraid of harming and losing this pregnancy and they may feel nauseated and unwell. The response is much the same for multiparous women, although they may be less concerned about potential harm to the baby.

In the second trimester, it is generally agreed that there is a marked increase in arousal, libido and performance, not only in relation to the first trimester but often also in relation to the non-pregnant state. There is a tendency to have a more intense incremental sexual response.

Sexual activity generally declines in the third trimester and this is very unlikely to be hormonal. The reasons are multiple and include physical awkwardness, fatigue and fear of premature labour. Women may also have been advised against sex on medical grounds. In addition to this, the male partner may be nervous, or may find his partner sexually unattractive in late pregnancy.

Post-partum

Sexual behaviour post delivery is closely related to previous sexual behaviour, and sexual desire returns post-natally often before the cycle returns, confirming again that a cycle is essential for neither libido nor sex. The response, of course, varies according to important physical factors. The suturing of a tear or episiotomy, the degree of lochia and discharge, tiredness, a degree of post-partum depression, anxiety about the baby and so on, all reduce interest in resuming the sexual life.

The reduced interest in sex post-partum usually continues for about three months, but there is evidence that women who breastfeed have a more rapid return to sexuality. Some who breastfeed get quite marked sexual stimulation from nipple erection and suckling. The release of oxytocin caused by suckling may cause uterine contractions similar to those of orgasm.

The whole subject of sex during pregnancy and the puerperium is complex. The psyche is more important than hormones and individual behaviour varies very widely.

SEXUAL RESPONSE IN THE MENOPAUSE AND AFTER

Until recently, ageing females have been an ignored group, but there is no reason why they should not desire and enjoy a fulfilling sexual life. As in all other phases in life there are wide variations in sexual activity in this group but, generally, if sex was happy and good before the menopause, it will continue to be so after the menopause. Some women, free from the fear of pregnancy, become more active; some, affected by physiological changes, become less active.

Data from Hite (1976) suggest that there is little change after the age of 60. Others, such as Pfeiffer and Verwoerdt (1972), suggest a gradual but steady decline in interest after the menopause. The data of Kinsey et al. (1953) showed regular intercourse and successful orgasm until 55, after which there was a decline related to age, but this is often closely associated with the health of the husband.

Physiological response

In the breasts, nipple erection remains an obvious and early response to stimulation. The breasts, however, are less elastic and more fibrous, and vasocongestion diminishes and does not occur after 60. Areola engorgement follows a very similar pattern.

The clitoris may shrink a little after 60, but remains a highly sensitive receptor and transformer of sexual stimuli. Tumescence occurs readily in the excitement phase and subsequent retraction also occurs. Vasocongestion of the labia does reduce progressively with age and the reduction in fatty tissue of the mons and labia does mean that the clitoris may be hypersensitive and painful in direct contact.

The epithelial atrophy which occurs in the vagina post-menopausally is well recognized, but there is also vaginal shrinking. Once five years post-menopause, the changes become very marked. The rapid youthful vaginal transudate response of less than 30 seconds gradually lengthens and after the age of 60 may take up to three minutes or even longer. This is partly because of reduced physiological responses in both female and male, but also because of actual vaginal tissue atrophy and low oestrogen levels. Enjoyment of regular intercourse after the menopause, even in the absence of hormone replacement, can prolong the efficiency of the lubrication response considerably. This appears to be true of all the other aspects of sexual response.

The elevation of the uterus and therefore also the expansion and ballooning effect of the upper vagina are progressively reduced after the menopause. Contractions of the uterus and of the orgasmic platform are fewer and, although the orgasmic phase is briefer, uterine contractions may be distressing and spasm may occur. This is associated with low oestrogen levels and is corrected by hormone replacement.

The resolution phase after the menopause is rapid.

Clinical considerations of the post-menopausal woman

Atrophy of the vagina leads to discharge, bleeding, dyspareunia and reduced lubrication. Associated with these symptoms may be urinary problems, such as recurrent cystitis and the distressing symptom of stress incontinence on orgasm. These symptoms naturally reduce libido. Hormone replacement will correct or alleviate the physical symptoms, make the female feel better about herself and is of great benefit in managing sexual difficulties after the menopause. Whilst the intensity of the sexual response does decrease with age, there is no decline in the ability to function, and the female can enjoy a very effective sexual life up to 70 and beyond. The response is sustained by hormone replacement, but is also maintained by regular sexual activity. Some women do go on producing reasonable levels of oestrogen even after the menopause, and those that have coitus regularly, especially if orgasmic, appear to maintain good lubrication and have less vaginal atrophy.

The decline in sexual activity with age is often more to do with the male than the female and the gradual development of impotence is important. Other reasons include boredom, the problems of sheer physical effort, sexual disinterest because there is no longer a reproductive potential and, in the case of the male, anxiety about performance. Cultural attitudes such as 'sex is for the young and beautiful only' are inhibitory.

Women who have lost a sexual partner in older age and have remained inactive for some time suffer from 'disuse vaginal atrophy'. It is much more difficult in later age to establish a new sexual relationship because of vaginal shrinkage and older women in this situation can be reassured that sexual activity does not always have to culminate in penetrative intercourse.

KEY POINTS

- The female sexual response is still poorly understood, the assessment being dependent on subjective reporting and crude objective observation.
- It is complex, involving local and central stimuli with very powerful psychosocial and environmental influences.
- It is able to be enjoyed from adolescence to old age.
- It is not strongly influenced by hormonal status, except post-menopausally when hormone replacement is beneficial.
- It is divided into four phases (EPOR) and a whole body response.
- Local stimuli are perceived through the sensory arm of the orgasmic reflex, the clitoris and anterior vaginal wall.

REFERENCES

Bancroft, J. 1983: *Human sexuality and its problems.* London: Churchill Livingstone.

Cutler, W.B., Friedman, E. and McCoy, N.L. 1996: Coitus and menstruation in perimenopausal women. *Journal of Psychosomatic Obstetrics and Gynaecology* 17(3), 149–57.

Hite, S. 1976: *The Hite report.* London: Talmy Franklin.

Hoch, Z. 1986: Vaginal erotic sensitivity by sexual examination. *Acta Obstetrica et Gynecologica Scandinavica* 5, 767–73.

Kinsey, A.C., Pomeroy, W.B., Martin, C.E. and Gebhard, P.H. 1953: *Sexual behaviour in the human female.* Philadelphia: W.B. Saunders.

Masters, W.H. and Johnson, V.E. 1966: *Human sexual response.* Boston: Little Brown.

Pfeiffer, E. and Verwoerdt, A. 1972: Determinants of sexual behaviour in middle and old age. *Journal American Geriatric Society* 20, 151–58.

Schulz, W.W., van Andel, P., Sabelis, I. and Mooyart, E. 1999: Magnetic resonance imaging of the male and female genitals during coitus and female sexual arousal. *British Medical Journal* 319, 1596–600.

FURTHER READING

Feldman, P. and MacCulloch, M. 1980: *Human sexual behaviour.* London: Wiley.

McCauley, E.A. and Erhardt, A.A. 1980: Female sexual response. In Youngs, D.D. and Erhardt, A.A. (eds), *Psychosomatic obstetrics and gynaecology.* New York: Appleton-Century-Crofts, 39–66.

2 Physical aspects of the male sexual response

Marek Miller

Disorders of the male sexual response, particularly erectile dysfunction (ED), are common and distressing. Attitudes to sexual behaviour have varied over the years, but workers such as Freud, Masters and Johnson, and Hite have contributed to liberalization, culminating in the 'sexual revolution' of the 1960s. Nevertheless, it is only comparatively recently that it has become acceptable to talk about male impotence. There has been an explosion in the basic science research effort devoted to this subject and knowledge of the physiological and biochemical events underpinning erection advances daily, bringing with it the possibility of formulating novel therapeutic interventions, if not also the advent of preventative measures.

The mechanisms of penile erection are complicated and, despite the intensive research effort, they remain incompletely understood.

The male sexual response and erection is dependent upon the integrated action of anatomical, vascular, neural, psychological and endocrine factors. There appear to be three main types of erection in man: reflex, psychogenic and nocturnal. It is the combination of psychogenic and neurogenic mechanisms that brings about normal erectile activity. Major advances have taken place over the past decade in our understanding of the physiology of normal erection and the pathogenesis of ED. The present chapter is concerned with the mechanisms of the normal male sexual response.

PENILE ANATOMY

The erectile tissues of the penis are found in the paired corpora cavernosa and the corpus

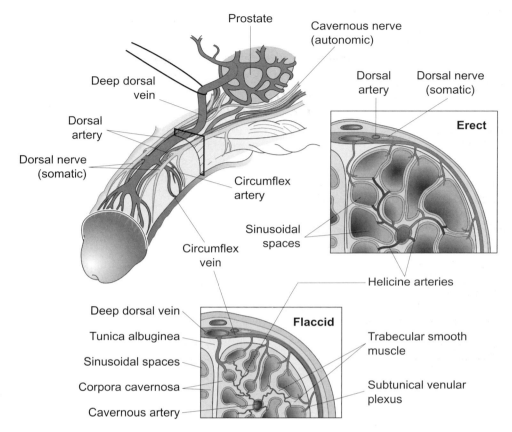

Figure 2.1   Penile anatomy and the mechanism of penile erection.

spongiosum (Fig. 2.1). The corpus spongiosum surrounds the urethra; distally it forms the glans penis. The corpora cavernosa are joined by a thin midline septum, they separate proximally to form the crura, which are covered inferiorly by the ischiocavernosus muscle.

Proximally, the bulb of the penis is covered by the bulbocavernosus muscle. Distally, each cavernosal body terminates within the glans penis, which thus forms a cap over them.

The corpora are encased by a fibrous sheath, the tunica albuginea, which is composed of collagen and elastin. The fibres of the tunica albuginea pass around each corpus cavernosum and unite medially to form the pectiniform septum of the penis. The septum is fenestrated distally, thus allowing for the free commu-

nication of blood flow between the erectile chambers. The outermost fibres of the tunica albuginea form a covering around both corpora cavernosa.

The corporeal parenchyma consists of a trabecular meshwork formed by smooth muscle fibre bundles, endothelial cells, fibroblasts and a collagenous extracellular matrix. This criss-crossing pattern creates the vascular spaces known as lacunar spaces or sinusoids, which are lined by endothelial cells and surrounded in turn by smooth muscle cells. It is this arrangement which accounts for the spongy nature of the penile tissues.

Electron microscopy of the erectile tissues has demonstrated gap junctions in human corpus cavernosum. These gap junctions are responsible for the rapid transmission of neural or hormonal stimulation, enabling the human corpus cavernosum to behave as a co-ordinated functional syncytium. This finding has added another layer of complexity to the understanding of the physiology of human penile erection.

Arterial supply

The blood supply of the erectile tissues is derived from the penile artery, a branch of the internal pudendal artery, in turn a branch of the internal iliac artery. In the perineum, the penile artery gives rise to: the spongiosal, bulbar or bulbourethral, the dorsal, and the deep or cavernous arteries (Fig. 2.1). Anatomical variation is not uncommon. In some instances the accessory pudendal arteries may be the only blood supply to the corpus cavernosum. Each cavernous artery penetrates the tunica albuginea and gives off multiple terminal helicine arteries, which open directly into the sinusoidal spaces.

Distally, the dorsal artery anastomoses with the spongiosal artery to form a rich arch, which gives supply to the glans. It gives circumflex branches to the mid-dorsal corpora cavernosa and, for this reason, bypass into a proximally occluded dorsal penile artery can improve flow into the corpora cavernosa.

Venous drainage

The penis has a rich venous drainage. The peripheral sinusoidal spaces of the corpora cavernosa are drained by small venules that coalesce to form venous plexuses beneath the tunica albuginea. A number of these subtunical plexuses unite and drain into the short emissary veins that pass through the tunica albuginea. Most of these then run into the deep dorsal vein to the internal pudendal veins. The glans penis and corpus spongiosum drains into both the deep dorsal vein and the internal pudendal vein. In the root of the penis, emissary veins drain into the cavernous and crural veins, and these drain in turn into the internal pudendal veins.

Nerve supply

The sacral autonomic innervation and higher centres that modulate the sexual reflexes are both essential for normal penile erection. For a fuller discussion of the central mechanisms of penile erection, the reader is referred to chapter 11 and elsewhere (Andersson and Wagner, 1995). Penile erection depends on the integrated action of the sympathetic and parasympathetic systems.

Sensory information from the penis is carried in afferents in the dorsal nerve of the penis, continuing within the pudendal nerve to enter the sacral cord via the dorsal roots of the second and fourth segments. Sensory information is then transmitted in ascending tracts. Afferent input via this pathway is important in eliciting reflexogenic erections. The cavernous nerves also contain somatic afferent fibres.

Somatic efferents to the bulbocavernosus and ischiocavernosus muscles originate within the cerebral cortex. They synapse in the ventral horn of the spinal cord, and large myelinated fibres travel via the anterior sacral roots (S2–S4) to join the pudendal nerve, which supplies the pelvic floor muscles. The autonomic pathways supplying the penis originate in the hippocampus, anterior cingulate gyrus and the thalamus. The fibres then pass down to the spinal erectile centres. A sacral parasympathetic erection centre lies at S2–S4 and a thoraco-lumbar sympathetic erection centre at T12–L3. From both these centres, fibres pass to the hypogastric and pelvic plexi, before fusing to form the cavernous nerves.

The cavernous nerves pass through the tunica albuginea to supply the corpora. These nerves are the final common pathway for both vasodilator and vasoconstrictor neural input to the cavernous spaces.

THE PHYSIOLOGY OF ERECTION

Penile erection and detumescence are haemodynamic events regulated by the state of relaxation or contraction of penile smooth muscle.

Trabecular smooth muscle and arteriolar relaxation are the key events that initiate and control erection; the precise mechanisms by which this occurs remain to be fully elucidated and much research effort has been invested into understanding the control of penile smooth muscle tone.

Arterial haemodynamics

During flaccidity, adrenergic sympathetic tone dominates and the terminal arterioles and sinusoidal smooth muscles are contracted. The key event in penile erection is a parasympathetically mediated (S2–S4) relaxation of the blood vessels and sinusoids of the smooth muscle of the corpora cavernosa, which produces a dilation and engorgement of the sinusoids. Muscle relaxation increases sinusoidal compliance and is thus able to cause elongation, expansion and erection of the penis. At erection the flow in the cavernous artery decreases as intracavernosal pressure rises. However, during full rigidity the intracavernous pressure rises above systolic and there is no inflow of blood.

The veno-occlusive mechanism

Dynamic vascular studies have shown that the restriction of penile venous outflow is an essential component for the initiation and maintenance of a rigid erection. It is thought that veno-occlusion is a passive, mechanical event. Dilation of the arterial tree and sinusoidal filling result in the compression of the subtunical venous plexus, hence increasing the resistance to blood flow and stopping flow in the emissary veins. Erection is maintained by this decreased venous outflow and rigidity is imparted by the subsequent rise in intracavernosal pressure, further aided by the contraction of the bulbocavernosus and ischiocavernosus muscles. With rigidity, the extra-tunical deep venous system is compressed by Buck's fascia. Defects in any of the components of this mechanism can lead to the inability of the penis to 'trap' blood effectively; this idea forms the basis of the concept of 'venous leakage'.

NEUROPHYSIOLOGY AND PHARMACOLOGY OF ERECTION

Erection cannot be regarded as the result of a simple balance between pro-erectile parasympathetic activity and anti-erectile sympathetic innervation. A large number of other substances have been demonstrated in perivascular nerves and are putative neurotransmitters.

The biochemical and neurophysiological events underpinning the erectile process have been subject to research activity, with major advances in understanding. A complex multitransmitter system is responsible. Nitric oxide (NO) has been implicated as being the final determinant in the erectile process (Burnett et al., 1992). Nevertheless, considerable effort continues into the elucidation of the contribution of other substances, such as vasoactive intestinal polypeptide (VIP), substance P (SP), acetylcholine (ACh), neuropeptide Y (NPY) and the prostaglandins (PGs) to erectile physiology.

Adrenergic mechanisms

The evidence for an anti-erectile pathway comes from experiments on the actions of drugs injected intracavernosally (Brindley, 1986). This pathway is continuously active when the penis is flaccid. The peripheral endings of this pathway release noradrenaline (NAd).

There also exists a pro-erectile sympathetic pathway. The hypogastric plexus contains efferent nerve fibres that cause erection. Electrical stimulation of the intact hypogastric plexus caused full erection in two out of nine patients and a conspicuous tumescence in the other seven (Brindley et al., 1989). Lesions of the hypogastric plexus are known to cause ejaculatory failure, but do not usually cause erectile dysfunction. Thus, the parasympathetic system itself is sufficient to cause erection. Loss of the parasympathetic erectile pathway, with survival of the sympathetic, is seen in men with complete lesions of the cauda equina or conus medullaris – a proportion of these men, though not all, are capable of full erection.

Adrenergic nerves have been demonstrated in trabecular smooth muscle as well as in the cavernosal and helicine arteries. In the flaccid state, the penile smooth muscle is kept contracted by NAd release acting via postjunctional alpha-adrenoceptors on the cavernous and helicine arteries, as well as on trabecular smooth muscle. Furthermore, NAd release is modulated by presynaptic alpha$_2$-adrenoceptors. Modulation of adrenergic activity seems to be one of the most important means by which the contractile state of the smooth muscle of the corpus cavernosum and the penile vasculature is influenced.

Alpha-adrenoceptor functions can also be demonstrated in circumflex veins and the deep dorsal penile vein.

Drugs such as trazodone influence penile erectile tissues by the blockade of alpha-adrenoceptors. Trazodone is a non-tricyclic antidepressant that was shown to have marked alpha-adrenoceptor blocking activity and was reported to cause priapism during treatment for depressive disorders. It has been postulated that in some cases impotence may be secondary to changes in alpha-adrenoceptor function. A small, but significant, difference was found between cavernous tissue from diabetic and non-diabetic patients with impotence. In contrast, no differences were found in sensitivity to phenylephrine between cavernous tissue preparations taken from impotent men with diabetes mellitus, alcoholism or Peyronie's disease, and men with no obvious condition causing impotence (Creed *et al.*, 1989).

No difference in the alpha-adrenoceptor function of isolated penile circumflex veins between potent and impotent men due to venous leakage has been found.

Cholinergic mechanisms

For many years the parasympathetic autonomic nervous system has been believed to be the sole effector of physiological erections. The results of early experiments showed that electrical stimulation of the nervi erigentes of animals brought about penile erection. This response was not abolished by atropine. It was later suggested that a balance exists between adrenergic anti-erectile and cholinergic pro-erectile activity, the function of cholinergic activity being to inhibit, via muscarinic receptors, the adrenergically induced penile flaccidity. However, the exact roles of cholinergic mechanisms are unclear; indeed, a considerable body of evidence exists to suggest that vasodilatation and hence tumescence and penile erection are not accounted for by a simple mechanism of acetylcholine (ACh) release, which then acts via muscarinic receptors.

Muscarinic receptors have been clearly identified in the human corpus bound to both cavernosal tissue and to endothelium. Acetylcholinesterase-containing nerves have been demonstrated in human penile tissue, as has choline uptake, ACh synthesis and release. It is known that atropine injection fails to block penile erection, and this led to the suggestion that muscarinic transmission plays no significant part in penile erection (Wagner and Brindley, 1980). ACh release and synthesis are found to be reduced in corporeal tissue from men with diabetes. The destruction of the endothelium effectively eliminated/attenuated the relaxation produced by ACh, a finding which suggests that, as in other vascular preparations, the effect of ACh is endothelium-dependent.

Parasympathetic activity does not equate to the sole actions of ACh; clearly other transmitters may be released from cholinergic nerves. There are three distinct mechanisms by which parasympathetic activity may affect erection and tumescence: (1) the release of NAd may be inhibited by stimulation of muscarinic receptors on adrenergic nerve terminals, (2) the postjunctional effects of NAd may be counteracted by muscarinic receptor-mediated release of relaxant factor(s) from the endothelium, and (3) the postjunctional effects of NAd may be counteracted by relaxant factors, such as NO and VIP, released from the parasympathetic nerves.

Overall, the findings suggest that parasympathetic activity may contribute to penile tumescence and erection by mechanisms that antagonize the anti-erectile effects of NAd. This is likely to include the muscarinic receptor-mediated inhibition of adrenergic activity as well as the generation of NO by the endothelium. Thus, much of the current research effort has focused on the role of other putative neurotransmitter substances and the term non-adrenergic non-cholinergic (NANC) transmission is used to describe these other processes that are responsible for the control of smooth muscle relaxation.

Non-adrenergic non-cholinergic mechanisms

There are a large number of substances included in the term NANC and the reader is again referred to the comprehensive review by Andersson and Wagner (1995).

1. The effects of nitrates on the vasculature have been studied for decades; however, that endothelial cells are able to release a substance which can cause vasodilatation was only discovered relatively recently. Shortly afterwards it was demonstrated that nitric oxide (NO) is formed by the action of an enzyme, nitric oxide synthase (NOS), present in the vascular endothelium but not in vascular smooth muscle cells. It was realized that NO was a secretory product of considerable import. It has since become apparent that NO is a truly remarkable molecule with a wide range of biological activities, which include neurotransmission, vasodilatation and cytotoxicity.

    Acetylcholine-induced relaxation depends on endothelial integrity and it appears that the endothelium plays a role in the regulation of local penile haemodynamics. Furthermore, it is thought that cavernosal endothelial cells may be directly innervated. This led to speculation that after the initiation of vasodilatation, an additional mechanism – mediated by the endothelium – is able to maintain tumescence. It is possible that the increased flow and shear forces provide the stimulus for such a mechanism to come into operation. An increase in flow has been shown to induce endothelial-dependent relaxation in a variety of vessels. In addition, SP, 5-hydroxy-tryptamine (5HT), ACh and ATP are all released from vascular beds and/or endothelial cells in culture under hypoxia-induced vasodilatation or shear stress.

    In disease states such as atherosclerosis, hyperlipidaemia and diabetes mellitus, there is endothelial cell dysfunction that may contribute to the pathogenesis of ED. In cavernosal tissue from impotent diabetic patients, decreased relaxation is found in response to electrical stimulation and this is associated with a lack of NO production.

    In addition to its effects on cavernosal smooth muscle cells to produce relaxation and vasodilatation, it is widely accepted that NO also acts as both a central and peripheral neurotransmitter. Thus, penile erection is an interesting example of NO functioning as both a neurotransmitter and a vasodilator. It is now thought that most penile NO is actually of neuronal origin.

    Nitric oxide diffuses into cells and activates soluble guanylate cyclase, raising the tissue levels of cyclic guanosine-monophosphate (cGMP). Thus, the intracellular levels of this important second messenger molecule are regulated by its generation via guanylate cyclase and its subsequent degradation by phosphodiesterase (PDE).

    It is interesting to note that NOS activity, and hence NO production, depends on O_2 tension. In the flaccid state a lowered O_2 tension leads to lowered NOS activity, and vice versa during erection.

    In summary, there is good evidence that NO is one of the most important neurotransmitters responsible for penile erection.

2. Vasoactive intestinal polypeptide (VIP) is a potent vasodilator consisting of 28 amino acid residues which inhibits contractile activity in many types of smooth muscle. It interacts with a specific receptor and its mode of action appears to be dependent upon the production of cyclic adenosine monophosphate (cAMP) and/or cGMP, as

well as the modulation of NO release. VIP is present in high concentrations in the erectile tissues of the human penis, in autonomic nerve fibres that have their endings around cavernous smooth muscle, penile arteries, arterioles and also circumflex veins. VIP has long been a putative neurotransmitter in the mechanism of erection.

3. A number of studies established that the human penis has the ability to produce and subsequently to metabolize prostaglandins (PGs). Perhaps this is not surprising as the sinusoidal spaces are lined with endothelium and smooth muscle cells. However, much of the research evidence about the action of various PGs is conflicting, and the role of endogenous penile PGs in normal physiological erection and erectile dysfunction remains uncertain, and has been specifically addressed in a review article (Miller and Morgan, 1994). However, of the various PGs, PGE_1 would appear to have the most appropriate profile of action for an erectogen. It is therefore somewhat surprising that there remains a lack of information about the ability of the human corpora cavernosa to produce PGE_1. Nevertheless, cavernosal PGE_1 receptors have been demonstrated in man.

4. Neuropeptide Y (NPY) is co-localized with NAd in adrenergic postganglionic neurones and may therefore participate in vasoconstriction with NAd in blood vessels. It has been demonstrated clearly both in the penile vasculature and in the corpus cavernosum. NPY has been found in reasonably high concentration in the human corpus cavernosum. NPY is also present in the fibres of the adventitia of both arterial and venous vessels and among smooth muscle cells. This peptide may be acting as a neurotransmitter or neuromodulator, and may contribute to veno-occlusion as it is found in the media of the deep dorsal vein of the penis. However, there are no effects of NPY on contraction of the corpus cavernosum or cavernosal artery to support its role in detumescence.

5. Calcitonin gene-related peptide (CGRP) immunoreactivity has been shown to be present in the nerves of the corpus cavernosum. CGRP has been shown to act as a potent vasodilator in a variety of human blood vessels and is believed to act via an endothelium-dependent mechanism. Erectile responses have been recorded after the intracavernosal injection of CGRP. If CGRP does indeed have a role in normal penile erectile physiology, then this role remains to be fully established.

6. Substance P (SP)-containing nerves innervating the human corpus cavernosum and penile vasculature are not dense. SP immunoreactivity is concentrated mainly in groups of nerve fibres underneath the glans epithelium. It is thought that the relaxation of contracted corpus cavernosum and the vasodilatation produced when injected intra-arterially may be the result of SP releasing NO and relaxation-mediating cyclooxygenase products from the endothelium. Overall, SP is not thought to play an important role in erection, but is much more likely to play an important part in penile sensory innervation.

7. Histamine is present in the vasculature and is synthesized by endothelial cells. Its presence has been demonstrated in the corpus cavernosum. Variable responses have been observed in human tissues *in vitro* in response to histamine administration; these include both contraction and relaxation. In experiments on the human corpus cavernosum and the circumflex vein, histamine had no effects on basal tension, but relaxed both tissues when they had been precontracted with NAd. These observations were not significantly affected by either H_1 receptor (mepyramine) or H_2 receptor (cimetidine) blockade. Nevertheless, the intracavernosal injection of histamine in humans was reported to lead to erection.

8. It is accepted that sympathetic adrenergic nerves are responsible for the maintenance of penile flaccidity; NAd may do this alone, but it is likely that a number of other factors

also play a role. Amongst the most important of these factors are the endothelins (ETs).

The endothelins constitute a family of peptides; ET-1 is known to be a potent, long-lasting vasoconstrictor and may therefore maintain penile flaccidity. An ability to synthesize and release ET appears to be a relatively specific function of the endothelial cells. ET-1 binding sites exist in the deep penile artery, the circumflex veins and in the cavernous tissues.

ET-1 induced contractions are greatly reduced by a calcium-free medium.

Muscarinic receptor stimulation and VIP both counteract the ET-1 induced contractions. In addition, the ET-1 induced contractions of human tissues are reversed by ACh. ACh and VIP are found in the same nerves. These findings provide evidence of an important anti-contractile action of VIP and NO in addition to the well-described pro-relaxant effects of these erectogens.

High ET concentrations may significantly contribute to both physiological flaccidity and erectile dysfunction, though the role of the ETs remains fully to be established.

9. Arginine vasopressin (AVP)-like activity is widely distributed, both in ganglionic neurones and in peripheral nerve fibres; AVP is also present in cavernous tissue in high concentrations. Its physiological significance remains uncertain.

10. 5-hydroxy-tryptamine inhibits increase of intracavernosal pressure induced by the stimulation of the sacral part of the spinal cord. It is thought that 5-HT exerts an inhibitory action on penile erection by a peripheral mechanism, an effect that may be mediated by vasoconstriction of the cavernosal vessels or an inhibition of the release of a vasodilator substance.

11. Adenosine triphosphate and other purines are shown to decrease both basal tension and phenylephrine-stimulated tension in the corpus cavernosum and relax penile arteries. It is proposed that ATP is a NANC transmitter in the corpora cavern-osa and that purinergic transmission may be an important component involved in the initiation and maintenance of penile erection. Its role may be in neuromodulation rather than neurotransmission.

THE ROLE OF SECOND MESSENGERS

It should now be apparent that corporeal smooth muscle tone is considered to be one of the most important factors determining the state of penile tumescence. A number of intracellular second messengers are responsible for the control of this tone. The most important of these are cAMP, cGMP, calcium, potassium and inositol trisphosphate. The mechanisms influencing the state of penile smooth muscle tone have their effects via complex intracellular second messengers systems.

Cyclic AMP and cyclic GMP were discovered more than 30 years ago. In the last 10 years much has been learned about receptor–cyclic nucleotide interactions and how GTP-binding proteins couple cAMP synthesis to receptor occupation. We have seen from the above that NO is active via the soluble guanylate cyclase. The importance of the phosphodiesterases in the control of cyclic nucleotide levels has been known for a number of years, but it is only recently that definitive work on their structure, function and regulation has been performed. It has become clear that different isozymes catalyse the synthetic and degradative processes and that more than one isozyme of adenylate cyclase can act as a catalyst. Furthermore, many different receptors can couple with cyclases.

Intracellular calcium concentration and bioavailability are among the most important determinants in the control of smooth muscle tone. Free intracellular calcium results in the events of contraction-coupling; therefore anything that will free this ion from intracellular stores will result in contraction. Membrane active compounds that increase calcium concentration will increase tone and lead to penile flaccidity, while those that extrude calcium ions and therefore lead to a decrease of calcium concentration will decrease muscle tone and therefore lead to penile erection.

The importance of potassium channels in the process of smooth muscle relaxation has been recognized. There is evidence that potassium channel openers relax smooth muscle cells. This is accomplished by the opening of potassium channels and the subsequent hyperpolarization of the cells. Hyperpolarization leads in turn to muscle relaxation by preventing the opening of voltage-dependent calcium channels. The mechanisms that regulate corporeal smooth muscle tone are shown in Fig. 2.2.

EFFECTS OF SEXUAL HORMONES

Androgens and testosterone, in particular, are necessary (although not sufficient) for sexual desire (libido) in men. The relationships between circulating androgen levels, libido and erectile function are incompletely understood. The peripheral effects of androgens on erectile tissues are similarly not fully understood. Testosterone is without significant effect on contraction or relaxation of human tissues *in vitro*.

It has been reported that treatment with oestrogens does not qualitatively change the response observed to stimulation and drugs. In contrast, *in vivo* work with castrated animals suggests that androgen deficiency has direct effects on the functioning of erectile tissues. It has been suggested that the observed reduction of noradrenaline release from adrenergic nerves might be the mechanism underpinning changes seen in testosterone deficiency. Animal studies show that castration reduces the erectile response and that this is reversible by testosterone. Workers conclude that the effect of testosterone is to enhance the erectile response to cavernous nerve stimulation at a site peripheral to the spinal cord and, more specifically, that it is the postganglionic parasympathetic neurones that are the target for androgen action (Giuliano *et al.*, 1993).

A study of the roles of both testosterone and prolactin in human sexual function suggested that both sexual behaviour and nocturnal erections were androgen dependent, but that different thresholds of serum testosterone concentration applied to these different aspects of sexual function (Carani *et al.*, 1996).

THE MECHANISM OF EJACULATION

There are three pathways of ejaculation: psychogenic ejaculation, reflexogenic ejaculation and nocturnal ejaculation. In the normal male sexual response, both the psychogenic and reflexogenic mechanisms are involved. The ejaculatory mechanism can be divided into three phases: the emission of semen into the prostatic urethra, closure of the bladder neck and ejaculation of semen.

The neural control of ejaculation involves both autonomic and somatic components. The first two phases are mediated by sympathetic discharge from a putative ejaculatory centre in the lower thoracic cord, neural impulses are transmitted via the sympathetic outflow, the hypogastric nerves and hypogastric plexus to reach the pelvic end organs. The last phase is thought to be mediated by somatic pudendal fibres that innervate the striated perineal and bulbocavernosal muscles. The afferent impulses for this reflex arise from the glans penis, travel to the pudendal nerve and then to the sacral cord. This reflex activity involving the spinal ejaculation centre is mediated by higher centres and specific areas in the medulla and thalamus have been described for its control.

THE INFLUENCE OF THE HIGHER CENTRES

For a discussion of the influence of higher centres in erection and ED, the reader is referred to chapter 11.

CONCLUSION

The quest for improving and maintaining male sexual function has been going on since time

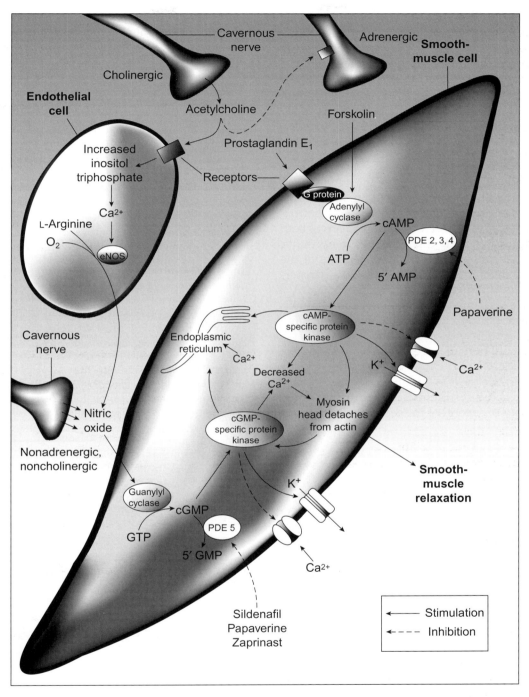

Figure 2.2   Mechanism for penile smooth muscle relaxation.

immemorial. Research and scientific endeavour have led to an increased understanding of the physiology and pathophysiology of the events that contribute to erection and to its failure. These advances have already afforded novel and effective therapeutic interventions for men with ED and will undoubtedly continue to do so in the future.

KEY POINTS

- The erectile tissues respond to neurogenic and chemical mediators as a syncytial entity.
- The autonomic erectile discharge involves both parasympathetic and sympathetic components.
- The neurophysiological characteristics of the autonomic erectile process are non-adrenergic non-cholinergic.
- Via several mediators, the calcium channels of smooth muscle cells are blocked, leading to relaxation and vasodilation.
- Sildenafil potentiates erection by blocking the degradation of cyclic GMP.
- Detumescence is sympathetically mediated.
- There is future potential in modulation of the activity of several of the second messengers.

REFERENCES

Andersson, K.E. and Wagner, G. 1995: Physiology of penile erection. *Physiology Reviews* 75(1), 191–236.

Brindley, G.S. 1986: Pilot experiments on the actions of drugs injected into the human corpus cavernosum penis. *British Journal of Pharmacology* 87, 495–500.

Brindley, G.S., Sauerwein, D. and Hendry, W.H. 1989: Hypogastric stimulators for obtaining semen from paraplegic men. *British Journal of Urology* 64, 72–7.

Burnett, A.L., Lowenstein, C.J., Bredt, D.S., Chang, T.S. and Snyder, S.H. 1992: Nitric oxide: a physiological mediator of penile erection. *Science* 257(5068), 401–3.

Carani, C., Granata, A.R.M., Faustini Fustini, M. and Marrama, P. 1996: Prolactin and testosterone: their role in male sexual function. *International Journal of Andrology* 19, 48–54.

Creed, K.E., Carati, C.J., Adamson, G.M. and Callahan, S.M. 1989: Responses of erectile tissue from impotent men to pharmacological agents. *British Journal of Urology* 64, 180–2.

Giuliano, F., Rampin, O., Schirar, A., Jardin, A. and Rousseau, J.P. 1993: Autonomic control of penile erection: modulation by testosterone in the rat. *Journal of Neuroendocrinology* 5, 677–83.

Lue, T.F. 2000: Erectile dysfunction. *New England Journal of Medicine* 342, 1802–13.

Miller, M.A. and Morgan, R.J. 1994: Eicosanoids, erections and erectile dysfunction. [Review]. *Prostaglandins Leukotrienes & Essential Fatty Acids* 51, 1–9.

Wagner, G. and Brindley, G.S. 1980: The effect of atropine, alpha and beta blockers on human penile erection: a controlled pilot study. In Zorgniotti, A.W. and Rossi, G. (eds), *Vasculogenic impotence*. Springfield, Illinois: Thomas, 77–81.

3 Psychological aspects of the sexual response

Janet Perrin

> Not the intense moment,
> Isolated, with no before and after,
> But a lifetime burning in every moment.
> T.S. Eliot

Definition of the sexual response

The normal sexual response

Anxiety and defences

Temperament. 'People vary...'

Emotional development: 'In the beginning...'
    States of bliss; separation and the finding of self;
    the importance of adolescence; the step into adulthood

The consultation as a mirror of the sexual response

Body fantasies
    Size matters; does it work? – 'troubled femininity';
    after surgery; on becoming a parent

Depression

'Sexual intercourse is a psychosomatic event'. This was the pivot of Dr Tom Main's seminar teaching and remains one of the basic tenets of psychosexual medicine. It serves to remind us that sex involves our minds as well as our bodies. It is about a delicate interplay between the physical and the emotional. It recognizes that powerful emotions come into play in sex, which influence the way the body responds. That these emotions may not be fully conscious and that the sexual response is strongly influenced by the subconscious has been recognized since Freud's work in the nineteenth century.

DEFINITION OF THE SEXUAL RESPONSE

The successful sexual response has been defined in physical terms (Masters and Johnson, 1966), in four phases: arousal, penetration, plateau and resolution. This has been described in more detail in chapter 1. However, the psychological definition of success belongs to the individual. To it the individual brings their own perception of sex with their own hopes, expectations and longings.

To every sexual encounter the individual brings their own personal mix of feelings, invested with differing importance and emphasis. Joyful feelings of love and warmth and happiness may be present, but feelings of anger, fear, grief and guilt may also be present. These, together with other related feelings, can be less than comfortable and can cause anxiety. Body fantasies are also present in this setting and may contribute to anxiety.

In the humdrum of ordinary, everyday life the mix of feelings in any individual is contained and controlled to a greater or lesser extent and rendered tolerable by a system of defences which are to a large extent developed in infancy and early childhood.

THE NORMAL SEXUAL RESPONSE

- It demands the arousal of feelings usually kept under control.
- It involves tolerance of the stirring of feelings not always fully conscious.
- It requires excitement of a powerful mix of emotion emerging through breached defences.
- It involves letting go and losing control in a vulnerable, intimate and exposed setting.
- It is at best a wet, messy and tender business and can put us in touch with the wet, messy and sensitive parts of ourselves, emotionally as well as physically.
- It is an event of total disarray of the self, a state of joy not easy to achieve for those who like everything orderly and tidy and in its place.
- It is not easy for those uncomfortable with showing emotion.
- It is not easy for those whose emotions feel dangerous or overwhelming.

ANXIETY AND DEFENCES

Anxiety may occur if uncomfortable feelings become overwhelming, or if letting go control of feelings becomes intolerable. Anxiety is a normal, healthy reaction to stress or danger. It is a state of mind influencing bodily responses and causing them to speed up in readiness for quick action. It can be helpful, e.g. for a student before an examination or a footballer before a match, to ensure they give of their best (Butler, 1985). However, high levels of anxiety can trigger defence mechanisms, which in the case of sexual anxiety can modify the sexual response causing difficulties for some people.

Defences are at work in everyone, helping to ease anxiety levels and enabling us to resolve difficult feelings gradually. They provide an emotional 'survival kit', always there for a reason, and in some instances life-saving, e.g. enabling us to remain cool in a crisis and not give way to emotion. The value of their presence must not be underestimated or dismissed lightly. Defences, not always conscious, may affect the sexual response and cause sexual difficulties.

These same defences, with the anxiety and emotion underlying them, affect the patient's manner and what they are like to be with, not only in the vulnerable, intimate sexual setting, but similarly in the vulnerable, intimate setting of the consulting room. It is this recognition which underlies the practice of psychosexual medicine and forms the basis for the study of the doctor–patient relationship (see chapter 6).

It is in the consulting room that defences can be identified and examined with the patient, and due tribute paid to them. Examining them together in the light of the sexual unhappiness may lead to a greater understanding by the patient of their difficulties. It also gives an opportunity for exposure of uncomfortable feelings, not always fully conscious, in a safe environment.

Because of the psychosomatic nature of sex, the delicate balance of anxiety, defences and the ability to let go control places the genitals at the centre of a sensitive emotional area. This is the basis of the psychosomatic use of the genital examination (see chapter 6).

This present chapter will consider the feelings of fear, anger, grief and guilt and some related feelings and explore the relevance of temperament and emotional development. Some clinical examples may then serve to illustrate and further explore their presence and the resulting anxiety in the sexual lives of patients and the disturbance that can be caused in the sexual response. It will include consideration of body fantasies.

Some examples will be given from the rich variety of defences encountered in the consulting room. A brief consideration of depression in relation to the sexual response will be included.

TEMPERAMENT. 'PEOPLE VARY . . .'

One of my main aims is to convey the uniqueness of the combination of feelings and de-

fences for each individual. It is this uniqueness which makes listening to and studying the response of the individual in the doctor–patient relationship, without any preconceived ideas, of such crucial importance.

In connection with this it is necessary to recognize that variations in temperament are as numerous as are individuals and upon temperament depends perception from the moment of, or before, birth, influencing emotional development and personal responses.

Professor Anthony Storr, in his consideration of solitude and temperament (Storr, 1997), writes 'Most psychiatrists and psychologists agree that human beings differ in temperament, and that such differences are largely inborn however much they may be fostered or suppressed by the circumstances of childhood or by subsequent events in a person's life.'

It was recognition of this which underpinned Dr Main's frequently repeated remark, 'People vary . . .' and his injunction to 'Scrub the tabula rasa clean and see what's left, now, in the room, in front of your eyes. You have a unique opportunity to see what this patient is like to be with, in the room, in front of you.'

I want also to make clear that no one feeling or particular combination of feelings and defences is specific to any particular sexual response. And no particular form of response will necessarily be seen as a difficulty, perception being all-important. It also follows that in writing about one aspect of the sexual response, other aspects will of necessity crowd in and overlap, since it is about letting go and losing control of a diversity of emotions with attendant anxiety and defences underpinned by temperaments as various as individuals.

EMOTIONAL DEVELOPMENT: 'IN THE BEGINNING . . .'

Emotional development in the human being largely takes place in infancy and early childhood and much of psychoanalytical literature has been devoted to its discussion, including, in regard to psychosexual medicine, Main (1992), Hinshelwood (1992) and Tobart (1992).

I want to refer to development in relation to the sexual response. Differences in temperament make themselves obvious from the earliest stage. Two infants given the same early environment will behave totally differently. One infant, for example, may either be sleeping peacefully or, on waking, pay immediate noisy tribute to its need for instant gratification, accompanied by beating of the air with fists, drumming of heels and puceness of face. Its milk will be downed with alacrity and, already asleep, it will rest until the next time when immediate demands for attention will be made. Another infant will awaken gradually and gurgle contentedly for 20 minutes or more before beginning to give vent to small indications of its need for attention. Often playful during feeding, it seems to conduct its life at a slower pace and appears a more contented child.

Thus do different temperaments reveal themselves, perceive the world around them differently and respond to their own inner impulses in their own unique manner. Rudimentary elements of fear and anger are in place to protect the infant against starvation and other dangers. These will be used, that is expressed or suppressed, according to individual perception of need, and gradually modified in response to their perceived reception by the mother.

Resolution of the conflict between the desire to love and be loved on the one hand and the power of anger and fear of abandonment on the other is one of the important tasks of infancy and disorders in this resolution can be reflected in the adult sexual response.

Rivalries and envies surface in relation to parents, as their separateness from the child and their togetherness with each other becomes clear.

As development proceeds, defences come into play as the need to bring raw aggression under a degree of control is appreciated by the child. Defences vary widely in their nature; some will be picked up from the family ethos, such as making a joke to conceal anger, laughing it off, dissolving into tears in a fragile manner or walking away to deal with it in a safe haven of one's own where it can be kept secret. All of these defences and very many more can be reflected in the adult sexual response and in the doctor–patient relationship in the consulting room where they may be usefully identified.

A sense of guilt may develop early if things are perceived as going badly wrong in the close family e.g. death, separation of parents. Together with feelings of grief with its concomitant anger, the child may feel to blame for, or to have failed in some way to prevent such a happening or feel inadequate to make things better. Feelings of anger, failure and inadequacy may persist into adult life in the sexual response with no recollection of their origins but only the evidence that this is what this person made of their early beginnings.

Interpretation of this evidence as it occurs in the doctor–patient relationship can enable some people to effect change in their attitude or their view of themselves or just to give up old responses which no longer apply. It is not always necessary to determine the original cause of such feelings and defences, although some patients will attach the cause to an event within their memory and through that give clear evidence of how they are feeling now, in the present.

In some people early burdens of grief, guilt and anger may give rise to depression, especially if these feelings are found too painful to be expressed. There are those who by temperament seem particularly prone to a depressive response and others who carry their burdens more lightly.

A clinical example may help to explore this further.

Case 1

Sex had been marvellous for Ms A for the first two years of her happy nine-year relationship. After the first two years something had happened for Ms A, she began to feel 'nervous' about sex and didn't experience her usual feelings of arousal. Penetration became painful and she felt inadequate. She sought help at the age of 33 years, first from her GP, where she saw a locum who suggested referral to a psychosexual doctor.

When she came to the clinic she was anorgasmic with no libido and had had no sexual feelings for the past two years. It had all begun when her partner became important to her, she recalled.

'Something had to come along and spoil it', she remarked bitterly. She was near to tears, the doctor noticed, but fought them back. She went on, 'When kissing gets passionate, I freeze off. I pull out of emotional investment, not to be hurt again. My partner's lovely, loving and nice, the one I want to spend my life with, but I don't feel good enough for him anymore.'

The doctor listened.

Ms A continued, 'I feel resentful and deeply unattractive, my body feels as if it doesn't work well any more. It feels violated. I feel very, very nervous.'

The doctor said: 'I noticed you said "something had to come along and spoil it", perhaps this has been a pattern for you?'

She moved now to childhood. Her dad had left when she was very young. She recalled feeling resentful and furious with him, although later she had realized he, too, was very young.

The worst part was that she and her mum had gone to live with her mum's parents and she found her grandfather dominating. Especially, she felt he had made her be thankful for every little thing. The doctor observed: 'You seem to have felt beholden and as if nothing nice ever came as of right', adding 'I notice you are often on the verge of tears, but you fight them back.'

'Everyone thinks I'm the strong one', she burst out, 'I'm sick of being strong, especially for my sister.' She was furious now.

The doctor said, 'I notice how strong you are here, fighting back your tears as though it's difficult to allow any weakness to show.'

She responded, 'I felt I had to be articulate, and do something about it, no good being a snivelling, blubbering heap.'

'And all that resentment and fury around important men in your life seems directed to your loved partner now he has become important', interpreted the doctor.

'I saw my grandfather dominating my mother, making her into something she didn't want to be.'

'And you seem afraid of that happening to you if you let go emotionally to your partner in sex or, indeed, to me here in this room, and becoming a snivelling blubbering heap.'

Now the tears came and she permitted them. She allowed herself to snivel and blubber, and afterwards she was calm.

A little was said about the appropriateness of letting go and allowing our wet, messy, weaker emotional side to show in sex as well as in the intimacy of the doctor's surgery.

Comment

This case seeks to show how important figures in a child's early life can become invested with anxiety. Echoes of this anxiety ('nervousness'), with its associated defences (in this case, controlling emotion, showing no weakness) can affect the adult sexual response, when another figure enters their adult life who becomes important.

The observation of the defence of fighting back tears and of needing to be strong in the room with the doctor, interpreted in the doctor–patient relationship, enabled the patient to lose control, let go of emotion and to recognize her anger and fear of domination with her partner in the present.

This was a recent first attendance and clues were given to other feelings which may require attention, e.g. guilt at her own inadequacy and fantasies about her body not working properly, both possibly contributing to her feeling 'deeply unattractive'.

The 'fear of domination' may have had earlier origins, predating memory, and surrounding the lone mother. Feelings may have been suppressed as too dangerous to encompass, for fear of total abandonment, and more safely projected on to the grandfather.

It is worth noting that the account given by the patient of their past is the patient's version of events as perceived by them and given the emphasis of their individual mindset. It is the patient's attempt to make sense of their present feelings in the light of remembered happenings. It is therefore not the story that is important, but the feelings that it portrays. These are the patient's feelings in the present, in their present relationship and colouring their sexual response. The same feelings are perceptible in the doctor–patient relationship, in the consulting room, and identifying them can free the patient to let go of these early restraints if they so choose.

States of bliss

Rudiments of joy and happiness are present in all babies in early infancy and, given reasonable emotional nurturing, will be the precursors of sexual happiness in the adult.

The newborn infant in the mother's arms, totally helpless and totally safe, presents a scene of infantile bliss of which a minimum is recognized to be necessary to every infant for healthy emotional survival. It is a picture of total, unguarded, helpless being with the mother of which the child feels itself to be a part.

This state has been linked with orgasmic states in the adult sexual response (Main, 1989). In his paper, Dr Main describes orgasm as 'a state of undefended mutuality, the body so used that the almost impossible requirements of infantile love are met – that the other's highest pleasure will be to look after my needs'.

He further suggests that 'this state of safe undefendedness requires a regressive journey via tenderness and trust into the primitive, infantile, abandoned relationship of utter acceptance and of trusting that one is accepted by another in uncomplicated, mutual fusion'.

He continues, 'In this state, adult-like issues of aggression, anxiety, carefulness, watchfulness are irrelevant and hampering' and concludes, 'Only the healthy adult dares to make this deeply rapturous regression without alarm, confident that he/she can emerge from it safely whole and unharmed.'

It would seem to follow that disturbance of the development of feelings of simple trust and acceptance, or early damage to these, may be areas where sexual anxiety can originate, affecting the achievement of total letting go sexually and possibly causing orgasmic or ejaculatory difficulties. Further anxiety surrounding the difficulty may lead to loss of libido or impotence.

Separation and the finding of self

The growing healthy child acquires within itself a security in the presence of the mother without anxiety about her sudden departure or about what may be expected by her.

This is a step towards security without her physical presence being constantly necessary. D.W. Winnicott has suggested it is also a step towards self-discovery and the beginnings of awareness of one's own personal impulses (Winnicott, 1969). 'It is only when the child has experienced a contented, relaxed sense of being alone with, and then without, the mother, that he can be sure of being able to discover what he really needs or wants, irrespective of what others may expect or try to foist upon him.' Winnicott contrasts this with what he calls 'A false life built on reactions to external stimuli.'

The importance of adolescence

The onset of puberty heralds profound change, physically and psychologically, in both sexes. It is a period of emotional upheaval that mirrors in many ways the toddler years as the young person takes their first tentative steps into adult life. Emotions are once more thrown into disarray, old envies and rivalries can resurface and a further opportunity is afforded for resolution of conflicts. That this is not quickly or easily achieved is well documented and requires psychological adjustments on the part of all members of a family.

Not only is there rapid growth and development, but boys experience their first seminal emission and girls the onset of menstruation. These significant happenings should be welcome as healthy markers of impending adulthood and a happy sexual life anticipated. The child who has gained an inner confidence in their own sense of being is most likely to welcome and delight in their burgeoning sexuality and gradually take their place as an adult in their accepting family. In other individuals, where there is still conflict between the need to love and be loved, or the intensity of emotion is feared, anxieties may be generated about mess or being out of control or loss of dignity.

Feelings such as these will affect the adolescent's attitude to their sexuality and may in time affect the sexual response. The adolescent's perception of family attitudes is important, attitudes about periods, masturbation, sexual wishes and about early sexual encounters.

Whether emotion is acceptably shown in the family and whether warmth exists between parents and in the family atmosphere are aspects unconsciously perceived and the way

the young person deals with them will inform the sexual response.

I have tried to indicate, but will note again, that for each individual their response depends upon their personal perception of an atmosphere or a situation, each of which may be perceived differently by someone else of a different mindset.

The step into adulthood

By the end of adolescence, the healthy young man or woman is ready to take the step fully into adulthood, owning their own sexual feelings, sexual wishes and their own genitals. They will have released themselves from the power of parental domination and from the need to rebel against it. The basis for their sexual response will have been forged.

Difficulties with taking this step are revealed in relation to the sexual response of many men, some of whom continue into adult life trying desperately to please women, fearing their disapproval and ultimate abandonment. Such men seem never able fully to dare to get in touch with their own impulses that contain so much of aggression and resentment, and which feel too dangerous to indulge.

This may lead to difficulties with commitment to any one woman or to a fear of sexual involvement at all, sometimes until the thirties or forties when they may experience impotence or premature ejaculation, possibly associated with depression.

One man experiencing difficulties sustaining his erection, after several sessions of psychosexual work, was able to encompass all his present feelings in an episode he recalled when he had entered the sixth form at school against his will but to accord with his mother's wishes. Unable to commit himself fully to the work, he had later 'dropped out'. It was then a relatively small step for him to recognize himself as a disappointer of women in sex, where he similarly 'dropped out', punishing them for their perceived domination as he had disappointed his mother in school. Recognizing this helped him begin to look at his own wishes and at his anger and resentment with women. Fear of being left alone if he incurred their displeasure gradually became clear.

Another man, who had made no satisfactory sexual relationships and was still living with his mother at the age of 54, attended the clinic when he met someone with whom he said he wanted to 'get it right'. His 'little boy' mode, subservient and avoiding responsibility for any work on his part, irritated the doctor, who felt cast in the role of fairy godmother, required to wave a wand to make his dilatory erection last. Interpreting this gradually and discussing it with him in relation to his partner and his mother, the first woman in his life, allowed him to get in touch with his anger towards women, including the doctor, suppressed for fear of the consequences.

A third man aged 40 and complaining of erectile dysfunction and premature ejaculation throughout his 18-year marriage, sought help six months after his wife left. He was wary of women, having felt hurt and rejected. Failing to stand up for himself, he feared his hopes would be dashed and also feared the damage he might do if his anger were ignited.

He felt himself to be on a 'cliff edge' of emotion, conscious of being very needy, but resorting to caring for others rather than risk allowing himself to be cared for. He was conscious of keeping a powerful control of his aggression, sometimes fearing he would turn it upon himself.

Sometimes the disorder in the sexual response is part of a wider pathology of depression, disabling anxiety and a sense of isolation one man described as 'amounting to an addiction'. This man, holding down a responsible job, was conscious of a deep, underlying anger, of being a pleaser of others but harbouring repressed feelings of guilt, shame and fear of failure. He projected a most pleasant manner, belying the resentment and fury beneath and acting as an effective defence against their access.

Some patients with very deep-seated defences may require longer-term psychotherapy than psychosexual medicine can offer.

THE CONSULTATION AS A MIRROR OF THE SEXUAL RESPONSE

By the end of adolescence, the adult mindset has been largely determined and will affect the manner and mode of being of the individual and the sort of atmosphere they create around themselves in adult life. What this individual is uniquely like to be with will be reflected in the sexual response and in the consultation.

Anxiety can be expected to be to the fore when a doctor's appointment is in the offing. Changes in the patient's usual pattern of emotion and defences can become evident in the car park, at the reception desk or in the waiting room, sometimes causing comment from the staff which can prove valuable.

Treasures can sometimes be forthcoming at the entry to the consulting room, which appertain directly to the sexual response. (Angrily) 'I wanted my husband to come with me. He came as far as the car park, and then backed off, dragging his feet like a small boy', or 'My partner brought me but the door with that big notice "Sexual Health" on it terrified him. He's sat outside.'

Such offerings represent the patient's version of the sexual response on entering the intimate setting of the consulting room and are worth noting by the doctor for possible use in discussion. Suppressed feelings are also present in the consultation and may become noticeable by their absence. They have been called 'the dog that didn't bark in the night'.

The manner and mode of being, and the effect on others of the patient complaining of, for example, premature ejaculation, can mirror the manner of their sexual response before the consultation has begun.

GP referral letters to the psychosexual clinic usually run to about an A4 page. For the patient complaining of premature ejaculation, the letter is usually a one-liner. The patient has already had an effect upon the GP.

The second contact with the clinic is when the patient rings in to make an appointment. For the premature ejaculator, no appointment is ever soon enough, he wants an appointment yesterday, and urgently and quick-about-it, leaving an irritated secretary in his wake.

The third contact is on arrival at the clinic for his appointment, when an agitated receptionist rings to say 'your next patient has come already, half an hour early . . .'.

And then the fourth contact, when the patient is called by the doctor from the waiting room. One young man was sat poised for action on the edge of his seat. On his name being called he sprang up, shot off past the doctor, through the double doors, nearly entering sister's office, saying 'Is it in here?' With a guiding hand gently on his arm, he was shown through the door of the consulting room. Only then did it become clear there was a girlfriend ambling along after him – completely left out of the whole proceedings – exactly as she was in sex.

And all this had occurred before the consultation had even started.

BODY FANTASIES

Body fantasies are present in the sexual setting and may contribute to anxiety. They make extra demands upon the clinician. They require an adjustment from the reality of their clinical observations into acceptance of the projection of the patients' feelings about themselves.

Feelings about the body develop as part of inner confidence about the self. Children are constantly measuring themselves up against their peers. Those children who are physically challenged or differently-abled or belong to a minority group may experience taunts or bullying. Feelings of their not being able to rely fully upon their bodies for proper functioning or of their bodies being abnormal may be confirmed in them and carried forward into adult life.

Size matters

With the onset of puberty and its varying rates of physical growth and sexual development, size may become an issue for any youngsters if they feel differently endowed. The media of the day plays its part in encouraging young people to aspire to conform to an artificially desirable standard.

Anxiety and fears and excitement about their newly emerging sexuality are normal in the adolescent as they compare themselves with each other and also compare the erect penis with the perceived size of the vagina. Fantasies of damage of the one by the other as excitement mounts are common in this age group. Hymenal fantasies of a tough membrane needing 'breaking in' with fears of pain and bleeding can cause caution in young girls but also in young men, some of whom back off from the damage they fear inflicting upon these perceived 'fragile flowers'.

Where early explorations are in fact experienced as painful, through insensitive handling, or through the tension of fear conveying itself to vaginal muscles, anxieties may increase, and fear of repeated pain may cause vaginismus and may go on to cause difficulties with consummation.

Vaginismus, tension of muscles at the introitus, causing tightness at the opening of the vagina, may also occur as a result of emotional pain, e.g. from the painful ending of a relationship, when anger and fear of further involvement may combine to create the defence of vaginismus.

The presence of vaginismus can also be painful physically for the partner, causing a less than enthusiastic response from him. It will also be painful emotionally for him, as he may feel rejected. He may go on to develop premature ejaculation or impotence and may present to the doctor stating that the vagina seems to be 'too small'. A young woman's complaint of a vagina that is 'too small' may, if she does not feel ready for sex, reflect feelings about her whole sexuality being as yet 'too small'.

Feelings associated with an early experience of rape or sexual abuse in a woman will usually engender sexual anxiety. Feelings of anger, intrusion, damage, dirtiness, powerlessness and hatred of men may occur and combine according to her perception and influence the physical response. Such a girl may complain of her vagina being 'too small', or of the engorged penis being 'too big' or 'threatening'. This vaginismus represents a defence mechanism triggered by the anxiety.

Boys or young men who feel they have been abused or raped may similarly experience sexual anxieties accompanied by feelings of powerlessness and lack of confidence in their sexual selves. This can develop into impotence or erectile dysfunction. Suppressed anger may cause fear of their sexuality which, failing to develop confidently, may make them feel 'small' and appear 'little boyish' and may be presented in the surgery as a penis that feels 'too small'.

Other common vaginal fantasies are of 'splitting' or 'tearing apart'.

To be big enough to accept an erect penis or to be delivered of a baby is something some women cannot envisage. Recently a patient told me her worst nightmare was of a delivery resulting in tearing, pain and wrecking of this whole genital area. These were her fantasies and she felt the same about sex and couldn't bring herself to experience it. I found myself explaining how stretchy and elastic it all was, and then suddenly 'Why am I telling you all this, you're a trained nurse'. These fears and fantasies have nothing to do with knowledge and need to be allowed out into the light of day and paid tribute to before they can be allowed to glide gracefully into the past.

Women sometimes request Caesarian section because of fear of terrible damage at a normal delivery.

Vaginal fantasies in men may include fear of being 'overwhelmed' or 'swallowed up' or 'totally engulfed'. These fantasies may relate to failure of resolution of infantile rivalries and feelings of domination by the mother. Such men may experience premature ejaculation or loss of erection on entry to the vagina and may go on to become impotent. A man's fantasies about his own 'manliness' may be reduced, e.g. by vasectomy.

Body fantasies about size in adolescence can give rise to a train of events that colour the sexual response well into adult life.

Case 2

Tina had reached the height of 6 ft by the age of 12. She found she attracted older boy friends. She enjoyed the attention, growing up quickly, dating and gaining entry to bars, no questions asked. She managed to avoid sex until she was 16, and then found it held no real enjoyment for her. She loved serving behind the bar in her local, recalling 'with two feet of wood between us' she could project a 'sexy' image. Sexually she remained a child, but no one would have guessed from her exuberant manner. She projected a big sexual image, a defence against a small sexuality. She grew to enjoy hugging her secret, private part of herself to herself, using it to tease, almost as a weapon.

When she came to the clinic, three years into her marriage, she came mainly for her husband's sake. She was a big girl at 30, her charisma seemed to fill the room. We avoided vaginal examination for several consultations. It was only after carrying it out that she seemed cut down to size, more of a person, more intimate.

She was delighted to read in a magazine in the waiting room of a well-known singer she liked who had a big sexy image too, but had admitted in the article to having sex rarely. She identified closely with her and recognized her own tendency to 'perform' to the excitement of others but without allowing herself any feelings.

She liked to give of her best and we wondered together how good she felt at sex and recognized the 12-year-old still hiding inside, feeling out of her depth. We puzzled too as to whether she may have been fearful that her unfettered sexuality may have been 'too big' if allowed to keep pace with her body.

Her need at 12 to find where she fitted in reminded me of the story of Goldilocks, the pre-pubertal girl trying everything out for size (Bettelheim, 1976).

Does it work? – 'troubled femininity'

Onset of menstruation is usually greeted with equanimity if the young girl is prepared for it in a sensitive manner. For some girls, feelings of mess and 'dirtiness' render the event less than acceptable. For those who experience severe dysmenorrhoea or menorrhagia or gross irregularities in cycle, this sexual part of themselves can be seen as messy, painful and out of control. Anxieties may occur and doubts arise as to the proper functioning of this important part of themselves, emotionally as well as physically. Fantasies of its being a troublesome rather than a pleasurable area can arise and affect not only the sexual response, but also other important events that depend on their womanliness.

For those who proceed to have problems with fertility, these fantasies may be further confirmed and in a proportion of these cases, resultant disorders in the sexual response itself may be playing a part. A fantasy of 'troubled femininity' may colour perceptions of pregnancy and childbirth, the latter another 'messy' event, which requires letting go control on the part of the patient.

Life events, which involve physical change in the body, e.g. termination of pregnancy, childbirth, hysterectomy, sterilization and the menopause, not unnaturally cause change in the woman's image of herself (see chapter 8).

Childbirth has to be one of the most important of these events. After a difficult delivery or Caesarian section, doubts may arise about her womanliness – how good am I at having babies, how good is my whole sexuality? Feelings of having missed out on a natural process, common in this age of 'birth plans', often give rise to unprecedented anger related to feelings of helplessness and loss of control.

Feelings of loss of dignity, of overexposure of what had once been private parts, or of irreparable damage having been done to the vagina, can cause sexual anxieties which delay the return to a normal sex life.

The anxieties may not be expressed until genital examination is carried out and the patient once again finds herself in a vulnerable and exposed position. If the doctor can combine the necessary physical examination with careful listening and observation, painful feelings can be shared and the woman allowed to take back control of her own body. One young woman, having bravely endured three days of attempted inductions, repeated examinations by different people, lamps ('like a mining lamp'), discomfort and exposure, ended up having an emergency Caesarian section. She was a nice girl who had looked forward to the delivery of her baby and felt cheated and bitterly disappointed. She hadn't been able to return to their normal happy sex life, her vagina feeling just 'there' now, unable to be used. Self-examination helped her to get in touch with the fantasy of the vagina having been rendered 'useless', since it had not been 'used' by the baby. Recognition of this, together with the feelings of its having been 'used' by so many strangers, helped her to own it again and begin to look at using it herself.

After surgery

Hysterectomy can leave fantasies of loss of womanliness, leading to grief reactions and in the susceptible, depression. Sterilization, for example, brings to mind a patient who felt like 'a convenient hole' afterwards.

Guilt and grief combined in one young woman who had had a kidney transplant, to shut out all ideas of sex with her husband.

Her feelings for the young donor, killed in a motorcycle accident, were uppermost in her mind, combining gratitude for her own life with grief for the loss of his, and guilt at being alive when he was dead. Determination to keep going, for his sake and for the sake of his family with whom she kept in close touch, dominated her emotional life.

Understanding of the intensity of these feelings, and the closeness she felt to someone whose organ resided in her body, helped her to put them into perspective and begin to enjoy her sexuality again.

One man complained of impotence after an operation for prostatic cancer. In a nutshell, he said the best things in life were 'a glass of port, a good cigar and a bad woman'. 'But you've been telling me how wonderful she's been throughout your whole illness', the doctor remarked. He realized then that he hadn't been able to think of her as 'bad' anymore, and an exciting marriage in which he used to sweep her off her feet had become altogether too

calm and peaceful. It was only when we were able to get in touch with some of the awful feelings of fear and anger, loss and mortality that he was able to begin again to indulge his usual fantasy of her.

On becoming a parent

The image of motherhood doesn't always sit happily together with the image of sexual partner. Breasts which had been for mutual pleasure may now be felt to belong entirely to the baby, husbands may feel neglected, rejected, disappointed and withdraw from sexual approaches.

'I was her total food and comfort for three months. I am not a baby making machine that can just switch off and become a lover', said one woman, unable to allow her husband to touch her since the birth of her daughter.

Sometimes the boundary between fantasy and fear can become blurred and requires sensitivity on the part of the doctor.

Case 3

Mrs B, who had had a normal sex life prior to the birth of her daughter, now 14 months old, had experienced pain and discomfort in her perineum in the weeks following the delivery. She knew she was different from her friends who were all up town with their babies, shopping and going for walks. She had had difficulty even moving about the house.

Sex had proved impossible and she felt there was something badly wrong.

At her post-natal examination she was told she had made a lot of scar tissue, which had blocked the entrance to her vagina 'like a ball'. She was very frightened, imagining something seriously grotesque.

Sent to a gynaecologist, he had exclaimed 'Oh! My God, I've never seen anything like this, just a moment while I take a photograph to show my students', confirming Mrs B in her belief that she was an out and out freak.

After surgical removal of the tissue, the reverse had occurred. She had been told 'everything's fine now', when sex was still exquisitely painful, and 'there is nothing more we can do for you' when she made her complaint. She presented at the psychosexual clinic a very angry lady indeed, and her fantasy of something appalling being present filled the room. The doctor wondered whatever she was going to find. On offer of a vaginal examination, the patient sent her husband packing and closed the window curtains. It took relatively little time for the doctor, who was willing to bear with the anger, to accept her fears and fantasies while examining the area and paying tribute to some soreness still apparent in relation to some neatly healed scars.

She sat suddenly, bolt upright, and said 'Thank goodness you can see something'; everyone else had said 'There's nothing to see, it's all fine'.

Paying tribute to the pain, emotional and physical, this fantasy which had filled the room was cut down to size and connected with reality.

DEPRESSION

Depression is characterized by a lowering of mood and vitality and sexually by loss of libido. It can occur at any time, but is most common at times of emotional change and turmoil, e.g. adolescence, and in association with loss. Losses, not only those that may affect the sexual image, e.g. hysterectomy, vasectomy, but also losses of job, good health, beauty and most commonly bereavement of a loved one, may affect sexual confidence and depress the sexual response. Infertility can be associated with depression in either sex, with feelings of failure and loss of procreative power.

Post-natal depression may be related to re-awakening of unresolved conflicts from the patient's own childhood. It is encountered most notably in those who doubt their ability to be a 'good enough' mother, who strive unrelentingly for perfection in mothering, and who have difficulty accepting help and support from others.

Withdrawing from sexual response, the better to devote their bodies entirely to the needy baby, their difficulties may be compounded by feelings of loss of identity, isolation, neglect and feelings of being a drudge. Remarks such as: 'My body belongs to my baby', 'The children are paramount', 'I give my all, and more', 'I'm a good mother, but everything else falls apart', pay tribute to their plight, and combined with 'No interest in sex whatsoever', may indicate the presence of depression.

Psychosexual work, with or without concurrent antidepressants, may benefit those with moderate depression. Severe depression usually requires more specialized help.

KEY POINTS

- Sexual intercourse is a psychosomatic event.
- People vary.
- Personal response depends upon individual perception.
- The genitals reside at the centre of a sensitive emotional area.
- The sexual response is mirrored in the manner and mode of being of the individual in the consulting room.
- We have minds as well as bodies.

REFERENCES

Bettelheim, B. 1976: *The uses of enchantment. (The meaning and importance of fairy tales).* Harmondsworth: Penguin, 215.

Butler, G. 1985: *Managing anxiety.* Oxford: Warneford Hospital.

Hinshelwood, G. 1992: On male sexual development, a psychological view. In Lincoln, R. (ed.), *Psychosexual medicine: a study of underlying themes.* London: Chapman and Hall.

Main, T. 1989: *The ailment.* London: Free Association Books, ch. 6.

Main, T. 1992: On female sexuality. In Lincoln, R. (ed.), *Psychosexual medicine: a study of underlying themes.* London: Chapman and Hall.

Masters, W. and Johnson, V. 1966: *The human sexual response.* Boston: Little, Brown.

Storr, A. 1997: *Solitude.* London: Harper Collins.

Tobart, A. 1992: Pregnancy childbirth and female sexuality. In Lincoln, R. (ed.), *Psychosexual medicine: a study of underlying themes.* London: Chapman and Hall.

Winnicott, D. 1969: The capacity to be alone. In *Maturational processes and the facilitating environment.* London: Hogarth Press.

4 Interaction of physical and psychological factors

Margaret Gill

The intimate connection

Physical and psychological factors in the doctor–patient relationship

The meaning and perception of pain

Psychological aspects of physical disease or bodily change

Physical expressions of psychological conflict or pain – somatization

The 'intimate connection' in action

THE INTIMATE CONNECTION

When my daughter was six, she came home from school one day obviously upset, yet unable to say why. As it happened, I had spent the afternoon at a workshop on child psychiatry and the place of drawing in work with children. At bedtime I invited her to draw the problem. She drew a head from which protruded a large tongue. At last she was able to say 'I pulled tongues at Mrs X in the playground'. Mrs X was a vindictive dinner lady. 'Then what?', I asked. She said 'If your Mum and Dad could see what you'd done they'd be so ashamed of you'. We both knew Mrs X. 'Well, darling', I said with a hug, 'I'd have pulled tongues at her too!'

We all know that there is an intimate relationship between our bodies, minds and emotions. What others do or say can have a profound effect on our sense of 'self'. This is especially so if it affects us in a vulnerable area such as the unformed identity of a child or the vulnerable nakedness of our sexuality. Yet down the centuries the physical and psychological have often been split apart, with the body considered inferior to the mind. The thread of dualism running through the centuries is beautifully illustrated in an article from the *Weekend Financial Times* in April 2000:

> We are peering here into a cavern that runs not just through modern medicine but through our culture. The mind–body split is normally traced back to Descartes, but in fact extends back through Christianity, which favoured the immortal soul over the sinful body, to Plato, who championed ideal forms over shadowy reality.
>
> What distinguishes modern western culture is that our philosophers and neuroscientists honour the body and regard the

mind as a sort of froth or epiphenomenon produced by the brain. (Burne, 2000)

In the introduction to *The Imaginative Body*, the editors quote Engel's summing up of this latter position (Erskine and Judd, 1994, p. 2):

> The dominant model of disease today is biomedical, with molecular biology its basic scientific discipline. It assumes disease to be fully accounted for by deviation from the norm of measurable (somatic) variables. It leaves no room within its framework for the social, psychological and behavioural dimension of illness. (Engel, 1977)

They go on to point out the danger of the psychogenic models, psychological reductionism.

Psychosexual medicine allows for the study of the body–mind connection in a unique way. The relationship of physical and psychological in the area of sexuality and sexual relating offers us glimpses into a 'space' which has qualities unlike any other. By this I mean that the balance and interplay of body and mind, with its 'fulcrum' the 'sexual self' (see Fig. 4.1), is focusing on one of the most creative and one of the most vulnerable parts of a human being.

The potential for life or death, shame or delight, denial or fulfilment is enormous. In working with another in this area we are, in a very real sense, treading on 'holy ground'.

In addition to the potential depth of this focus, we are also faced with its potential breadth. No wonder we try to break it up into its parts. Yet being body–mind doctors means finding a way to hold the dimensions together. It means protecting and holding the breadth of the space in which the physical and psychological overlap and interact in a person's sexual relating. To 'watch this space', to reflect on it with our patients and to try to understand what is presented to us is to make change possible. But it is hard. We and our patients may well swing backwards and forwards in the delicate balance between the body and mind, focusing on one and ignoring the other (Fig. 4.1).

The 'sexual self'

If we consider a person's 'sexual self' or sexual identity, it will be made up of many physical and psychological factors. Body image, for example, combines reality (slim with long legs or short and stubby, straight red hair, big eyes, crooked teeth, etc.) with ideals and perceptions. Clearly, many of the possible influences in Fig. 4.2 play a part here.

> Most researchers seem to concur that the fundamental sense of self as embodied and differentiated – the body self – is related to emotional and cognitive aspects of self-perception. Also implied is an assumption that the multifaceted body-image operates as a totality of interrelating levels of body experience filtered through social reality. (Erskine and Judd, 1994, p. 14)

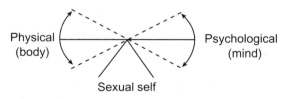

Figure 4.1 Physical and psychological balance and imbalance in the 'sexual self'

Life experiences affecting the sexual self

A couple came together, the wife complaining of her husband's lack of initiative in love-making. He looked embarrassed and awkward. In the course of the discussion, looking down at his large hands, he said 'I've always been cack handed'. He was told this as a child and it went deep. When his wife was asked if he was 'cack handed' in his lovemaking, she said 'No, he is gentle and tender when he touches me'. His fantasy needed to be confronted by her truth.

A whole variety of life stages and life experiences affect a person's sexuality. Many involve loss of some kind. The experience of ageing of the male body with loss of firm erections can lead to a feeling of being 'less of a man'. In an older woman, there can be loss of arousal and even of orgasm. A hysterectomy can have similar effects, though for other women results can be more positive. Loss of the capacity to have children can result in feeling less of a woman and therefore less desirable and desiring, sexually. Loss of a partner through death or desertion can result in loss of previously good erections or loss of libido in either sex, for similar reasons. Loss of status and value through redundancy is another common cause of lowered libido.

'Potential space'

So where does this interchange between the physical and the psychological take place and how can it be influenced? One way of seeing it is as a 'potential space' in which body and mind meet and relate. This space is obviously not physically separate from either body or mind but is, perhaps, the area most open to fresh understanding and change. It could be said to contain the 'sexual self' as it is at the present moment. It is the psychological connectedness of body and mind that works alongside the neurological and physiological connectedness within the body. This concept is somewhat similar to Winnicott's idea of transitional space – a space for 'experiencing'. Here the inner world of the person connects with and relates to their outer world.

> An intermediate area of "experiencing", to which inner reality and external life both contribute...a resting place for the individual engaged in the perpetual human task of keeping inner and outer reality separate and yet inter-related. (Winnicott, 1953, p. 90)

A simple example of this is of a young woman with vaginismus. Her vagina is registering

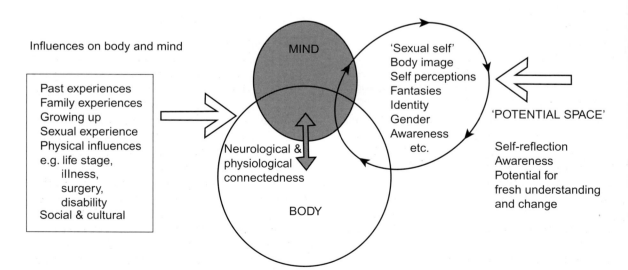

Figure 4.2 Interaction between physical and psychological factors

pain on any attempt at penetration. Her mind concludes that she has a tiny opening there. In the potential space, these two perceptions merge into a fantasy that she is 'too small' for sex, physically and emotionally. This probably taps into an unconscious fear. She is blocked from further progress until the fantasy

is recognized and reconnected with the mind and body perceptions that are then open to change.

When one person's 'sexual self' encounters that of another, the complexities multiply! This may bring a good sense of relatedness and affirmation or it may deepen the difficulties.

A young man had been teased in the school changing rooms for being bigger than all the rest, genitally. He chose a dainty petite girl with vaginismus as his partner. His uncertainty about whether it was 'OK' to have a big penis was deepened by his girlfriend registering such pain at his attempts to penetrate her. Both needed attention to their anxieties and fantasies about their genitals. It is interesting to wonder whether their choice of the other as a sexual partner might have been an unconscious attempt to resolve their difficulties about genital size.

PHYSICAL AND PSYCHOLOGICAL FACTORS IN THE DOCTOR–PATIENT RELATIONSHIP

We have seen that the 'sexual self' includes both conscious and unconscious aspects. It is also, in a sense, open to reflection by the individual. It is as if we are both inside and outside of ourselves in the 'potential space'. It is a part of us and we can stand outside and examine it. The main block to doing this alone is that much that is crucial and problematic is also unconscious. A trained psychosexual doctor can help in that reflective process by giving focused attention to what the person offers, within the space they share together, the doctor–patient relationship. Some of what is unconscious can then become available for consideration.

In Fig. 4.3 the doctor–patient relationship is shown as overlapping 'potential space' between doctor and patient. The discipline of the doctor allows some contact between the 'sexual self' of the patient and what we might call the 'therapeutic self' of the doctor. Other parts of the doctor, the more personal, are excluded. In practice this is far from clear cut or easy, and only experience, training and exposure to critical examination of the work by others help in this discrimination. It is not something that can be learnt from a textbook

because it involves learning from mistakes as well as successes. It is about real life human contact, albeit within therapeutic boundaries. Where the doctor is open and unafraid of examining his or her own reactions and responses and is basically 'for' the patient, there is a place, I believe, in this messy discipline for 'good enough' doctoring. I will come back to the therapeutic boundaries of the doctor–patient relationship at the end of this section.

'Whole body' doctoring

Just as there is an intimate connection between the physical and psychological in a person's sexuality and sexual relating, so there is in psychosexual doctoring. The doctor needs to bring body and mind together in the disciplined and professional use of looking, listening, feeling, thinking and touching (examining). These skills are examined in detail in chapter 6, but it is relevant to note here that as well as giving attention to the body–mind of the patient, the doctor needs to learn to use body and mind in an integrated way as a listening tool. Feelings, thoughts (however 'irrational'), impulses to examine or not to touch and self perceptions may arise out of the doctor–patient relationship and can be vital clues as to what is going on in the patient's sexual life.

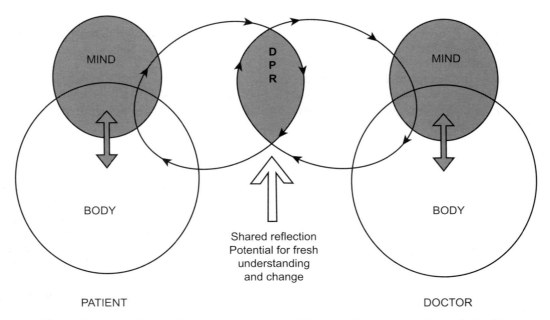

Figure 4.3 Interaction of physical and psychological factors in the doctor–patient relationship

A thin, pale young man rose in the waiting room when his name was called. As he looked at the doctor he seemed to flinch. She thought 'he thinks I'm going to hit him'. Reflecting back to him later her sense that he was expecting the encounter between them to hurt him in some way, she learned of his long history of abuse by the women in his family.

Shared potential space

Just as Donald Winnicott described transitional space in a person – an area of 'experiencing' between inner and outer reality – so the doctor–patient relationship can be looked at as shared transitional or 'potential' space. Here the inter-relatedness of body and mind can be explored in relation to the patient's sexual life and new ways of responding can be tried out in safety. Winnicott related his ideas to the worlds of religion, art and creative imagination in the adult. The body–mind link is implicit in the origins of the transitional phenomena starting with the baby and the breast.

In its mother's arms every infant experiences the earliest psychic blueprint (and perhaps a corporeal imprint?) of sexual and love relationships to come. (McDougall, 1995, p. 10)

The breast is replaced by a loved transitional object. As he grows older, the child's transitional space widens to include other transitional objects and then concepts and ideas. In the sexual focus we have a different adult field to study, but nonetheless exciting in its potential for creative shared 'play' (Winnicott, 1953, p. 91).

If the patient's psychological space is holding his inner and outer reality, so in the doctor–patient relationship, he meets an outer 'reality' in the doctor who is offering his/her own potential space as a kind of dynamic mirror. The patient can encounter his own reality in a new way by encountering it in relation to the doctor's. Unlike the relationship between two sexual partners, the focus remains on the patient. Connections between physical and psychological, which are blocked in the patient and affect the sexual function or libido, can safely be made with the doctor's help. The doctor holds in awareness the messages from the patient's body and mind which seem either too frightening, exciting or even shameful to allow to co-exist. In doing so he/she dares to suggest to the patient that they do not have to be kept apart. Some of these are in the patient's unconscious, but the doctor can sometimes 'read' them and bring them into consciousness at the right time.

A person feeling shame and anger about childhood sexual abuse might deny any feelings of arousal, even pleasure. In the shared space of the doctor–patient relationship, perhaps during examination, these apparently conflicting and even unspeakable feelings can be owned. This allows the patient to take their feelings of sexual arousal back into consciousness and to have some choice about using them in non-abusive sexual relating.

> Taking off one's clothes is such a revealing action, exposing those hidden areas of our bodies, laying ourselves open to the possibility of ridicule or disgust. Does the survival of such an experience give us the confidence to reveal other vulnerable feelings? (Skrine, 1997, p. 120)

The process may sound straightforward, and indeed the 'moment of truth' may be quick in itself, but it will only happen if such trust is built between doctor and patient that these immensely vulnerable moments of exposure of body to mind and vice versa can be risked at all. Even after such an insight is reached, the time needed to take it on board and make it a part of the 'sexual self' can be considerable, especially after abuse.

The 'intimate connection' between doctor and patient

There is a professional 'intimacy' in the interaction of doctor and patient, body and mind in this way. It may be that the shared awareness of a sexual 'spark' between the two, when available for comment and not denied, may be an important turning point in the work. Shared qualities between this kind of doctor–patient relationship and the sexual encounter between partners are:

- Depth and a light touch.
- Seriousness and playfulness.
- Firmness and gentleness.
- Pain and pleasure.
- Nakedness and cover.
- A sense of fulfilment at the end.

In this sense the doctor is like a skilled 'lover', attending to the sexual needs of the patient. *But* – and it is a very important *but* – there are different boundaries here, which, if not held firmly by the doctor, can easily result in abusive rather than creative work. These depend on:

- Focus – on the patient's 'sexual self' and the problem.
- Touch – sanctioned for examination not for arousal.
- Sexualization of the consultation must be examined.
- Clear boundaries of time and space for clinical therapeutic work.

Psychosexual doctors are familiar with the 'sexualized interview'. Some patients attempt to seduce the doctor with hints of personal attraction or erotic material. It is often a much-needed defence, a way of avoiding more vulnerable or shameful feelings or of ensuring continued interest. The doctor may feel annoyed or engaged. Certainly, he or she will feel out of control of the work and 'de-doctored' by being treated like this. However, it may need to be confronted in a prompt and matter of fact way, without blaming the patient, who may be doing it unconsciously. By bringing it to consciousness, the reasons for it and the underlying feelings can be examined together.

It is no accident that the physical and psychological so often fly apart! They are a potent mixture, especially in the sexual area. To keep the relationship in focus and to allow for new integration, the inner space of the patient must be protected and respected. It must be handled with great care, with the doctor's own integrity of body and mind and not with collusion. With such protection, and possibly because of it, psychosexual medicine can sometimes yield amazing results in a few sessions of brief therapy.

THE MEANING AND PERCEPTION OF PAIN

Pain does not exist until you feel it, and you feel it in your mind, Bertrand Russell got it right when he went to the dentist with a toothache. "Where does it hurt?" the dentist asked. "In my brain, of course". (Brand and Yancey, 1993, p. 52)

Whatever we might conceive of as 'pain' occurs in the mind. One of the clearest points of inter-relatedness of physical and psychological factors is seen in our perception of pain. Pain from a known source is far less frightening (though it may be more intense) than pain from unknown causes. Which doctor has not interpreted their own persistent headache as a brain tumour or abdominal pain as appendicitis on occasion? The sensations we feel as 'pain' are transmitted, like all other sensations, in electrical impulses along the neurones to the brain. A sort of 'neutral dot dash Morse code' as Dr Paul Brand, the famous leprosy surgeon, calls it (Brand and Yancey, 1993, p. 46). The brain supplies the interpretation and the emotional response. It is here that there is great scope for variation and adaptation.

One woman may get thrush, with its intense irritation and pain, and simply get treatment and get over it. For another, it may be the 'proof' that there is 'something wrong' with her sexually and the pain on intercourse will persist after all signs of thrush are gone. For yet another, it provides an ideal (if subconscious) excuse to avoid what is not pleasurable anyway – and again the pain persists. In all cases the pain of thrush is a physical reality, but the meaning and perception of it will differ.

Intensity of pain sensation can also be affected by its perceived meaning. We all know that if we stub our toe or jam our fingers in a door it feels as if our whole body is in pain, as that sensation floods out all others for a while. Similarly, a small cut on the hand can seem very large as it keeps 'shrieking' at us when pressed or knocked. In such cases the 'noise' gradually dies down and our body map returns to normal.

Why do some patients present us with what seems to be an ongoing sensitivity to pain in the genitals? Slight pressure on the vulva may be described as 'stinging', 'stabbing', 'burning' and accompanied by grimaces, tears and even physical withdrawal. A trigger that should be received by the brain with equanimity sets off a major emotional reaction that is not receptive to ordinary reassurance and rational explanations. What seems to happen is that the discomfort of pressure in the vulva (often felt for the first time in using tampons or attempting penetration) keys into a pre-existing fear of penetration as damaging – a fear which in itself is irrational and possibly unconscious. Sometimes there is a message lurking in the background from parents or school friends about the 'tearing of the hymen' or bleeding. Often there is no accessible reason for the fear. Perhaps a person's 'sexual self' is still small and vulnerable and in need of the brain's protection in this way.

One further aspect of pain in the vagina is worth mentioning. Generally speaking, pain is a signal of impending damage to the body. The greater the pain, the greater the damage. Defensively, the body acts to protect itself and minimize the pain. Paradoxically, by relaxing vaginal muscles in vaginismus the pain is eased. Such a response usually has to be learned in conjunction with the exploration of any underlying fears and fantasies about penetration. It helps, when a patient is beginning to believe that penetration could be possible, just to be alerted to this 'body–mind' need for retraining.

Why do women seem to present with more genital pain in psychosexual disorders than men? Is it because the hiddenness and mystery of the vulva and vagina lend themselves to a psychological interpretation of pain far more than the penis, where a cause for pain can be more readily seen for what it is? Conversely, perhaps emotions and feelings, the traditional preserve of women, are more acceptable in men when converted into physical symptoms such as premature ejaculation (anxiety about performance) and loss of erection.

PSYCHOLOGICAL ASPECTS OF PHYSICAL DISEASE OR BODILY CHANGE

We have seen that no change in our body happens without its psychological impact. But the way an individual reacts to bodily change, whether through disease, surgery or life stages, depends on many things – notably their context, history and temperament. Equally, the impact on the 'sexual self' of such change is unique to the individual, even with the common changes of the life cycle, such as puberty and ageing. The work of psychosexual medicine is to study the unique process for this individual patient that is causing difficulty, in order to find out what change is possible. The range of potential interactions from body to mind is vast, but a few examples will be offered here as illustrations.

Physical changes after childbirth

A beautiful, slim Asian woman presented in a Family Planning Clinic 10 months after her first pregnancy, complaining of lack of orgasm. Her delivery had been fine and her general libido was good, but she noticed that she felt 'baggy' in the vagina and was slower to orgasm than before. Asking more about the 'bagginess' during examination, the doctor was shown a slight gaping of the labia to expose a small vaginal opening. 'It was never like that before, maybe it needs a stitch'. Something had changed in her body image on seeing this slight vulval change. Now she was 'baggy' – too loose to orgasm easily except in certain positions. She needed to acknowledge the change with the doctor and mourn the loss of her tight vulva before she could accept that it was normal and make adjustments in her lovemaking. Shyly she then said she had discovered that her clitoris was 'very pleasurable' and her husband had started to give her a climax that way.

Surgery and invasive procedures

Any surgery, even minor operations, will have psychological impact for a time. Surgery that materially affects the person's sense of self as a man or woman can have profound and long lasting effects. Hysterectomy, oophorectomy or orchidectomy and surgery to the breasts or penis are obvious starting points for sexual difficulties in some people. Others survive such procedures with their sex lives surprisingly intact. What is not so often recognized is the effect of invasive diagnostic procedures that penetrate the body's boundaries in an intimate way with some parallels with the sexual act.

A young man developed ulcerative colitis in his university years. He was a non-ejaculator, except in his sleep. Although his illness was mostly a very unpleasant and painful experience, he did acknowledge eventually that his feelings about the necessary endoscopies had included some sexual arousal and excitement. He shared his embarrassment and fear that he would have an erection as the nurse was touching his perineum.

A woman in her late thirties, who had a good sex life previously, had an endoscopy to investigate rectal bleeding. The pain was intense, yet the doctor persisted for 20 minutes, telling her roughly to 'relax'. She was humiliated and felt as though she had been raped and yet could do nothing about it, as 'the doctors must know what they are doing'. This experience had left her with dyspareunia and avoidance of sex for some years. Recognizing within the doctor–patient relationship that she had felt 'raped', yet unable to say so, led to a satisfactory 'disconnection' of that painful memory from her vagina and from her sex life – which she then resumed without difficulty.

Illness

Illness, which does not directly affect the sexual parts of the body, can still have profound effects on the person's sexuality. Often it leads to a feeling of vulnerability, fragility and being in need of protection. A coronary thrombosis or cardiac bypass, for example, may leave a person feeling very frightened of strenuous activity long after the medical need for such caution has passed. Their whole identity has been affected and the 'sexual self' is part of that. Suddenly life and the body are finite and not 'immortal' after all.

A very successful businessman in his mid fifties suffered a serious coronary thrombosis whilst on holiday. Not long beforehand his business partner had forced him out. He lost a great deal of money, together with the sense of being successful all his working life up till then. The profound shock of this combined emotional and physical onslaught made his libido plummet for the first time in his life. He was potent when he did make love, but he could not see himself as the successful lover any more, having lost so much of what gave him his identity – success and physical fitness.

Disability

Disability and its effect on a person's sexuality is a large and complex area, but one which deserves at least a mention in this consideration of the relationship between body and mind. Disablement in a previously fit person comes into the category of effects of illness, but there are people who live with disability from birth whose sexual difficulties may also need attention. It requires very careful listening on the part of an able-bodied doctor, especially, to hear what is relevant and irrelevant and to be able to empathize accurately with a disabled patient. Sometimes the doctor is so taken up with the obvious physical difficulties that an otherwise 'ordinary' psychosexual difficulty can be missed. At other times there can be a collusion in 'normality'. Mrs X was at pains to reassure the doctor that her spina bifida had nothing to do with her sexual problem (secondary vaginismus) at all.

Mrs X had 'gone numb' about a year before. She was in her mid thirties, married for the second time, with two children of seven and nine. She had developed secondary vaginismus and just 'froze' if penetration was attempted. Otherwise sex play was fine. She knew her body, she told the doctor, and it had caused her no problems sexually – after all she had two children. When she was eventually examined vaginally she could barely feel the doctor's fingers. She really was numb. Over the years her limited walking had worsened and she was virtually confined to a wheelchair. Now it seemed as though there was a change in her vaginal sensation too. Doctor and patient struggled in the face of this physical fact and its significance. Did she perhaps realize, subconsciously, that there had been a change and been unable to face it until then?

These examples are just the tip of the iceberg in looking at how bodily changes, especially unwelcome ones, affect the mind in psychosexual work. Now it is time to turn our attention to looking at the same entity – body–mind – from the angle of the effect of the psychological on the physical.

PHYSICAL EXPRESSIONS OF PSYCHOLOGICAL CONFLICT OR PAIN – SOMATIZATION

Sometimes psychological conflict or unacceptable feelings are so unbearable that they are transformed into physical symptoms, which *can* be borne. Such patients can present to a whole series of doctors, convinced that their sexual difficulty has a physical cause and cure, if only it can be found. No amount of reassurance that there is 'nothing wrong' seems to help. Their very resistance to a psychological explanation tells us that the cause is buried in the subconscious and not accessible to rational thinking. We have already met the woman who is 'too young' or 'too small' for sex, emotionally. She develops the fantasy of a small vagina, which is impenetrable, and presents with primary vaginismus. Some such patients even persuade gynaecologists to operate to widen the vaginal entrance with no physical cause apparent; they are so convinced and convincing.

Feelings of smallness or inadequacy in a man can lead to a fantasy of a small penis, which can be deeply held to, even though genital examination reveals one of normal size. Physical symptoms from impotence and premature ejaculation to inability to have any arousal with a sexual partner can be presented. Often there is difficulty with passing urine in public too. If the anxiety is mild, the patient may respond to a chance to share his anxiety and be reassured as to his normal sized penis. The fact that another person (the doctor) sees it and says it is normal may be enough. With greater degrees of anxiety, he may remain unconvinced and these are the men with body dysmorphic disorders who seek penile augmentation with all its risks and disadvantages. It seems as though the body, or in this case the penis, has to bear the mind's burden whatever the cost.

Conflicts of desire

So often in this work, the cause of the physical symptom is a conflict of feelings in the psyche. A man may be both attracted to a particular woman and overwhelmed by her, leading to impotence. The woman's own sexual difficulties may make her demanding of a hard penis to satisfy her, though she seems to be sexually exciting and desirable. The penis literally 'downs tools' to resolve the conflict. Similarly, a man who has been left by his wife with whom he thought he had a satisfactory sex life may be impotent with his new partner. His fear of further rejection renders him impotent when he most wants to be potent.

'Sexual depression'

Unexpressed anger is a well-known cause of depression. Unexpressed sexual anger can likewise cause sexual depression in the form of loss of libido and the avoidance of sex.

A woman with grown-up children seeking a career change was turned down for a job she really wanted and felt she could do well. The rejection went very deep and though her husband knew she was disappointed, he failed to listen to her long enough to hear how hurt and angry she really was. Her anger at the job rejection was compounded by her anger towards her husband, but she only recognized her hurt feelings consciously. Suddenly she switched off sexually and couldn't bear any touch at all. Mystified, she sought help and was amazed at the flood of feelings triggered off as she talked, nine months later, about the job interview. She was able to re-establish verbal communication with her husband and normal sexual relating followed.

'Sexual denial'

Unacceptable feelings can be even more deeply buried, yet yield to a psychosexual approach.

> An intelligent professional woman was unable to consummate a 12-year-long relationship with a man who was highly controlled emotionally. In other respects, he was an 'ideal' partner. Doctor and patient had worked hard over some weeks without any real progress. One day, when the doctor was examining her again, the patient cringed and said 'it feels as though I'm going to be stabbed'. The doctor interpreted this, saying 'that sounds as though you do not feel you have an opening at all'. The patient recognized that, unconsciously, that was how she felt. Rationally, of course, she knew she had a vagina. She had been unable to resolve her conflict of feelings in this 'ideal' relationship. At one level it was a great success, but at a deeper level she felt unfulfilled. Her body expressed the block for her with its 'no' to consummation. When that partner left in anger and frustration, this patient found a new partner and was able to consummate quite quickly and with pleasure.

THE 'INTIMATE CONNECTION' IN ACTION

The following case illustrates the interaction of body and mind in both patient and doctor. The doctor paid attention to the connection between the two in her own perception. This helped the patient to make the necessary connections herself and to resolve her sexual difficulty. Not all cases resolve so easily or present so clearly. This one is chosen, not because it is necessarily typical of psychosexual work, but because it is a clear illustration of the theme of this chapter in action. The case report is interspersed with reflective comments.

Case 1

> Mrs A was referred to a Psychosexual Clinic by her GP. She had a good sex life for the first four years of her marriage until her first pregnancy ended as a ruptured ectopic pregnancy at four months. She was very ill at the time and had the affected tube and opposite ovary removed, the latter because it was cystic. Later surgical attempts to bring the remaining tube and ovary together had not led to the hoped for second pregnancy. Mrs A came with her husband, 18 months after her pregnancy. She had not cried about it at all and her family had not discussed it with her in any detail. Gradually, her sex life had deteriorated from loss of lubrication and apathy to vaginismus. In the last six months she had had such severe vaginal spasm that intercourse had become impossible. The GP thought that she was afraid her husband would hurt her. The couple came together. This lady presented in a striking way. She was wrapped in a white fur coat and wore a maternity smock. She could not understand why she felt such panic when her husband approached her.

Comment

The doctor, looking at the white fur coat, thought, 'she looks as though she's wrapped in cotton wool'. Not knowing whether this thought was relevant or not at the time, the doctor simply 'logged it' and continued. The presenting symptoms of vaginismus and panic at any approach by her husband seemed to suggest that examination would be both difficult and potentially rewarding.

An examination was offered and the patient somewhat reluctantly accepted. At her request, her husband left the room. She said, 'I feel sick at the thought', but with encouragement climbed on to the couch. The doctor gently touched her vulva and asked how she felt. She looked anguished and said 'I want to crawl up the couch to get away'.

Comment

A patient looking anguished and wanting to crawl up the couch to get away triggers off feelings in a doctor about being damaging and hurtful to the patient. It is quite hard to recognize that these feelings are coming from the patient and are not personally directed at this particular doctor. They need to be reflected back for consideration, rather than acted on by a doctor retreating into reassurance and finishing the examination abruptly.

The doctor commented to the patient that she seemed to feel disgusted, even ashamed of her vagina and wondered why that was. Crying, the patient talked of her anger that she had lost 'most of what made her a woman', her resentment towards the baby that had caused it to happen and her fear that there might have been something wrong with her in the first place to make it go wrong. She said, 'even the parts left don't match up'. She felt a complete mess inside. How could she allow physical contact feeling like that? It had been impossible for her to acknowledge her resentment of that baby even to herself. Everyone in the family thought she only felt pain at its loss. Not wanting to make her pain worse, they had 'wrapped her in cotton wool' and avoided discussion of what had happened.

Comment

By reflecting back to the patient what the doctor saw of her bodily reactions, this woman was enabled to voice some of her feelings, which had become blocked since her ectopic pregnancy. The doctor did not know, until she was told, what these feelings were. She might have been able to make some guesses about them, but she probably would not have been correct. The particular mix for this patient, of resentment towards the baby that was so much wanted and the feelings of being a mess inside, were unique. No wonder, with that degree of conflicting feeling, the family had avoided the topic almost entirely.

Over the next two sessions there was a dramatic change in this patient. Somehow having verbalized her unpleasant feelings and the conflict that these created in her, she could let go of her bodily defences against intimacy. She came out of her cotton wool wrapping, lost weight and began to look attractive and sexual again. Soon she admitted to feeling her vagina and finding it roomy and pleasant. She was able to resume intercourse and enjoy it. Later on she reported that she was considering IVF, which she had not been able to face before.

Comment

This patient presented with an intense but short-term difficulty. Previously, her sex life had been good and healthy. Perhaps that laid the foundation for her ability to work quickly and effectively when she met a doctor who was not thrown off the scent by the degree of her panic and spasm. Some defences go much deeper and tap into earlier patterns of dislike or avoidance of sexual intimacy. Whilst a doctor might take the same approach, these would not necessarily yield to interpretation so rapidly.

The process can only go a step at a time and at the patient's own pace.

KEY POINTS

- The 'sexual self' includes inter-related physical and psychological dimensions, conscious and unconscious, which are changing and changeable.
- The doctor–patient relationship is a shared 'potential space' in which reflection can occur, connections between a person's physical and psychological expressions of sexuality can be understood, fantasies uncovered and new connections made.
- Physical pain can persist, if it has psychological meaning for the patient, after the original cause has been treated.
- All physical changes in the body have a psychological impact. Life stage changes, childbirth, surgery, illness and disability can all affect the 'sexual self' and lead to psychosexual problems.

- Psychological conflict, shameful and unacceptable feelings relating to the person's sexuality are sometimes converted into physical symptoms which are easier for the psyche to bear, though not easy for the patient who cannot find a physical cure.

REFERENCES

Brand, P. and Yancey, P. 1993: *Pain, the gift nobody wants*. London: HarperCollins.

Burne, J. 2000: Getting real about the brain. *Weekend Financial Times*, 22–23 April.

Engel, G. 1977: The need for a new medical model. *Science* 196, 129–36.

Erskine, A. and Judd, D. (eds) 1994: *The imaginative body. Psychodynamic therapy in health care*. London: Whurr.

McDougall, J. 1995: *The many faces of Eros*. London: Free Association Books.

Skrine, R. 1997: *Blocks and freedoms in sexual life*. Oxford: Radcliffe Medical Press.

Winnicott, D.W. 1953: Transitional objects and transitional phenomena. *The International Journal of Psychoanalysis* XXXIV(2).

5 Presentation and management

Gill Wakley

Patients presenting to health professionals

Sex and the consultation

Hidden problems

The timing of the presentation

The direct approach

Investigations

Referral to a specialist clinic

PATIENTS PRESENTING TO HEALTH PROFESSIONALS

The health professional never knows quite what the next patient will bring. In secondary or specialist care, the referral will indicate the speciality – although patients sometimes give quite different histories by the time they attend the specialist. In Sexual Health or Family Planning, the consultation is going to be something to do with sexual behaviour. In Primary Care, the next patient could bring anything. A few doctors and nurses say that they 'never see any sexual problems' or that 'I see too few patients with sexual problems to do an audit' (taken from a survey on why doctors had not attended further education on sexual health). An anonymous general practitioner (Anon, 1998) writing a comment on sexual health discussions in surgery stated 'I usually have at least one consultation on sexually related matters per surgery and on some days as many as four or five'.

If health professionals feel less than confident in managing sexual problems, it will be more difficult for them to pick up the clues. Some consultations are more appropriate than others. For example, a consultation for acute lower abdominal pain by a married woman with two children is not the best time to make a psychosexual exploration of her reply that she has not had sexual intercourse for several months.

Women attend primary care more often than men. It is often easier to obtain a sexual history because they attend for contraception, pregnancies and intimate examinations, such as cervical smears. It is more important to seize the moment with men, especially the 16–50 age group, who attend primary care infrequently.

Men in this age group often attend for urgent conditions, such as accidents and intercurrent infections. Enquiries or advice on sexual health may be inappropriate at such consultations (unless clearly related to their sexual lives, such as a sexually transmitted disease), but they can be asked to attend for a well person check.

Many patients clearly wish to bring their problems to their ordinary medical care. A questionnaire survey of 500 randomly selected patients in general practices (Dunn *et al.*, 1999) found that the prevalence of one or more defined sexual dysfunctions was 44 per cent in men and 36 per cent in women. Only 5 per cent had received help for their problem from their general practitioner, but 42 per cent would like help. The commonest choice of professional help was the family doctor, followed by the family planning clinic. Half the women wanted help from a female professional, but only 27 per cent of the men specified that they would prefer a male professional. This large cross sectional study indicated that sexual problems cluster with self-reported physical problems in men, and with psychological and social problems in women. It implies that effective health promotion and sexual therapy could have a broad impact on health in the adult population.

Self-referral

Self-referral occurs either with an openly presented problem, or as a hidden problem (see below). The patient has chosen a health professional, rather than to consult a relationship therapist, counsellor or religious adviser. Patients who consult doctors and nurses expect holistic care, including an examination of mind, body and social circumstances.

Referral by the patient's partner

When patients remark that their sexual partner has told them to attend, it is important to establish whether they perceive it as a problem too. A man or woman whose partner complains that he or she is always wanting sex, or never wants sex, may not see it as their own problem at all. Does the absent partner expect or hope that the doctor or nurse will tell the patient to change? You may need to see the partner instead, but it is important to be careful that you are not colluding with the patient in front of you into blaming the other one. You may end up with two people each blaming the other for the difficulty.

SEX AND THE CONSULTATION

Discomfort with the area of sexuality can discourage practitioners from even approaching the subject. The more often you signal to patients that you are prepared to talk about sex, and that you are comfortable with the subject, the easier it will be for them to share their concerns.

Sexuality and its problems are more likely to be encountered when cervical cancer screening, contraceptive advice, mammography or testicular self-examination are being discussed. The prevention of transmission of common infections such as chlamydia, the prevention of pelvic inflammatory disease in young women and the detection of sub-clinical sexually transmitted diseases in men are challenges which health professionals have barely started to tackle.

Taking a sexual history uses the same skills as other history taking, but there are extra difficulties. Both the patient and the health professional may be embarrassed because of unfamiliarity with discussing these matters openly. If the history is not taken in a competent way, inaccurate or misleading information may be recorded.

The language used for sexual anatomy and sexual practices may not be common to both parties. Particular care must be taken to establish whether you and the patient are talking about the same things. 'Making love' can be anything from caressing, kissing, to penile penetration of the vagina. Which does the patient mean? 'Sleeping with' someone may mean sexual intercourse to you, but just sleeping in the same bed to someone else. 'Vagina' means something quite specific to a health professional, but to a patient it may mean the vulva, the opening of the urethra or even the uterus.

Assuming that the sexual partner is of the opposite sex is another pitfall. If it is not obvious from the name or the context, find out which it is by asking directly. Pat or Lesley could be either. 'Is Pat male or female?' signals to the patient that you are not likely to be shocked by the answer.

It may also be necessary to explain to a patient why you need to know about their sexual history. It may not be obvious to the patient why you are inviting information on sexuality, if it is not in response to an overt presentation of a sexual problem. For example, 'Some people find that going on to treatment for blood pressure affects their sexual life. Have you noticed any difference since you started on this treatment?'

In a busy practice it is not possible to take a 'full history' from everyone. We all learn at an early stage in our training to focus on the presenting complaint and ask for information relevant to that complaint. The history taking which we learned as students, going laboriously through each system, is simply impractical. If you listen without interrupting, most patients will tell you about the problem in between one and three minutes. Then, as with any other problem, checking that you have understood the problem and making supplementary enquiries completes the history.

If the problem is clearly described, few questions are necessary. A mental checklist helps to ensure that the patient has not missed out anything pertinent. For example:

'When did the problem start?' (Lifelong or acquired?)
'Did anything else happen at the time it started?' (Any trigger factors?)
'Does it always happen or is it connected to a particular situation or person?' (Situational?)

If these factors did not emerge while the patient was giving the history, the reasons for the omissions need to be considered. Perhaps the man did not divulge that the problem only happens with the wife because he thinks you will disapprove of him having sex with another woman. The woman may not tell you that she had exciting orgasmic sex with a previous partner if she is afraid that her present partner will discover that she compares him unfavourably. You may not be told something significant that happened at the time the problem started because it seems too trivial, or too terrible, to mention.

It is important that you are an active listener, who notices what is not said, rather than just being a passive receptacle for information.

It is usually inappropriate to consider taking a sexual history from the very young. If you suspect sexual activity, for example because of vaginal discharge or perianal warts, this may have child protection or legal considerations. You may need to think of referral at an early stage. Explaining that you do not have the necessary skills to sort out the problem which needs investigation is just as routine in this case as it would be for any other field in which you do not have expertise.

The older the child, the more appropriate it becomes. To omit taking a sexual history from a teenager with cystitis, vulval or penile soreness, or a genital rash might be negligent.

Most adults are not offended if you ask if they are sexually active as part of a general enquiry.

The perception of the elderly as being sexually active changes with age. Teenagers cannot believe that anyone over 40 years old could be still sexually active, but the older we become, the more we realize that sexuality may continue into extreme old age. Most pensioners are pleased to be asked, although their activities may be restricted through lack of available partners or infirmity.

People with physical disabilities have the same rights to fulfilling and safe sexuality as everyone else. For young people with disabilities, sex education, information, family planning and advice are less accessible. Access to surgery premises and clinics is frequently difficult. Carers are protective and often treat the disabled as children with no sexual needs or desires. It may be difficult to arrange a private consultation with someone with a disability when the carer brings him or her into the room, and stays to assist, preventing private conversation.

Opportunities such as well person checks, the registration medical for new patients or a consultation for travel immunizations may provide the perfect opportunity for dealing with sexual health promotion or sexual health problems. It is relatively simple to add sexual health screening questions to a general medical history taken in the context of a well person check.

In women, information often flows naturally from questions about contraception, pregnancies or gynaecological conditions. In men, urological complaints or bowel disorders may provide a useful start. If no information has been obtained previously, an enquiry such as those following can be helpful:

'How is your sex life?'
'Have you a sexual partner at present?'
'Have you noticed any changes in your sex life since (your periods stopped/you have been on this treatment/etc.)?'

The importance of observation and listening to the body language and words is explored further in the following chapter.

HIDDEN PROBLEMS

Patients are often unsure of what reception they will receive from the health professional and may try out various strategies to establish if it is acceptable to mention their problems.

The visiting card

Doctors are familiar with the feeling of bafflement at the end of a consultation, of not understanding why the patient had attended.

Case 1

Mrs M rarely attended the surgery now her family had grown up. She made a routine appointment to see the doctor with a pain in her abdomen. It had occurred several times, lasted a few minutes and gone. No other symptoms were elicited. Examination was normal. The doctor was puzzled at the sudden presentation of a trivial ailment and asked if she was concerned about anything else. Mrs M looked uncomfortable and said 'No not really'. The doctor waited a little, but Mrs M gathered up her things and left saying 'So everything's all right then'. Two weeks later, she re-attended. This time she was able to tell the doctor that she was having painful intercourse and that it was gradually getting worse since her periods had stopped three years previously.

The hand on the door

Similarly, patients unsure of their reception may postpone the presentation of their sexual problem until they are on the point of leaving. The patient complains of a problem and the health professional deals with it. Then, just as the patient is leaving, he or she blurts out a question about a sexual difficulty. A flight path is open for either the health professional or the patient. If the question is met by an annoyed or alarmed look, the patient can say something like 'Oh, never mind', or 'I'll ask about that another time' and leave. The doctor can put up a defence – look at the clock and remark 'I can't deal with that today'. If there is time, it can be dealt with then and there by inviting the patient back to the chair to start again. If time is pressing, then an acknowledgement of the patient's difficulty such as 'I can see this is important for you – it's difficult to ask about isn't it?' and a firm arrangement to return to discuss it further, is more appropriate.

The oblique approach

Similar to the visiting card, these patients drop clues into the history. The health professional asks about contraception and the patient replies 'Oh, I don't need any' – that could mean anything from not having intercourse (and she wants to talk about that) to trying to become pregnant (and she wants to talk about why she isn't). The patient asks about his poor stream of urine and then says 'All sorts of things change as you're getting older don't they?' The doctor or nurse could just agree, or could pick up the clue and ask what is meant.

Somatic complaints and surrogate markers

Almost any somatic complaint can be presented as a lead to a concern about sexuality. If you ask 'Does it affect your sexual life?', patients can be helped to express their worries more openly. Sometimes the patient has not made the connection between their sex life and the somatic complaint, such as vaginal discharge, pelvic pain, contraceptive problems, tiredness or irritability. The health professional needs to think 'This patient has just made another excuse for not having a cervical smear'. Or 'This is the fourth method of contraception she has had. Is there a hidden sexual problem?' The interaction between the body and the mind has been considered in more detail in the previous chapter.

THE TIMING OF THE PRESENTATION

Valuable information can be gleaned from noting the timing of the consultation. The urgent appointment may mean that the complaint is urgent (like premature ejaculation) or the attention needed is urgent (the girlfriend is leaving if he doesn't get it sorted). Sometimes it is a sign of ambivalence; the patient only wants to spare a short time, or knows that the health professional will only have a short time, so that there is plenty of opportunity for flight.

The very 'not-urgent' appointment can also indicate ambivalence ('I'm not sure that I want to look at this so I will have an appointment in six weeks time'), or a low self-esteem ('I know you are too busy to pay attention to my silly needs').

The 'special' appointment is interesting and often irritating when the health professional realizes that the patient has successfully manipulated them into arranging to see him or her outside normal consulting hours or for much longer than usual. Even more irritating, but in need of understanding, is the specially arranged appointment that is not attended. Is it ambivalence, a sense of worthlessness, more manipulation, anger or just plain forgetfulness?

It is always worth asking why someone is presenting at this specific time. A factor, not appreciated by the patient as significant, may then become apparent. Some 'rites of passage' are likely to precipitate a complaint of sexual difficulties. These will be discussed in more detail in chapter 8, but for now I will highlight those moments when it is particularly likely that problems will emerge.

Beginning sexual life

The start of sexual activity can be very confusing as well as exciting. Young people sometimes feel pressurized into behaving like all their friends when they as individuals want to do something different.

Case 2

C attended a family planning clinic for the results of some swabs. She was supposed to go back to the young people's clinic where they were taken, but turned up at a morning clinic in the same building. Her notes were found; the swabs were all clear. The doctor noticed that she looked close to tears when she heard the results and asked what was worrying her. After some initial reticence, she poured it all out. She hated going to the young people's clinic; it was full of girls she knew. She could not understand why having sex was so painful unless she had too much to drink – 'It shouldn't be like that' she almost wailed. She knew her boyfriend was more experienced than she was, so she thought he had given her an infection. When she came to a halt, the doctor wondered aloud why she cared so much about seeing girls she knew in the clinic. C replied that they would know why she was there. 'Because you are having sex like they are?' posed the doctor. There was a silence, and C looked wildly round the room. The doctor took pity on her and started off a conversation full of generalizations about girls not being sure that they are ready for sex, or not being sure that this boy is the one she wants . . . and then said 'But what about you; what do you want?' More slowly, C talked, thinking as she went. She did not want a serious relationship; she wanted to work hard and get some qualifications. She wanted to put sexual activity on hold for a bit; she did not like the pressure that her boyfriend put on her to be fun and be out all the time. She sat in silence for a moment, and then said she thought she would finish with him. She added that she would return to the clinic if she needed more advice in the future.

Young people mature emotionally at different rates. A teenage boy may wonder if he is homosexual – but he has not yet made the transition from preferring to go out in a group of the same sex to wanting to be alone with an individual. Both sexes worry about when to ask or agree to sexual activity and what the other person will think, or, worse still, say, about the performance.

Now we are three

The change from being a couple to having an intrusive demanding baby can precipitate sexual problems. Research shows that there is a gradual return to sexual activity (Von Sydow, 1999) during the post-partum year with wide variability. Very little of the research looked at the attitudes or feelings of the male partners. One recent study that included both partners (Byrd et al., 1998) showed that few couples (19 per cent) had resumed sexual activity at one month, but 90 per cent had by four months post-partum. Another study (Barrett et al., 1999) showed that of those with sexual problems in the post-natal period, only 19 per cent discussed this with a health professional. Discussion about possible changes in sexual feelings after delivery and enquiries at post-natal visits would enable more preventive work to be done.

New beginnings

Changes in the relationship with the partner may be another trigger. The wife who returns to work and makes a career after the children is no longer so dependent and can be seen as a threat. Her husband does not recognize this 'new woman'. The wife or husband of the newly slim fitness fanatic, or indeed the partner of a convert to any all-enveloping enthusiasm, may complain of similar problems.

A new relationship after divorce or widowhood may provoke feelings of guilt at the betrayal of the old relationship or comparisons, imagined or real, between present and past partners.

Losses

Bereavement reactions can affect the closeness between a couple. The loss of parents, redundancy or the loss of health can all precipitate a crisis in the relationship. The depressed state of mind and the desire to protect oneself from further hurt can shut out a partner.

Is it all over?

Ageing, or fear of ageing, is a subject often raised obliquely in a consultation. It is easy to absorb the messages from television, films and advertising that sex is for the young and beautiful. There are still health professionals who just do not see older people or people with disabilities or illnesses as having sexual needs or desires, and it is difficult for patients to raise their concerns with such a professional. No wonder they so often try out the doctor or nurse with hints of 'Of course, I'm not the man I was' or 'What age do you stop having smears then?' The doctor or nurse may need to introduce the subject in a matter of fact way to allow any problems to be discussed. For example the health professional can ask a woman who has returned for a check-up after a hysterectomy 'How is the sex life then?' as part of the general enquiry, and make sure that it is in the same tone of voice as the question 'What about the waterworks?'

Old damage

Problems like sexual abuse or rape may re-emerge to cause distress because of new reminders. A woman may watch a film that unexpectedly includes a rape scene and be taken back to her own distress. A man hears a radio programme about others complaining of the sexual abuse they suffered as children in care. His own damaged childhood comes flooding back. Sometimes the memories, more bearable in adult life, can provoke them into seeking help for the first time.

THE DIRECT APPROACH

An increasing number of patients are able to present their problems openly. They complain of

- Lack of desire.
- Lack of performance.
- Lack of satisfaction.

It is important to establish exactly the nature of the problem. Some examples of the difficulty with language have already been given. Other muddles relating to the specific complaint can

occur. If the patient complains of 'impotence', he may mean that he does not want to make love, but you are likely to presume he means failure of erection. Similarly, a woman may complain of 'not wanting to do it' and you assume that she has loss of desire, when she actually means that she does not have an orgasm on vaginal penetration and prefers clitoral stimulation.

It is very important not to assume that you know what the problem is. Ask the patient to describe the problem in more detail, reflect back what you think has been said, until it is quite clear between you that you are both talking about the same problem.

INVESTIGATIONS

Just as in any other condition, investigations should be guided by the history. A sudden onset of impotence in a healthy young man whose partner has been unfaithful does not require investigations. A blood sugar is essential for a man of 44 with a gradual onset of erectile difficulties and vague ill health. If abnormal results are found, they are not necessarily aetiological and may only be part of the problem. A man with a normal testosterone level feels just as keenly that he is 'less of a man' as another with a low result.

Screening tests

Some authorities would propose that a battery of tests should always be done, others that only those indicated by the history should be carried out.

If practitioners initiate *screening* procedures they should have conclusive evidence that screening can alter the natural history of that disease in a significant proportion of those screened (Cochrane and Holland, 1971).

The following criteria should be kept in mind when considering a screening test:

- Is the condition for which you are screening important?

- Is the natural history well understood?
- Is there a recognizable early stage?
- Is there a suitable test?
- Is the test acceptable?
- At what intervals should you repeat the test?
- Are there adequate facilities for the diagnosis and treatment?
- Is treatment at an early stage of more benefit than treatment at a later stage?
- Are the chances of physical and psychological harm less than the chances of benefit?
- Can the cost be balanced against the benefits the service provides, against other opportunity costs and benefits?

Low desire

Occasionally disorders of desire can be linked with hormonal problems or secondary to physical illness. It is worth screening for these because they are treatable and sometimes serious, difficult to differentiate on the basis of history alone, easy to detect with a blood test and not costly compared with not testing. Patients often expect a hormonal cause for their problem and cannot move on to discussing other factors until you have dealt with this possibility.

A random testosterone is normal in a high proportion of patients. If a low result is obtained (laboratory normal ranges vary) then further tests are indicated:

- Testosterone level at 9 am: low levels in the morning usually suggest hypogonadism.
- Serum hormone binding globulin to calculate the free androgen index (if available).
- Luteinizing hormone level: low levels suggests pituitary problem, a raised level suggests testicular failure.
- Prolactin level: raised levels may be iatrogenic or indicate a pituitary problem. If only mildly raised, it may not be significant. The test should be repeated.

Other tests suggested by the history may include:

- Follicle stimulating hormone and luteinizing hormone to establish whether a woman is menopausal (especially if the patient has had a hysterectomy or has amenorrhoea under 50 years of age).
- Thyroid hormone and thyroid stimulating hormone levels.
- Liver function tests (if drug or alcohol abuse is suspected).
- Biochemical screen or full blood count (e.g. in complaints of fatigue to exclude physical illness such as leukaemia or Addison's disease).

Performance disorders

The major reason for arranging investigations is for erection dysfunction. The *ABC of Sexual Health* (Tomlinson, 1999) suggests that measurement of blood pressure and glucose are mandatory, but that other tests should depend upon the history.

If erectile dysfunction is combined with low desire, see above for possible tests. If it is thought vascular function may be compromised, arrange additional investigations such as arteriography, doppler ultrasound or the response to injected drugs.

Opinions differ as to whether measuring nocturnal tumescence is reliable or useful. A portable monitor such as a Rigiscan is available for use by patients at home, but it is difficult to establish how reliable are the results or even what place nocturnal tumescence plays in the evaluation of erectile dysfunction.

Any neurological symptoms should be confirmed, if possible, by physical examination.

Specialist referral may be required if the condition is not already evaluated.

Lack of satisfaction

Unless the lack of satisfaction is secondary to any of the conditions above, further investigations are unlikely to be helpful. The history should be the guide.

REFERRAL TO A SPECIALIST CLINIC

Ideally, referral onwards occurs when the patient and the health professional agree to seek a specialist opinion, or for more specialist investigations or treatment.

Patient request

Patients may not wish to discuss their private sexual life with someone they see for other physical complaints and ask for a referral for this reason. They may have concerns about confidentiality or confusions about your role as a friend or professional (especially if you live in the same locality and meet them socially). They may feel that you will not have the expertise to deal with the problem. However, it is still important to establish what the problem is, and who is the most relevant professional to help them.

Flight from the problem

Health professionals may have their own fears or difficulties with confusion of roles, especially if they know patients socially. It can be a sensible conclusion to refer if it would cause awkwardness, but it is worth trying to understand your own motives. If you could cope with knowing other sorts of secrets about a patient, but not the sexual ones, the problem may be yours not the patient's. You may also be anxious about not being competent, not having the 'answer' for the patient. You may be underestimating the help you can give by listening, and at least helping the patient to feel that their pain in this private and difficult area of their lives is understood.

The referral

The work that can be done in a special clinic depends to some extent on the way the referral is handled. Due weight should be given to the patient's problem.

If the patient is in full agreement with the referral, the main difficulties are the expectations of the referrer and the patient. The doctor in the special clinic is put into the position of an expert who will have the answers, rather than the professional who helps the patient to unravel the complexities of his or her own problem.

If patients are not aware of the reasons for the referral, or feel rejected by the original person in whom they confided, or think they should not have been referred in this way, barriers are created before the start of the consultation.

Case 3

Mrs W had been referred to the psychosexual clinic after being sent to a gynaecologist. She had complained that her husband said he could not get inside properly since her hysterectomy earlier in the year. The gynaecologist had found no structural abnormality, concluded that there was a psychological problem, and told her that she was being referred for her sexual problem to another clinic. She arrived looking tense and angry. At first she did not want to talk, and looked as if she expected to be attacked. The doctor encouraged her to say what the problem was for her, and how was it affecting her. She started by saying 'It's not in my mind you know. That gynae man hardly looked at me, just got me up on the couch, said it looked all right and told me it was in my head. He couldn't get me out of the room fast enough'. After listening to the history, the doctor was no further forward. The problem had started after the hysterectomy, but the patient could shed no light on why it happened. She was certain that something had been done during the operation. The doctor re-examined the patient, taking her time and talking her through it. There was a long silence while the patient and the doctor contemplated why the clinical examination was so easy, but vaginal penetration by a penis was not. It took four more sessions before enough trust had been built up between them for the patient to reveal her anger at her husband. He had been unable to understand why she had been upset when a hysterectomy had been proposed. The patient's grandmother, to whom she had been very close as a child, had died suddenly after 'having it all taken away', but her husband had dismissed her fears, telling her that everything was different nowadays.

You can only refer for expert help if you know who the experts are. Meeting and talking with the staff from the range of facilities in your area is the best way of being able to discuss with patients who would be the best choice for their particular difficulty. You cannot meet them all, but you should at least know what type of treatment is on offer.

Secondary care facilities such as urologists are easy to find – but do you know whether they offer treatment for impotence? Some urologists offer a dedicated clinic with nurse practitioners or a joint clinic with the psychosexual specialist. Others refuse to see anyone with erectile problems. Your local genito-urinary medicine clinic may offer an erectile dysfunction service that is just for physical treatment, and you will have to continue to see the patient to help him through the psychological effects of the impotence.

Your local Relate service may offer specialist sexual counsellors, or have only generalist counsellors for relationship problems. You may have an excellent facilitated group for rape victims, or a group taken over by vociferous campaigners with a vested interest. The psychosexual service (if one exists) may offer a behavioural psychologist, a cognitive therapist, a nurse practitioner trained in psychosexual nursing or a doctor who has an interest in sexual problems but no accredited qualifications in sexual medicine. On the other hand, you may have a clinic with doctors or nurses trained and accredited by the British Association of Sexual and Relationship Therapists, the Institute of Psychosexual Medicine or other specialized training.

Your duty of care to the patient includes referral to someone competent to deal with the type of problem, if this is at all possible. If it is difficult to find a suitably qualified person with whom the patient can work, or if the patient is unhappy about referral, it is worth remembering that the support of the person to whom the patient first presented the problem may be all that is acceptable or required.

KEY POINTS

- Patients may try you out with trivial problems or mention the real reason for the consultation at the last moment.
- Sexual problems may be disguised by physical complaints.
- People are pleased to be asked about their sexual life as long as they understand the reason for the enquiry.
- Most patients can explain what the problem is in their own words in less than three minutes.
- Noticing what has not been said in the history can help to unravel hidden difficulties.
- Ensure that you and the patient are talking the same language. Words about sexual activity and sexual anatomy can mean different things to different people.
- The timing and nature of the presentation can often help the health professional towards an understanding of the problem.
- Investigations should be guided by the history.

REFERENCES

Anon, G.P. 1998: Perspective. *Trends in Urology, Gynaecology & Sexual Health* 3, 49.

Barrett, G., Pendry, E., Peacock, J., Vicotr, C., Thakar, R. and Mayonda, I. 1999: Women's sexuality after childbirth: a pilot study. *Archives of Sex Behaviour* 28, 179–91.

British Association of Sexual and Relationship Therapists, PO Box 13686, London SW20 9ZH.

Byrd, J.E., Hyde, J.S., DeLamater, J.D. and Plant, E.A. 1998: Sexuality during pregnancy and the year post-partum. *Journal of Family Practice* 47, 305–8.

Cochrane, A.L. and Holland, W.W. 1971: Validation of screening procedures. *British Medical Bulletin* 27, 3–8.

Dunn, K.M., Croft, P.R. and Hackett, G.T. 1999: Association of sexual problems with social, psychological and physical problems in men and women; a cross sectional population study. *Journal of Epidemiology & Community Health* 53, 144–8.

Institute of Psychosexual Medicine, 12 Chandos Street, London W1G 9DR.

Tomlinson, J. (ed.) 1999: *ABC of sexual health*. London: BMJ Books.

Von Sydow, K. 1999: Sexuality during pregnancy and after childbirth: a metacontent of 59 studies. *Journal of Psychosomatic Research* 47, 27–49.

6 The skills of psychosexual medicine

Anne Smith

Observing and listening

The sexual history

The hidden agenda

The doctor–patient relationship

The psychosomatic genital examination

The use of chaperones

Is training (in Psychosexual Medicine) for the acquisition of knowledge or the development of skill? Knowledge can be taught – by a scholar to a pupil. Skill must be acquired – by daily practice with efforts to improve it. (Main, 1989)

By inference, these skills cannot be learned from a book – they have to be developed through practical work. The following pages therefore are to stimulate interest in the skills of psychosexual medicine, rather than to teach it. Much of what is discussed will be familiar to those who have developed good communication skills through their training as GP Registrars.

OBSERVING AND LISTENING

The essence of practising modern medicine is on sharing decisions with the patient and informing them fully of potential side effects, whether this is of medication or surgery. Psychosexual medicine takes this sharing to a further dimension in that it focuses on sharing and interpreting the emotions detected during the interaction between doctor and patient or, when a couple presents, on those emotions observed and felt between the couple.

All doctors use the basic method taught in medical school of:

Phase 1 – taking a history.
Phase 2 – asking relevant systemic questions.
Phase 3 – physically examining the patient.
Phase 4 – ordering investigations to prove the diagnosis.
Phase 5 – treatment for the disorder.

All this is done from a position of knowledge of diseases and their symptoms – it can be taught by a scholar to a pupil.

Working with possible psychological causes of sexual dysfunction needs a different approach. The variety of causes for the problems experienced by patients defies simple analysis and therefore has to be approached from a position of ignorance. This different approach is not instead of the regular medical model but superimposed on, and incorporated into it. It consists of:

Phase 1 – listening to an uninterrupted statement of how the patient views the problem.

Phase 2 – noting the effect the patient and his presentation has on the doctor.

Phase 3 – understanding the patient's body language.

Phase 4 – noting the effect the doctor's interventions have on the patient.

Phase 5 – investigation of the feelings the doctor has noted.

Phase 6 – interpreting all these observations back into the patient's sexual life.

The observations and feelings noted during phases 2, 3, 4 and 5 apply to the whole of the consultation, but most importantly to the time during examination. When examination is not accepted, performed or even offered, it is equally important to observe and think about phases 2, 3 and 4. It is at this most intimate moment that the patient and doctor may understand for the first time the underlying cause of the patient's dysfunction. This moment of realization has been called the 'moment of truth' in psychosexual medicine and can be the most therapeutic time of the consultation.

In the early part of her book, *Blocks and Freedoms in Sexual Life*, Skrine (1997) details body–mind doctoring in a general way as well as in a genital examination.

One of the key points of this therapy is that the doctor must be prepared to listen and not make assumptions about the patient's problem. The effect of constructive listening and working with a patient to understand the problem is significant in helping the patient to come to terms with and accept their problem. Only then can the patient deal with it. This means that the patient cures himself with the help of the doctor. The doctor is the agent of cure, but does not prescribe a cure.

Psychosexual medicine differs from the general practice of medicine in that it is centred around observing, listening and interpreting what has been seen and heard rather than progressing to physical investigations and treatment. The latter, of course, can also take place if necessary.

Physical diseases such as diabetes, neurological damage during operation or injury can cause sexual dysfunction. However, as well as the physical reason, the doctor must not forget that the patient will have emotions about his loss and the psychological overlay on a physical problem can be immense. Erectile dysfunction in diabetics can be helped with prostaglandin intra-cavernosal injections, intra-urethral alprostadil or oral Sildenafil, but the patient should still have help with his emotions regarding his loss of normal function if he is to get sufficiently positive results with the treatment. It is no good giving the man the ability to have an erection with physical means if he has psychological reasons for not wanting one! (Fig. 6.1).

As humans we are created with two ears, two eyes and one mouth and, in the practice of psychosexual medicine, those organs should be used in that proportion. There will be

Psychosexual problems: body–mind doctoring

Physical – by knowledge	Psychological – by ignorance
• history	• listen to patient's story
• relevant questions	• note effect on doctor
• examination of body	• doctor's effect on patient
• investigations	• observe body language
• treatment	• investigation of feelings
	• interpretation

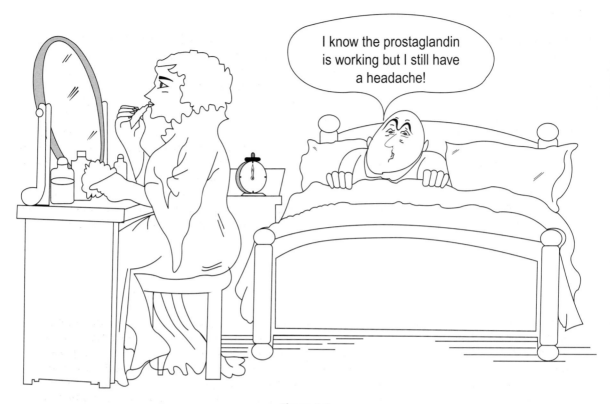

Figure 6.1

times when the doctor finds himself talking a lot or questioning the patient. What does this mean? Is the patient so passive that he is 'not giving' and, if so, is he like that in his sexual relationship? Is the doctor so embarrassed or uncomfortable with this patient that his anxieties are controlling the encounter? (A doctor's defence against work.) Is that the doctor's feeling or is it being projected from the patient?

It is only after observing and hearing the interaction, along with some thought, that the mouth comes into play and then only to clarify what has occurred or to interpret what has been shared.

• Observe and listen

> You have two eyes, two ears and one mouth
> – use them in those proportions

Observing and listening are therefore two very important aspects of the skills of psychosexual medicine. Just as important are the natural curiosities humans show and the power of thought. For instance, when a patient presents with a psychosexual problem curiosity as to 'why now?' can be informative. Sometimes the problem has been present for months or, in some cases of non-consummation, years before help is sought. What has happened to precipitate the request for help?

How did the patient come to have the consultation, i.e. is he motivated for his own satisfaction, was he sent by a complaining partner, did he see another professional who referred him (in which case another professional has chosen the doctor and not the patient himself). Thought about all these matters and discussion with the patient can help the understanding of his behaviour and perhaps his difficulties.

The effective use of silence

Listening becomes impossible when the patient falls silent! Observation, however, becomes paramount, along with thought. The natural tendency during silence in a consultation is for the doctor to break the silence, but it is worth thinking before speaking. Identifying what has occurred just before the silence, as well as trying to understand what kind of silence it is, should aid the doctor as to whether to break the silence or not. If the doctor breaks the silence, it needs to be done in a therapeutic way and not just to ease discomfort. A thoughtful silence is best left to the patient to break, as only he knows when his thoughts are concluded. An uncomfortable or sad silence could be remarked upon, such as 'Something we have just discussed seems to have made you feel very uncomfortable/sad'. The doctor's observation and 'testing' of the emotion he thinks he has witnessed allows the patient freedom to verbalize those uncomfortable/sad feelings and also shows the patient that the doctor is aware of his feelings. It allows the doctor and the patient to move the encounter forwards as equals. Perhaps the most obvious silence is that when the patient sounds and looks sad.

Case 1

A 37-year-old married lady came to see the doctor, complaining that she no longer wanted to have intercourse or any intimacies with her husband. This had been present for two to three years. She talked freely about her marriage and how much she had enjoyed sex previously. This was the only time during her narrative that she seemed alive and pleased. Her husband was losing patience with her, although he had been very understanding until the last few weeks. The disgruntlement he was showing had caused her to make the appointment. All the while she talked, the doctor felt extremely sad that this lovely lady had lost her special sexual life, yet was surprised that Mrs A was businesslike and unemotional in her presentation of her problem. Mrs A also stated that she had no idea why her feelings had changed. There followed a long sad silence which the doctor allowed to continue for quite a while, then she remarked to Mrs A, 'Your words were describing a loss but without any emotion and yet you made me feel very sad while you were talking'.

Suddenly Mrs A had tears streaming down her face as she sobbed quietly. Through the tears came the sadness of losing her womb because of adeno-carcinoma shortly after her first (and only) child was born. The sobs became louder as she talked on about her father going out to do some shopping for her after the hysterectomy. He went out but never returned, having had a heart attack in the shop and dying instantly. She had felt as though she had grieved at the time, but as she talked realized that her husband's words of comfort had annoyed her. She felt he did not understand the guilt she had at having a diseased uterus and having it removed, which stopped them from having further children and, as she saw it, also being the cause of her father dying.

As the doctor and she discussed these feelings, Mrs A realized that she had not linked her physical losses with her emotional losses, as the latter had occurred some time after the events themselves. They were also too painful for her to feel and she existed in a businesslike way to protect herself from them. This, however, also shut out her husband and her own sexual needs, which could have provided comfort in her hours of loss.

• Silence

> Silence can be thoughtful and therapeutic – do not always be the one to break it

Observations made are 'tested' with the patient for their validity.

In the above case history, the doctor allowed the silence to stay while she thought about the interactions between herself and the patient. This gave the patient thinking and feeling time also. The verbalization of the effect the patient's presentation had on the doctor released the patient's tears, sadness and innermost guilt. It

was also a 'test' by the doctor to see if the feelings the doctor had been made to feel by the patient were valid.

• Is it mine or is it yours?

> A doctor's feelings may be his own, or it may be projected into him from the patient – check it out!

Interpretation of an angry silence allowed a patient a similar freedom to express his innermost feelings.

Case 2

> Mr B attended with his second wife and was complaining of problems getting an erection. The more he talked, the angrier the doctor felt and the more uncomfortable his wife appeared. Eventually he stopped and there followed a long silence, during which the doctor felt extremely angry, yet recognized that it was not her own anger she was experiencing. After a seemingly long time of thought the doctor 'tried' out her feelings with the couple. 'As you talk you seem to be very angry and upset.' His denial was controlled anger, so the doctor tried again. Mr B bristled with indignation as his wife said 'I have felt his anger for a while, but not been able to help him with it'. The doctor felt very uncomfortable, as there were now two females remarking upon this man's angry persona. He stood and, for a few seconds, the doctor thought he was going to pick up a chair and hit her with it. However, he just leaned over the chair back and shouted in rage about how his wife (first wife, not the one with him now) had taken his family, his house and – even his balls! He then collapsed sobbing in the chair much as he had described his throbbing penis collapsing during his lovemaking.

The anger had not been in the room before he entered, it had developed as he talked, therefore it had something to do with him. He was so frightened by it that he denied it initially and behind the anger was a man in great pain – small and helpless like his genital organ. Strong feelings need to be tolerated, contained and accepted by the doctor rather than avoided during this sort of work.

• New feeling in doctor during consultation

> A new emotion felt by the doctor since the patient entered must have something to do with that patient

THE SEXUAL HISTORY

Do doctors in general practice, family planning and busy hospital outpatient clinics have time to take a detailed life history – even if it were useful? Time is precious to both doctor and patient and should be used efficiently.

The first few moments of the doctor–patient relationship provide the doctor with clues to the patient's difficulties and an opportunity for the doctor to create an atmosphere of trust in which the patient can reveal his true feelings and fantasies. These same few moments are important for the patient as they can provide the patient with a model of a type of consultation that they may not have previously experienced. It is perhaps during these moments that the doctor can become aware of whether the patient is motivated for change in himself. If so the prognosis can be good. However, if he has been sent by his partner and is attending to 'keep the peace' and look as if he is 'doing something about the problem', then the prognosis is poor.

Dr Tom Main observed that, militarily, a manoeuvre known as deep penetration on a narrow front had been very successful in infiltrating enemy lines during the war. This same technique is used in psychosexual medicine – not as a physical invasion, but as a psychological investigation into the here and now of the patient's problem. In other words, the doctor enables the patient to focus on the narrow front of their last sexual encounter and together they try and understand the feelings behind that behaviour. It is a means to infiltrate the defences of the patient and get to the core of the problem.

Patients bring to the consultation their life events. Attitudes developed and gained from parents, peers, teachers, the church, the media etc. have made the patient what he is now. The effect of those attitudes is real and alive in front of the doctor and they also have an effect on the doctor.

The sexual history then is a detailed look at what is happening now in the patient's life as described by the patient, rather than through a questioning technique by the doctor.

• Doctor being active

> If you find yourself questioning repeatedly, is the patient making you do all the work and does he do that in his relationship?

The doctor has to try and create an atmosphere that enables the patient to talk about the most intimate part of their life. He must endeavour to focus on the last attempt at lovemaking or the last time sexual contact was avoided. Often the patient will reveal their avoidance behaviour by digressing on to other subjects and show the doctor a live display of his behaviour with his partner at home. This can be commented on to try and demonstrate the effect he is having on his partner and may help him to see himself as he really is, rather than as he likes to think he behaves.

It must be a very difficult thing for a patient to bring intimate sexual problems to a doctor. Sexual life is private and should remain so, but when there are problems it needs to be shared. The doctor plays an important role in creating an atmosphere so that the patient can feel more at ease. The mere observation of the patient's reticence to say what is bothering him is often enough to free him to disclose the problem. He will often struggle to use medical terms or vague phrases, in an attempt to put himself on a level with the doctor. A doctor who feels comfortable with his sexuality can help the patient by using everyday words for the genital organs or intercourse.

The doctor in the consultation may feel that he is afraid to progress with the patient or afraid to voice certain sexual phrases or language. Is the patient feeling the same? Verbalizing the discomfort can often free the patient to share feelings that have been suppressed for weeks or years. Sometimes the emotion released (as demonstrated in case 2) is like a volcano erupting and sometimes like a gentle stream rippling down the mountain (as in case 1). Whatever the emotion, and however the patient displays it, it is interesting, it is clinically significant and in skilled hands can be very therapeutic.

THE HIDDEN AGENDA

General Practitioners are in an ideal position of trust with patients, so that the very nature of general practice, i.e. family medicine, can produce an atmosphere where sexual problems can be discussed. There are many opportunities. Contraception, pregnancy, post-natal visits being the most common scenarios where sexual matters can easily be broached by patient or doctor. Routine reviews of hypertension etc. produce encounters where discussion of drug side effects can allow the patient to bring forward any sexual difficulties. The GP often knows the spouse who is being complained about and may not perceive him or her in the same way as the patient. However, with discipline and focused work those perceptions can be put aside and the spouse seen through the eyes of the patient.

The nature of general practice also gives the patient an opportunity to test out the doctor and he may use another illness to 'assess' the doctor's attitudes (using a calling card). It may be at the last minute as he makes for the door that he says 'By the way doctor . . . '. He is ready for escape through the door if his enquiry or complaint is not received appropriately.

Vaginal discharges may be complained about on numerous occasions with nothing being found on examination or on swabs. This can be a covert way for the patient to say 'There is something wrong with my vagina sexually', but it is dressed in a physical overt complaint because the patient feels unable to complain directly about her sexual life. The doctor's ears, eyes and thought processes have to work overtime to pick up the hidden clues as to the real reason for the visit.

Short appointment times, pressure of work and his own embarrassments regarding sexual matters can be a great defence to not hearing the covert, or even the overt, presentations patients sometimes make regarding their sexual dysfunction.

Why has the patient presented now? The problem may have been present weeks or years but now he presents it. Why? This can be an irritation to the doctor if he has been seeing this patient regularly and especially if other consultations have been less pressurized and the present one is running late. There may be a threat of the relationship breaking up, a desire for a child, a new partner after bereavement or after failure of relationship, a role change as in from girlfriend to wife etc. The reasons can be endless, but if thought about and discussed with the patient it can be useful to therapy.

Doctors are taught in medical school not to get involved with patients emotionally (essentially this is important doctrine), but doctors cannot escape the fact that patients cause emotions in them. There are those patients where he is content to extend the consultation and those where he cannot finish quickly enough. Some make him sad, some angry, some irritate and some puzzle him. It has to be accepted that patients trigger all sorts of feelings within the doctor, including those of his own sexual standing and personal awareness as well as those of sympathy, guilt and sadness. The doctor is there to work with his patient and not himself. He must not discuss his own circumstances with his patient, even if it were to gain empathy.

The doctor, because of the Pandora's box syndrome, may also ignore the hidden agenda – should he take the risk, freeing the patient to share his sexual difficulty, and try to work with these problems? What if he unleashes emotions he cannot control? Or what if the patient decides to leave his or her relationship – has he been the cause of the break up? These are all natural dilemmas when beginning to work in this way with psychosexual medicine problems. Doctors seem to take more power on themselves than is justified. The aim of therapy with these problems is to help the patient understand what is going on and it is only he or she who can actually do something positive about it, not the doctor.

THE DOCTOR–PATIENT RELATIONSHIP

Dr Tom Main defined the doctor–patient relationship in psychosexual medicine as follows

> In orthodox medicine, the doctor is knowledgeable and the patient is ignorant. His job is to be fairly passive while the doctor questions, examines, investigates, makes the diagnosis and then gives advice. With emotional upset both parties are ignorant. The patient is not passive and the doctor is not a teacher (doctor means teacher) but a

listener. His relation to his patient is much more one of equality, co-ignorance and co-endeavour. The two set out as partners trying to understand the problems, with the doctor ignorant but willing to understand. He listens and offers his understanding to the patient somewhat tentatively and then observes how his patient uses it.

It is, therefore, a fluctuating, developing live event with each party having an effect on the other. At times it may be as equals, at times one partner passive, the other active, one of parent with child or even sexualized by the patient. Each change is fascinating and meaningful, as it is effected by that patient at that time, live, i.e. here and now. Focusing closely on how the interactions change and the effect one has on the other can throw light on the interactions that patient has on his partner back in his sexual life. The two relationships, doctor and patient, and patient and partner are in parallel.

Berne (1968), in *Games People Play*, looks at the interactions of child relating to adult, adult to adult, etc., and demonstrates that negotiated work can only take place when the adult to adult model is attained.

The effect of patient on doctor

It never fails to surprise doctors how many patients present with a long list of complaints about their partner, but have never managed to speak about these feelings that they have kept hidden for years. They seem to think their partners are thought-readers. Exploration of these complaints may reveal anger towards the partner, and the patient can be helped to understand how difficult it is to become aroused in the presence of such strong negative feelings. It is often a tremendous surprise that the lack of arousal is due to their own emotions and not due to their partner's behaviour or attitudes.

Certain emotions arise in consultations that can paralyse the doctor. Vulnerable, childlike behaviour can make the doctor overprotective, so that he stops thinking about the meaning of what is happening. He may also modify his interpretations to avoid hurting the patient emotionally and find himself being weak and ineffective. Flirtatious behaviour or sexualizing of the interaction by the patient becomes frightening and blocks work, unless the doctor can step back with thought and find a way of interpreting the behaviour back to the patient. The patient who feels better at the end of the consultation, but who has left the doctor feeling worse, has managed to 'dump' the problems on to the doctor, leaving them as his responsibility to sort out.

The effect of doctor on patient

The effect of the doctor on the patient has been described as a 'dose of the doctor' (Balint, 1986). It easily can be forgotten that how a doctor behaves in a consultation can have beneficial or disastrous effects on a patient without their being any conventional medication or treatment given.

A patient behaving like a spoilt child with the doctor may behave the same way with their sexual partner. The partner may give in to prevent sulking. The doctor can notice this, remark upon it and give a different model of behaviour to the patient. The patient may have had a domineering mother and, if the doctor is female, she could give a relaxed 'mother' image, moving the consultation to equal adult interaction, instead of mother with daughter. These changes of interaction can be novel to patients, stimulate them into new ways of thinking and help them to move forward with their sexual behaviour.

The live events occurring in the consultation, the 'here and now' happenings, are significant and parallel to those live events which occur between the patient and their partner.

Doctor–patient relationship may be doctor and couple

It has been made clear that this form of therapy relies on working with the interaction between the patient and the doctor. The doctor learns to use this interaction to interpret to the patient an understanding of their problem back in their sexual partnership as well as excluding physical causes by the standard medical model of treatment.

When a couple present together, as they often do with non-consummation of marriage, the interactions in the consulting room are more numerous.

1. The man and woman interact with each other (or do not, as the case may be if there are great communication difficulties between them).
2. The man interacts with the doctor.
3. The doctor with the man.
4. The woman interacts with the doctor.
5. The doctor with the woman.

It is much more difficult to 'keep one's eye on the ball' of whom is feeling what. A different approach is therefore needed. Dr Tom Main stated that

The way a patient presents should be accepted at face value, not queried, not reformed, not altered. If a couple come together, the doctor should accept this, but work out by listening how it was they came together and not separately. The doctor should not decide *ab initio* to see a single patient only or couples only but should face whatever difficulties the presentation creates.

Now the doctor listens and observes the interactions occurring between the couple rather than the interaction occurring between one of the partners and himself. How the couple behave together is a glimpse of how they interact elsewhere, i.e. sexually. Their behaviour in the consulting room can be interpreted to show them how they are affecting each other in their sexual lives also. Naturally the doctor will feel drawn to one or other at different times of the consultation and this also can be utilized.

Case 3

Mr and Mrs C both attended the surgery. They were in their thirties and had several children. Mrs C did most of the talking. Suffice to say the words she presented and the picture they presented together with their body language is shown in Fig. 6.2.

Listening to them and observing them together showed the doctor a very graphic account of what was happening in that family. Sadly they were not aware of it themselves. The doctor found herself pulled towards empathy for the man and his exclusion from the family unit, as well as sadness at his relegation to the end of the day's chores – i.e. if she was not too tired by then she might allow him intercourse. He felt used, neglected and unnecessary. At other times the doctor was pulled towards the woman as she exuded love, warmth and closeness with her children. The doctor could understand even more the feelings of the partner who wanted desperately to be part of this close knit unit and wanted his wife back as a sexual person.

It was only when the doctor remarked on these observations and feelings that a glance was exchanged between the man and the woman – the first piece of positive interaction so far. Mrs C looked astounded and Mr C began to look hopeful. From then Mrs C began to wonder about his feelings and not just those of the children, whilst he expressed his resentment of how he had been treated.

This couple were motivated and attended together. The doctor's observation of their behaviour in the room freed this couple to understand and care about the other. They modified their interactions and Mr and Mrs C became the 'unit with attachments' instead of

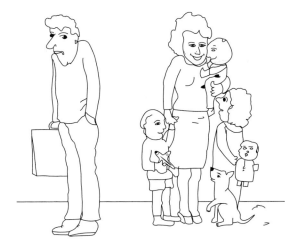

Figure 6.2 The 'couple'

the unit being Mrs C with the children and Mr C as attachment. Their progress towards recovery of a satisfying sexual life was speedy, as each of them wanted change when realization of their behaviour became conscious.

THE PSYCHOSOMATIC GENITAL EXAMINATION

The moment the doctor chooses (or decides not) to examine the patient needs careful thought and understanding. It can be a most revealing 'moment of truth' in therapy, as patients discard many defences along with their clothing. Conversely, they may lie on the couch still clothed – all defences kept in place. Again this is interesting behaviour and tells the doctor something about their feelings. Genital examinations are the most intimate moments for patient and doctor and can be the time when hidden fantasies are shared for the first time. Observing the body language offered by the patient, noting what that patient is making the doctor feel and finding the words to put those observations back to the patient in the context of their sexual life, can be the moment when patient and doctor first understand the causes of the problem. The genital examination is not just a physical event to exclude physical disease but a combined one of body–mind doctoring.

• Behaviour at examination

> The body is expressing a feeling that the patient cannot express directly, verbally or emotionally

Fantasies are many and varied. Some of the most common are listed below, but this list is far from exhaustive.

• A vagina so small that it will split, tear, bleed and be painful.
• A vagina blocked by tough skin, or other kinds of blockage.
• A vagina with a hole at the top so that anything put in will disappear among the bowel.
• A vagina which contains a tomb – i.e. the womb where a baby died – by miscarriage, termination or stillbirth.
• That the penis is so big it will destroy the vagina.
• That the vagina has teeth and therefore is not a safe place to insert the penis.
• That the penis is so powerful it can inflict pain and damage.

The lady on the couch who disappears up the bed and clamps her knees shut at the moment of vaginal examination is not behaving like that just to annoy the doctor, but is demonstrating some emotions to him that she is unable to put into words. It is possible that if she behaves this way with the doctor, she behaves in the same way with her partner. She is clearly demonstrating that she either wishes to keep the doctor out, or protect what is inside. Her anxiety may be about her body, her emotions or a mixture of both.

When asked to drop his trousers for genital examination, it is interesting to see if the man does just that or puts himself up on the couch for examination. In the former, he is confident about himself and on equal status with the doctor. The man who opts to lie on the couch may be putting himself in a passive role. His choice shows the doctor his feelings during that intimate moment of genital examination and

When all else fails!

"I have ways of making you feel!"

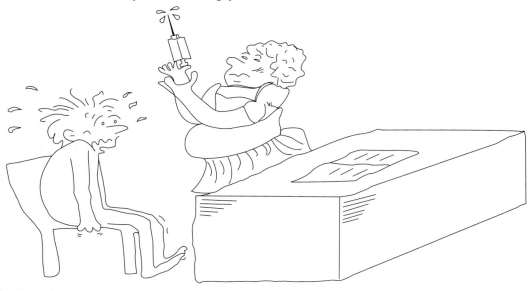

Figure 6.3

may reflect his thoughts about his sexual relationship at home. The doctor can then tentatively offer an interpretation of this behaviour to help the patient understand his own difficulties.

On one such occasion, the doctor was trying to work with a man whose erectile dysfunction was psychogenic. The history, examination (both physical and psychological) and the investigations proved negative, but he was resistant to a psychological approach for his problem. There was a moment of stalemate. After discussion, he asked to try Alprostadil in injection form, stating 'I must have something to give me an erection'. The doctor mixed the injection, explained the procedure and asked the man to lean back against the couch (not lie on it). To give a test dose of Alprostadil, and to train the patient to use it, the doctor had developed the technique of letting the man lean against the couch. In order to protect her back and to enable her to see his facial reactions

while giving the injection, she knelt on the floor. On this occasion the patient, previously non-emotional and factual, relaxed, smiled, blushed and began to get an erection before the injection was administered. Discussion of these happenings (the most valuable being the fact that the patient was towering over the kneeling doctor and the female doctor was medically about to give him an erection) allowed him to release his anger at his partner for no longer making love to him, for always 'towering over him' and for belittling him. He never needed the injection – it was just a route to his inner protected feelings (Fig. 6.3).

At the moment of truth, there is an intensity of feeling for both the patient and the doctor. The doctor must handle this with great sensitivity because the patient has exposed himself to the doctor, and more importantly to himself. It is vital that the doctor does not run away from the moment into giving reassurances because, if he does, the patient may become frightened by his own feelings. Equally, the doctor should not allow the patient to run away from his feelings either. The doctor's role therefore is not to diagnose or prescribe, but to act as a catalyst to help the patient realize his true feelings. On occasion, it is the doctor who contains the patient's emotion until the patient is ready to feel it for himself.

The doctor is privileged by the patient to share his innermost thoughts, those that he had not even allowed himself to see or hear consciously: thoughts that, had the doctor realized them and stated them, might have been rejected by the patient. At the moment of truth, the patient 'surfaces' those thoughts, states them, feels them consciously and knows them to be true. They are his most innermost feelings. It is his moment of truth.

Sexual orgasm produces intense emotion, followed by contentment and an emotional, as well as physical, closeness. This is followed by physical withdrawal, which gives way to a sense of well-being and confidence to face the immediate future. The psychosexual consultation containing a moment, or moments, of truth is similar. An atmosphere has been created that allows the patient to feel intense emotion and, as with orgasm, physical withdrawal is essential. The patient especially (also the doctor) needs space to think through and feel what he has just experienced. Consequently, the consultation is often concluded soon after the intense feeling. Many thoughts and feelings will have been stimulated in the patient's mind and he will require time to withdraw and think about them.

All psychosexual medicine consultations do not contain a genital examination. Some are simple problems and genital examination is unnecessary. However, it is very important to think about a consultation after it has occurred to determine if examination was really unnecessary or was there some interaction occurring that prohibited the doctor from suggesting it, or was it suggested and refused by the patient. If so, why?

A non-consummated couple may present as 'a delicate china doll lady' with a very caring and protective man. The interaction between this sort of couple is a parallel between the individuals and the doctor and consequently the doctor may also fear hurting or breaking this vulnerable lady. Yet thought about those feelings can reveal that she is a very powerful lady rather than a delicate one.

A patient who flirts during a consultation may make the doctor feel it is too risky to offer genital examination, even in the presence of a chaperone. This is an especially difficult situation for a male doctor with a flirtatious female patient. Observation of her behaviour, especially if she is having sexual difficulties of dyspareunia etc., can give insight into how teasing her behaviour could be to her partner.

As with all psychological medicine, there is not a definitive list of reasons for behaviour, fantasies or symptoms. Every patient is unique and must be thought about in a fresh way, based on what has been presented and the interactions occurring live in the consultation between doctor and patient at that moment of time.

- Doctor–patient interaction.
- Why now?
- Here and now.
- Psychosomatic examination.
- Moment of truth.
- Interpretation.

THE USE OF CHAPERONES

Is there a need to have a chaperone?

Much controversy is heard regarding this topic. There is little doubt that if psychosexual medicine could be practised in an ideal world, then a chaperone would not be used. It introduces a third party to the consultation and therefore must alter the interactions between doctor and patient.

Difficulties caused by the presence of a third party include:

1. If medicine dictated that chaperones always be present during intimate examinations

there would be concern that necessary examinations would be neglected because of unavailability of a chaperone – yet another defence in psychosexual medicine against working with the emotional problem.

2. The genital examination provides an opportunity for confiding deeply sensitive information about sexual abuse, previous terminations, miscarriages, domestic violence, lack of sexual feeling, dyspareunia, premature ejaculation, body image distortions etc. The presence of a chaperone may lower the doctor's acuity in detecting the non-verbal signs of distress and inhibit him with interpreting what he finds to the patient. The chaperone's presence may also stop the patient from behaving or verbalizing feelings that he might have been able to share with a doctor he trusted.

3. The cost of employing a nurse to fulfil the role may also be a difficulty for small or charitably funded clinics.

4. The patient may wish to have a family member as chaperone – this could reduce the likelihood of disclosure of sensitive information and delay the development of self confidence in young men and women.

Advantages of a chaperone include:

1. This is the ultimate safeguard for the patient against abuse during the examination and great emphasis is given to it, but abuse during examination is probably very rare.

2. It would protect the patient from perceived abuse and safeguard against the doctor causing unnecessary discomfort, humiliation or intimidation during the examination.

3. The chaperone may provide reassurance to an anxious patient – the psychosexual doctor though would wish to understand what the anxiety was about rather than reassuring against it.

4. The presence of a chaperone protects the doctor from false allegations of sexual abuse.

RCOG guidelines regarding chaperones for genital examinations

The above advantages and disadvantages are outlined in full in the RCOG's Report of a Working Party on Intimate Examinations (RCOG, 1997). Perhaps the most valuable sentence they include in their report on chaperones is

> It is acceptable for a doctor to perform an intimate examination without a chaperone if the patient and doctor agree. The Working Party considers that a chaperone should be offered to all patients undergoing intimate examinations in Gynaecology and Obstetrics irrespective of the gender of the gynaecologist. If the patient prefers to be examined without a chaperone this request should be honoured and recorded in the notes.

Perhaps the most sensible attitude regarding chaperones in psychosexual medicine is to establish early in the consultation that the patient is in fact suitable for this sort of brief psychosomatic interpretative therapy, i.e. is not paranoid.

CONCLUSION

The skills of psychosexual medicine are complex, practical and not factual. Each interaction is unique. It may have similarities to previous consultations, but offering the patient ready-made solutions or good ideas learned in the past must be avoided. Each individual is the product of different life events and needs to be seen with fresh eyes and heard with a fresh ear if therapy is to be successful.

It is satisfying work for patient and doctor alike when successful. As the skills are practical ones, they are learned through the seminars organized by the Institute of Psychosexual Medicine.

KEY POINTS

- Observing and listening are more important than asking questions.
- Silence can be used effectively.
- Overt and covert problems have to be recognized.
- Understanding the effect of the patient on the doctor and the doctor on the patient.
- Using the genital examination as a psychosomatic event.
- Interpreting the doctor–patient relationship as a means of insight into the patient's problem.

REFERENCES

Balint, M. 1986: *The doctor, his patient and the illness.* London: Churchill Livingstone.

Berne, M.D. 1968: *Games people play.* London: Penguin.

Main, T. 1989: The ailment and other psychoanalytic essays. In Johns, J. (ed.), *Training for the acquisition of knowledge or the development of skill?* London: Free Association Books, 220–34.

RCOG, 1997: *Intimate examinations: Report of a working party.* London: RCOG.

Skrine, R. 1997: *Blocks and freedoms in sexual life.* Oxford: Radcliffe Medical Press.

7 The relevance of past history

Susan Walker

Family influences
    Unconscious choice of partner; the threat of intimacy; the past, the body and the relationship

Past traumas
    Psychological trauma; past relationships; sexual abuse

Case 1

Peter, age 58 years, came to see me because of problems with erections. He had separated one year ago from a 10-year marriage. They had mutually decided it was not working and the parting had been amicable. Since then he had had several relationships, but to his disappointment they had all been short lived. He was sure this was because of his sexual problem.

This situation is not unusual, and my thoughts were of his loss, although a sense of loss was not immediately apparent as he told his story. I suggested that his grief could be most apparent at moments of physical intimacy (his sex life with his wife had been good) and might be getting in the way. We talked about performing and achieving and he went on to tell me about his older brother who had always been so successful with women. He remembered how they used to share a bedroom and how often his brother had thrown him out of it in order to have sex with the latest girl. It never happened the other way round. He grimaced. He had felt bullied, intimidated and inferior. He had turned to academic achievement as a marker of his own success, but had never felt good about himself when it came to women or, I suggested, as a potent man. He went on to explain that his brother remains unmarried, always on the lookout for a new relationship. 'I think his early years have stayed with him' he said. 'And yours with you', I replied.

This case history demonstrates the common finding in psychosexual medicine of a link with a relevant aspect of the past. For Peter, the past was not just a broken marriage and the grief not felt at the time, but a lifetime of believing himself to be unsuccessful with women, unable to perform in bed, unlike his brother. The failure of the marriage seemed to confirm his inner beliefs, and his sexual potency disappeared, as it had done at times when he was younger.

His earlier background was of domination by an alcoholic father who was violently abusive to his mother. To stand up to his father (and brother) meant to be like them, angry, dominant, a bully. 'But potent?' I wondered aloud. A difficult dilemma. He remained passive and silent in the consultation, his feelings locked in, just like they had always been.

In this way the past continues to exert an effect on how we live our lives, how we relate to others, especially those close to us. It affects the way we behave, often consciously but always unconsciously as well. Patients come to us as human beings with a life history of experiences, feelings, beliefs and expectations. Thus the past is always present in the room when doctor and patient meet. The doctor's past is of course also in the room, and will influence what happens, consciously and unconsciously.

So how can we discover the relevance to any individual patient? It can be useful to think about this influence by structuring the past in time.

The immediate past

The influences of the immediate past include the feelings the patient has about the appointment. How did they come to be referred? Why have they presented now? This question is of special interest if the problem has been present for some time. Were they sent by a spouse, or because the person who originally heard the problem thought it a good idea? Have they talked with anyone else about the problem and what are their expectations of the psychosexual consultation? The relevance of the immediate past for the doctor might include how she felt when reading the referral letter. Perhaps she feels inexperienced with this particular problem or, if the referral is from a colleague who has previously 'failed' with this patient, she may even feel in competition, that she will be able to do a better job.

What is happening in the lives of doctor and patient currently that may interfere with the understanding of the problem?

The intermediate past

The intermediate past can be thought of as the history of the presenting problem. What sort of relationship is the patient in and what is its history? When did the problem arise and what else was happening in the patient's life at the time? The relevant past personal history will include previous relationships, in particular past sexual relationships and major life events, births, deaths and marriages. There may also be past traumas, both physical and psychological.

The distant past

The distant past history can be thought of as that which includes family and childhood influences, and how these have shaped the individual and their way of relating to others. These influences will, of course, be present in both patient and doctor, but only those of the patient will be discussed in the consultation as and when they arise. The doctor's past will influence her own beliefs and expectations of relationships. They will also affect the way she perceives her professional role, and unconscious blocks may make it difficult for her to receive all of the patient's history with an open mind. The more she can be aware of her own blocks, the freer she will be to react to the patient in a useful way.

So all of the past, of both doctor and patient as described above, is in the room so to speak, at the moment of meeting and during the consultation. Any one influence may predominate at any time. How then can the doctor discover which aspects of this patient's past are relevant to the presenting problem in the 'here and now'? Traditional history-taking teaches us to ask questions – how long have you had the problem? When did it start? Are there any other, associated symptoms? We attempt to form a diagnosis, assisted by investigations of various kinds that we hope will assist us in categorizing the symptoms and signs into a diagnostic box, one that has a known management plan. The problem with this approach is that it imposes restrictions on what the patient tells us, and on what the doctor chooses to consider as relevant or irrelevant. The traditional approach is often unhelpful in informing us how patients feel about their difficulties, and what fears or fantasies they may have about them. It is here that the art of listening becomes so important. In the consultation important factors in the past history may be spoken about, but inevitably some will not be mentioned. These unvoiced feelings commonly turn out to be some of the most important, but they are denied, unknown or forgotten for a variety of reasons. Understanding which aspects of past history are relevant will develop more freely if the doctor allows the consultation a freedom to flow wherever it needs. Balint (1957) suggested that the doctor should be able to notice and tolerate emotional factors active in the patient that have been ignored or rejected previously. The doctor must learn to accept them as worthy of her attention. This requires the doctor to hear not only the content of the patient's conversation, but also to focus on the way doctor and patient respond to each other. This is the doctor and patient relationship, and its study can prove to be a crucial source of information. Awareness of the interactions between doctor and patient, and in particular the doctor's awareness of her own emotions, can allow the doctor to perceive influences of which the patient may be unaware.

FAMILY INFLUENCES

The family is where we all begin. It is where we experience what relationship to another means. This starts from the earliest relationship, that of infant to mother, and moves on to include father, siblings, the wider family and then the community around us: school, friends and finally sexual relationships. We form patterns of learned behaviour within relationships based on our pasts that become our inner models of expectations and beliefs. It is here that our beliefs about ourselves and our potential are shaped. Within the consultation the doctor is experiencing and trying to make sense of any patterns that emerge.

The child develops a sense of trust and comfort with intimacy from the early years of relating to mother. From this develops the child's sense of himself as loving and loveable. Where there has been severe disruption of this trust, the child is liable to grow up with a low self-esteem.

Unconscious choice of partner

Unless we are able to love ourselves, we are not in a strong position to love others. If we believe somewhere that we are unlovable, we mistrust and may reject anyone who tries to show us otherwise. They do not fit with our learned patterns. In order that the blueprints should match, as it were, we are liable to find a partner who offers us the opposite, that is unloving behaviour and rejection.

Case 2

Sarah, 39 years, arrived looking hesitant and subdued. She told me how she had lost her sex drive years ago following her sterilization. I felt the sense of loss about this and asked her about her children. She talked fondly about each of her five children, two by her first marriage and three with her present husband. She went on to tell me about the termination she had nine years ago. The pregnancy was unplanned and her husband had been adamant that they should not have another child. Reluctantly she had agreed to have a termination, feeling that there was a risk that her husband would leave if she did not go along with his wishes. She had ended up going to the appointment alone and had decided to have a sterilization at the same time.

I felt angry towards this husband who seemed so uncaring, and wondered aloud whether she too had been angry with him. She went on to tell me about their life together and as she talked it struck me how very controlling he was of her. He had never been physically violent, but was always too busy running his own business to help much with the children. Anyway, she felt it her duty to run the house, put meals on the table and look after the children. I said it sounded like a full-time job and asked if she ever had any time to herself. She said that occasionally she went out with girlfriends, but her husband didn't like her to. He would make it difficult, she said. 'Difficult', I reflected. She told me how, whenever she had been out, he would check her pants for stains when she arrived home, looking for evidence of her having been with another man. She said she thought it was because he loved her so much.

I could hardly contain my angry feelings, but I was also curious. What made her so ready to put up with this, and why did she feel it was a sign of love? I commented that she seemed to feel reassured by his behaviour. She went on to talk about her mother and how as a teenager she had rarely been allowed to go out, especially not with boys. If she did go out, her mother had gone with her. Most of the time she had stayed at home cooking for the family. Her father had left when she was a baby and her mother had never gone out with another man. One day in her late teens she had rebelled and decided to leave home and her mother had not wanted to have any further contact with her.

She went back to talking about the marriage, her first husband had been the same, she said, but had left her for another woman. 'I've a mother of a husband now.' She laughed. I smiled inwardly at the hidden verbal abuse in the statement. She then cried about how unloved and unwanted she felt. The tears turned to anger as she talked about how she felt unable to refuse sex, but resented it so much. We talked about her inability to stand up to him because she felt he would reject her, and she made the connection to how she had felt at home with her mother. I said that perhaps it felt safer to do what she had always done.

I saw her again and thought she was clinically depressed. She had started antidepressant treatment from her doctor. She cancelled the following appointment and I thought that I would not see her again, but she came back several months later. She said she did not need any more appointments, as she had decided to leave her husband. She had seen a solicitor and was planning to get divorced.

For Sarah the controlling and demeaning behaviour of her husband was a repeat of her mother's control of her evolving independence. However, his behaviour felt familiar, and reassured her of his love. She had not known about an alternative way of relating, and felt unable to express her anger about it until finally she felt it was too late and she left, just as she had left home years before.

The threat of intimacy

Sexual behaviour is a powerful way of expressing feelings in a relationship. The positive aspects of this are the expression of love and the maintenance of physical and emotional closeness. But if negative feelings, especially fear of rejection, are avoided they may reappear in the sexual relationship as difficulties with desire or arousal, or in physical symptoms such as dyspareunia, vaginismus or erectile dysfunction. An inability to sustain an erection or to allow penetration becomes a very effective means of keeping a partner at a distance, preventing intimacy and the risks felt to be associated with it.

In the consultation the doctor often feels unable to get in touch with the real person and is kept away from the difficult feelings involved. This pattern of relating often follows a family history of lack of closeness, or early feelings of being subsumed within a relationship. Patients frequently report a lack of physical closeness within the family, and a subsequent inability to feel comfortable in close physical contact with another. It is as if they have never experienced the intensely pleasurable feelings of being in another's arms. For others, the family has been a source of physical closeness, but there was little emotional comfort. The adult then feels a sense of unease with emotional intimacy. The past experience results in an expectation of dis-comfort and leads to avoidance of intimacy at all costs. Relationships may always be short lived or deteriorate at the time when circum-stances require a fuller commitment.

A common presentation is that of the man or woman who has no sexual problems whilst the relationship is new or superficial, but who go on to lose their desire or ability to have sex as soon as the relationship becomes important.

Case 3

Christine's parents divorced when she was 12 years old. The marriage had always been difficult. Her father had left several times before. Her mother had looked after the children as well as she could, but she had to go out to work leaving the children alone at home, and in any case earned very little money. Christine remembered feeling abandoned and angry with her mother as well as her father. She felt that her mother had deprived them not only of a father, but of all the material things her friends had. She met Jim, who 'was different to other men'. About one year into the relationship, soon after they had spoken about their desire to spend the rest of their lives together, she suddenly went off sex. Much to her sur-prise, they subsequently married and her husband stayed loyal to her. 'I'm perfectly happy with a sexless marriage, I've told him to leave several times', she said. We looked at her unexpressed anger and her expectation that she too would have a marriage in which her husband did not remain faithful to her, and that it would ultimately end in divorce. She dis-covered how envious she was of her husband's ability not to worry about money and of his happy, plentiful childhood, and through this how she was unintentionally destroying the relationship.

Patients who are phobic about commitment withdraw at the point when they sense that to give more of themselves would result not only in greater intimacy, but would risk the pain of the loss of such closeness in the event of rela-tionship breakdown. Early satisfying family relationships build a secure basis for the ability to trust another. To feel close we have to let ourselves be known and trust the other not to reject us. A family history of parental loss through bereavement or separation in child-hood can so often result in the child losing their sense of security. At this time, children may not only lose a loved parent but possibly siblings, a home, school, friends and contact with rela-tives. In addition, they may have to deal with the emotional unavailability of the resident parent who is overwhelmed by their feelings of loss at the time. The child feels angry at this rejection, and subsequently guilty and ashamed of these feelings. With no outlet for these emo-tions, the child is left to cope alone, and the experience becomes one that leaves a perman-ent scar, with fear of future repetition. The adult then becomes someone who, usually at an unconscious level, feels unable to trust in the love of another and avoids true commit-ment and intimacy. This way of relating is then justified by seeing the pattern of their broken relationships as proof that 'it's not worth get-ting too involved'. The expectation of relation-ship breakdown and repeated rejections thus reinforces the beliefs derived from childhood.

Parental loss in childhood may not be appar-ent as such in the history, but the parent may have been unavailable to the child for other reasons. These may include factors such as overt illness, or because of the parents' own upbringing, so that damaging ways of relating reverberate down the generations.

The past, the body and the relationship

Psychosexual problems often present at times of stress in the relationship, and are often blamed for the difficulties in the relationship. As with other psychosomatic presentations, patients often cling to the hope of a physical treatment, or may expect the doctor to simply solve the problem for them. Occasionally, symptoms may be offered as an acceptable presentation of emotional difficulties. This is surprising given the difficulty most people have in discussing details of their sex lives, but perhaps it reflects a societal change in which sexual problems are seen as legitimate and valid.

Case 4

A 29-year-old woman presented with a history of severe dysparuenia. At examination she cried out with groans of pain, although I had only put a finger at the introitus. Her screams brought her otherwise detached and disinterested boyfriend rapidly to his feet, rushing to comfort her. The pain continued for some time, although I had ceased touching her, and I found myself offering the same comfort verbally as her boyfriend was doing. The screams had reminded me of a woman giving birth, and with time we understood how much she needed him to look after her, and her fear that he wouldn't. He noticed how difficult it was for him to show tender feelings at other times when he felt unwanted, and as they began to communicate more openly about their feelings her symptoms disappeared.

Feelings about sexuality, physical closeness, nakedness and our bodies are all part of our childhood experiences. What we experienced in our early years is, at one level, what we are most comfortable with. This may of course contradict an expressed conscious desire to do things differently. Patients often describe how they felt embarrassed, uninformed and ashamed about sexual matters within the family, and how they planned to give their own children a different experience. They are then surprised that it is so much more difficult to do than they had imagined.

Sexual inhibitions that have arisen as a result of strong religious or moral teaching about sexual matters are particularly difficult to counteract. Women may feel unable to initiate sex, which would be an open admittance of sexual feelings. Such inhibitions may lie behind difficulties with masturbation or orgasm. The man is then cast in the role of sole seeker of sexual pleasure, and both partners may then feel that he has to take his partner's body, rather than be given it.

Years of relating in this way results in increasing resentment on both sides. He feels angry at having to press her for sex, and she consciously or unconsciously disapproves of his desire and withdraws even more. Some time later the couple may present with the common story of her loss of libido, and his frustration at having to try to persuade her. Neither feels loved or understood and the relationship deteriorates.

Family influences may merely set a pattern of difficulty in discussing sexual issues openly. The ability of the doctor to talk openly about the subject within the consultation often triggers a parallel openness in the relationship, with early resolution of difficulties.

PAST TRAUMAS

What is meant by trauma? It can be defined as any event that leads to feelings that overwhelm the sense of self; a disintegration, falling apart, a threat to survival.

Trauma can conveniently be divided into physical and psychological, although it will often result in both. It is certainly possible to undergo psychological trauma without any overt physical trauma, but the very common physical symptoms that we see are, I suggest, the bodily manifestations of psychological trauma. Similarly, it is hard to imagine a physical trauma that does not deliver an equivalent blow to the psyche. This may be the case even when the physical trauma is not obvious. Trauma that is felt as a threat to survival can result in a protective emotional withdrawal that may present with psychosexual disorder, because penetration has an emotional equivalence of getting inside the self.

One patient presented asking for help because of her inability to have a cervical smear. She had no difficulties with sex. After discussion, she linked this with her memory of frequent visits to the dentist as a young child. Although she had not had any extraordinary dental work done, she remembered the terror she had felt when the metal instruments were in her mouth and she did not know what would happen next. She remembered that her mother had not been allowed into the room with her on these occasions. On the morning on which we had agreed to do a vaginal examination, she had vomited three times from anxiety.

Obvious physical traumas include physical assault, accidents, severe illness or operations in the past. Gynaecological operations, especially hysterectomy, often result in psychosexual disorders. Patients may feel inhibited about discussing these issues with their surgeon. A patient presented with bladder problems and during vaginal examination revealed that she had not had sex since her hysterectomy five years previously. Her fantasy was that the end of her vagina was open because her womb had been removed, and she was afraid of the damage that a penis, and particularly ejaculation, would cause inside her.

Physical assault, in particular rape, invariably results in some degree of psychosexual dysfunction. Unfortunately, if reported, this may be made worse by the inappropriate actions of the police and medical services.

Childbirth is physically traumatic. Women are so vulnerable at this time and may sustain extreme physical trauma ranging from bruising and tearing of the vagina and vulva to episiotomy, forceps delivery or caesarean section. These physical traumas, along with the vulnerability, fear and feelings of not being in control, combine to leave psychological scars long after the physical scars have healed.

Vasectomy and circumcision can cause similar psychological scars in men.

Physical trauma that results in a change of body appearance or function can undermine confidence in oneself and the body. Mastectomy and orchidectomy are especially difficult in this respect. Spinal cord injury with sexual dysfunction or direct genital injury have obvious relevance to psychosexual problems.

The effects of past physical trauma are individual, and the severity will depend on numerous factors, including age, degree of trauma or severity of disease and the psychological vulnerability of the patient.

Psychological trauma

Psychological trauma can have an effect on sexual function because of the way it interrupts the complicated interactions that sexual relating requires on both the physical and psychological level. Bereavement of any kind, the loss of a loved partner, a child or a job is such a trauma. External circumstances that involve major life changes, or a change in one's role or sense of identity, become a potential source of difficulty.

Psychological trauma is a concomitant of physical trauma and may or may not heal with the physical healing. The emotional consequences of childhood loss, rejection or separation have been explored earlier in this chapter. The same trauma also applies to adults who suffer loss. Patients commonly present with sexual difficulties after rejection or separation from a previous partner. The difficulty may only become apparent with a new partner, when the pain of the loss is re-evoked. The helplessness felt becomes expressed in a physical impotence.

Other emotions can also become overwhelmingly unbearable and result in fixed physical symptoms.

Case 5

A woman presented with a 3-year history of recurrent pelvic pain and attacks of cystitis for which no organic cause could be found, despite intensive investigation. At our first meeting she described how she had had her first sexual experience after getting drunk at a party. The kissing had lead on to more and whilst trying to say no she had suddenly felt the penetration. She felt guilty, ashamed and 'dirty'. Her parents had insisted she go the genitourinary clinic to be checked for infection. She did not link this event to her physical pain. She had a firm belief that her symptoms were due to infection that the doctors had somehow missed, until she remembered, quite suddenly, how she had glimpsed the face of this man in a large crowd. It was after this that the pain had started and her sexual problems developed. We understood together how the psychological trauma of the event had been awakened, but not at a conscious level, resulting in her pain being felt in the 'wrong' place, her body.

Past relationships

The possible effects on future relationships of the psychological trauma of rejection or loss in previous relationships has been mentioned in the last section. In addition, previous relationships, especially when sexual, can alter our expectations of new ones.

Early sexual experience and first sexual intercourse may have long lasting effects on future sexual activity. At puberty the sex hormones stimulate sexual arousal, and the adolescent is driven towards more intimate relationships and sexual experimentation. Early experiences of difficulty or rejection can result in extreme feelings of embarrassment or inadequacy and may inhibit further exploration. The avoidance may become established as a pattern, which seems to confirm the feelings of non-acceptance.

Early homosexual experiences can have similar effects. In one study 10 per cent of adolescents had had homosexual experiences. These early experiences may cause guilt and confusion, and may inhibit future heterosexual relationships unless there is reassurance that it is often a part of sexual exploration at that age, and is not necessarily indicative of final sexual orientation. The ability to discuss sexual feelings with a trusted adult or peer can be vital. Lack of support at this stage is likely to lead to emotional withdrawal.

A young woman presented with non-consummation of her marriage secondary to severe vaginismus. She was convinced that this meant she was a lesbian and should never have married. Some time later she revealed that during her adolescence she had intense feelings towards a girlfriend, and although there was never any sexual contact she had always feared this meant she would be unable to have a sexual relationship with a man. This belief then became a self-fulfilling prophecy.

For others, it is the loss of control experienced during intense sexual arousal in first experiences that is subsequently feared. For women, this can result in a need to control any sexual feelings at all, so much so that all feeling is lost and sexual desire cannot be felt. For men, the loss of control from intense arousal, which may result in premature ejaculation, can become a source of performance anxiety or a fear of the vagina itself.

The usual experience is that of continuing teenage experimentation under the drive of the sex hormones. This is a time of insecurity and uncertainty, whilst finding a sense of identity: who we are, where we fit in and what kind of relationships we want. Most teenagers are therefore more focused on themselves than on the actual relationship, discovering the subtle signs and signals that communicate sexual attraction. For some, these interactions are so difficult that the move from a social relationship to a sexual one becomes fraught with difficulty. They withdraw from any further attempts at sexual contact with a belief that they are incapable or abnormal, and may become stuck with this view of themselves. Low self esteem and insecurity combined with ignorance or mistaken beliefs about the body or its functions compound the problem.

Erectile difficulties on attempting first penetration are surprisingly common, and for some become part of a lifelong anxiety about sexual performance. These difficulties are usually present on a background of general feelings of inadequacy. The failure to perform as expected, and the associated feelings of embarrassment, maybe even shame, are an attack on his sense of manhood, and can lead to extreme anxiety that predisposes to a cycle of failure and ever increasing performance anxiety.

In my experience, many patients who present with sexual difficulties have an expectation that sex 'just happens'. They interpret the normal stage of 'fumbling' as a sign that things are not as they should be, and feel inadequate and incapable as a result. It is as if they believe that there is no learning phase in the process of finding out about sexual relating.

The transfer of feelings and knowledge about a previous partner on to a different one may also cause problems. Anxiety about performance or a self-centred way of relating may lead to the assumption that there is a right way common to all relationships, and such beliefs can cause communication problems and mutual resentment. It also prevents the creative coming together in a new sexual relationship that will inevitably be different each time.

A man married a woman who was sexually 'frigid' and unavailable. After they had separated he assumed the same would be true of his new partner and never gave her the space she needed to express herself sexually. She held on to her resentment silently, feeling pressurized and unheard, and slowly lost all desire for sex. As the years went by she became the sexually unavailable woman he complained about.

Sexual abuse

The incidence of childhood sexual abuse in the general population is unknown. Figures suggest levels of 15–30 per cent, but will depend on definitions of abuse. Childhood sexual abuse can be defined as the exploitation of a position of trust or authority when the child is being used for sexual stimulation by the adult. This is an abuse of the child's needs for love and affection. The abuse may or may not involve direct physical contact and often includes threats of punishment on disclosure.

The effects of childhood sexual abuse are unpredictable and individual, although it has been suggested that some factors are more psychologically damaging to the child. Those acts that include penetration and those that have occurred over a long period of time are thought to be particularly harmful. Subsequent disclosure with police involvement and family break up may add to the trauma experienced. A study by Jehu (1991) of women who had experienced childhood sexual abuse found that 94 per cent of the study population described sexual problems.

Intimacy with the doctor is particularly threatening for these patients, with the fear of exploitation within the helping relationship where the doctor is felt to be more powerful. The nature of the psychosexual consultation, that includes not only an emphasis on sexuality and the feelings involved, but also potentially a genital examination, makes it inherently difficult.

Examining patients can provoke strong emotions in both patient and doctor. This is particularly true in patients who have been abused. Awareness and acknowledgement of these feelings reduces the likelihood of them interfering with the consultation, and can give the doctor a greater understanding of the patient's problems.

I have found it useful, on occasions where even the suggestion of a genital examination is too threatening to the patient, to try to explore the feelings and fantasies about it as thoroughly as possible. Although there is always the potential for abuse in which the doctor may inadvertently get caught up, provided this is kept in mind there is also, in my view, great potential for healing.

In clinical practice, however, there are no constants. One person might suffer lifelong problems as a result of what might be seen as a relatively minor incident, whereas another who has suffered long-term penetrative abuse has managed to form good relationships with less degree of impairment of sexual enjoyment. The difference is probably the result of other stabilizing factors within the individual.

Emotional and sexual difficulties are common effects of childhood sexual abuse. Feelings of guilt and low self-esteem, often from a sense of having encouraged the abuse or because the child was in reality blamed for it, can be overwhelming. The damage may be exacerbated if there is memory of having enjoyed it. The enjoyment may have been emotional, because it was a way, possibly the only way, to feel close to and loved by the abuser, or physically because of bodily arousal. Guilt is often profound because of childhood sexual curiosity and fantasy, including unconscious sexual wishes. The child may also have benefited materially from the abuse, being offered rewards of some kind.

The secrecy and social stigmatization surrounding the issues of childhood sexual abuse increase the sense of shame, which is also a common feature in adults presenting with such a history. This can be sufficiently threatening to prevent disclosure completely, or not uncommonly may lead to non-attendance for help after disclosure. Feelings of self-blame and low self-esteem are common and may result in a continuation of abusive relationships into adult life.

Anger towards the abuser and often also towards those adults who did not prevent it can persist either consciously or unconsciously, when it may be turned against the self and incorporated into self-loathing.

A sense of difference from others, of not knowing how to be in relationships, and an inability to receive sexual pleasure is a common complaint. The sexual difficulties or physical symptoms seem to confirm the idea of being abnormal.

Patients often report flashbacks during sex. Occasionally, a specific sexual act leads to retrieval of memories of abuse.

A patient presented with a sudden onset of dyspareunia, which had started after her husband had masturbated her whilst she was sleeping. She woke at the point of orgasm and this triggered the memory of her father touching her under similar circumstances.

Another patient, who had been abused by an unknown babysitter, summed up her inability to form a relationship with a man when she said 'I always think of every man over a certain age that I meet, that he might have been the one that raped me'.

CONCLUSION

This chapter has focused on the relevance of past history as it relates to patients presenting with psychosexual problems. The multitude of past influences, and the forgotten or unconscious nature of so many of them, poses difficulties for doctor and patient alike as they attempt to unravel the threads of the story. Observation of the doctor–patient relationship provides real understanding of the patient's patterns of relating. Traditional history-taking limits the potential of the consultation to lead to relevant issues, and restricts the development of a shared space in which real therapeutic change can occur.

KEY POINTS

- The immediate, intermediate and distant past all influence present behaviour and feelings.
- Denied, unknown or forgotten aspects of the past will emerge more easily if the consultation is allowed freedom to flow wherever it needs.

- Our beliefs in ourselves and our potential are shaped in our earliest family experiences.
- Intimacy can be threatening if trust had not developed in secure early relationships.
- The body is often used unconsciously to express emotional difficulties.
- Early sexual experiences and first sexual intercourse can have long lasting effects on future sexual activity.
- The effects of physical trauma and childhood sexual abuse depend on the psychological vulnerability of the individual.

REFERENCES

Balint, M. 1957: *The doctor, his patient and the illness.* London: Pitman Medical.

Jehu, D. 1991: *Clinical approaches to sex offenders and their victims.* Chichester: John Wiley, 243.

FURTHER READING

Crowe, M. 1998: Sexual therapy and the couple. In Freeman, H., Pullen, I., Stein, G. and Wilkinson, G. (eds), *Seminars in psychosexual disorders.* London: Gaskell Royal College of Psychiatrists, ch. 4, 59.

Doyle, G. 1998: Sexual abuse. In Freeman, H., Pullen, I., Stein, G. and Wilkinson, G. (eds), *Seminars in psychosexual disorders.* London: Gaskell Royal College of Psychiatrists, ch. 6, 101.

Malan, D.H. 1979: *Individual psychotherapy and the science of psychodynamics.* London: Butterworths.

8 Problems with life events

Margaret Denman

Adolescence

Pregnancy and childbirth

Ageing

Disability

Terminal illness

Bereavement

ADOLESCENCE

Fears and fantasies about sexual matters can start at an early age. Changing hormone levels, alterations in bodily function and configuration can be both confusing and exciting at this stage of life. In this new century, the pressures on young people in the western world to be 'sexual' have never been so great. These pressures come from the media and equally importantly from their peers. Guilt and shame associated with sexual activity outside of marriage is becoming less as the influences of religion and culture wane. Today's adolescents are generally less likely to believe that masturbation could make them blind, although they may still be made to feel that it is 'dirty' and it may leave them with feelings of guilt. Contraception is available to all and abortion is virtually obtainable on demand.

On the other hand, HIV and other sexually transmitted diseases are openly discussed by the media, both in documentaries and soap opera. Confusion over sexual orientation may

start in adolescence. Homosexuality is ostensibly becoming more acceptable and is certainly discussed increasingly. Whilst dramas containing sexual encounters between members of the same sex are now more prevalent in films and on television, the old prejudices still exist and teenagers will hear derogatory terms used against gay people. This can be confusing as an adolescent struggles to find his or her own sexual identity.

The National Survey of Sexual Attitudes and Lifestyles in Britain asked about age at first heterosexual sexual intercourse (Wellings *et al.*, 1994, 37–54). People of age 16–59 were surveyed. The age of first intercourse decreased with each age group surveyed. Women aged 50–54 at time of interview had a median age of first intercourse of 21 years, whilst those aged 16–19 at interview lost their virginity at a median age of 17. Figures for men were 20 and 17, respectively. As well as the decline in the median age, there was an increase in the number of males and females experiencing sexual intercourse before the age of 16. This decline in the age of first intercourse is disproportional to the decline in the age of menarche, which is the most easily measurable parameter of sexual maturation. Interestingly, the percentage having their first sexual intercourse before the age of 16, particularly amongst the female group, was much lower in the groups from the Indian sub-continent than any other ethnic group. This may reflect cultural as well as religious influences.

Most individuals surveyed were able to recall with ease the timing of their first intercourse, testifying to the importance of the event. Losing one's virginity is memorable, and the circumstances can often take on long-term significance. Wight *et al.* (2000) surveyed 7395 Scottish teenagers from a whole range of social groups. The survey population had a mean age of 14 years 2 months. Eighteen per cent of the boys and 15.4 per cent of the girls reported experience of heterosexual intercourse. A large number of both sexes reported regret that it had happened. Thirty-two per cent of girls and 27 per cent of boys thought that it had happened too early, whilst 13 per cent of girls and 5 per cent of boys stated that it should not have happened at all. For both sexes any pressure surrounding the event was associated with regret and with girls lack of prior planning with their partner was also significant.

Many events during adolescence can affect future sexual functioning. Girls whose periods start at a very early age or those who start very late may feel 'marked out'. Big breasts, small breasts and weight problems fill the pages of agony columns, whilst boys may worry about penis size. Both sexes worry about acne. I recall a young man who came repeatedly to the family planning clinic to show his penis to a series of female doctors, saying that it was too small. It was finally, when he described his humiliation by his stepsister in front of her friends, that he came to understand that he felt 'small' as a person. He gradually came to believe that his penis was 'big enough'.

As with all aspects of human sexuality, surveys and statistics do not always help with the problem in hand, as human behaviour and experience do not fit into neat categories. A theory about the cause of a problem may not be helpful when faced with an individual in the consulting room. Presenting symptoms cannot always be taken at face value. Difficulties that initially seem to be related to a physical problem may in fact be associated with depression or general low esteem, and a holistic approach must be taken.

PREGNANCY AND CHILDBIRTH

Pregnancy and childbirth are amongst the most dramatic events in a woman's life. As well as the physical changes, there are enormous social and emotional upheavals. These events and the circumstances surrounding them can have a great influence on sexuality and relationships. Men may also have altered sexual feelings towards a woman who is pregnant, a woman who has given birth or a woman who is now a mother. Being a mother or having sex with a partner who has now become a mother may present a problem. The effect of a baby and children on a relationship and on lifestyle is multifold. Circumstances surrounding the conception, which may for example not be planned or at the other extreme may be the end result of years of infertility, may have an effect on the subsequent relationship and sex life. Post-natal depression is common and is often related to loss of libido.

Dixon *et al.* (2000) studied 131 couples following childbirth. Approximately 50 per cent of first-time parents in this study described their sex life as 'poor' or 'not very good' eight months after the birth of their baby. Twenty per cent of them said they would like help for this. First-time parents also reported a rise in the incidence of problems in their general relationship, with a rating of 'poor' or 'not very good' increasing from 1 per cent before pregnancy to 20 per cent eight months after childbirth. Not surprisingly, the changes in the general relationship and the quality of sex life were associated in these couples.

Altered body image may make a woman feel unattractive during pregnancy and after the birth. Delivery can be traumatic, leaving the woman with vaginal tears, scars and pain. There may be altered bladder or bowel function and dislike of the body that has not resumed the pre-pregnancy shape. Men may also have fantasies about the effect of the delivery on their partner's anatomy, even more so as they are now expected to be present in the labour ward. The fear that their partner may have to go through another awful experience if she became pregnant again may sometimes be a cause of impotence.

The demise of the routine post-natal vaginal examination has left many women without that reassurance that their body has now returned to normal and is ready and able once again to receive a penis. Although no medical examinations should be done 'routinely', a careful assessment at the six-week post-natal check up can identify those women who would benefit from a genital examination. General questions about 'returning to normal' or 'any other worries' can sometimes elucidate these problems. An examination can help to dispel fantasies about tight stitches, painful scars or a lax vagina before the problem becomes entrenched. This can be seen as a form of preventive medicine and may stop the development of long-term problems that are much harder to treat.

Some women need 'permission' from the health care professional to resume intercourse or reassurance that it is fine not to feel like sex when your breasts are bursting with milk and you have had no sleep for weeks. It is impossible to generalize, as some women will resume intercourse as soon as possible, even before the post-natal visit, whilst others wait for many months.

Case 1

Barbara brought her five-month-old baby Alice to see me at the well baby clinic at my surgery. No appointments are needed for this session. I had already met her daughter several times at her eight-week check and earlier immunizations. I knew Barbara from the past and had dealt with a breast abscess that had appeared four weeks post-partum. Her large, red-haired mother, also my patient, had phoned me at this time and arranged for me to see her daughter as an emergency. I knew her forceful mother well, having helped her with her own sexual discomfort after her menopause.

Barbara showed me a tiny patch of dry skin on Alice's arm. Whilst doing this she asked me for more contraceptive pills, and with the same breath, asked if it was usual for sex to be sore this long after the birth of a baby? I said no, it was not usual, and that it would be best if she made an appointment to see me in my general surgery time so that I could examine her and discuss her problems further. I would be able to prescribe the pill then. We discussed the baby's minor skin problem and they left.

A couple of weeks later they turned up at a routine morning surgery. I was now able to review her notes. Since her confinement, she had seen three doctors in four visits. The notes relating to the first appointment mentioned a 'lump' in the perineum, for which she had been reassured. The second was her visit to me for the breast abscess, then there was the routine post-natal check and the comment in the records was that her episiotomy was well healed. She was prescribed the contraceptive pill. A fourth appointment a month later was for more pills. I worked out that she could not have really needed more pills at that stage.

Alice quietly amused herself in the pushchair and was not intrusive. It did not feel like a three-way consultation and the atmosphere between the patient and myself felt quite intimate, as if we knew each other well. As she had complained of soreness, and alerted by the previous mention of 'lump in the perineum', I suggested immediately that I examine her. She got on to the couch readily and I did a vaginal examination. She was a little bit sore on one side. There was a great deal of white discharge. I took a swab and confidently diagnosed 'thrush'. Great, I thought to myself, this might be a quick consultation after all. I discussed the treatment.

As I was dealing with the specimen, I felt something unspoken hanging in the air. I went and sat on the edge of the couch as she was still lying there, having made no move towards getting up or dressed. She said, 'Actually doctor, I have completely gone off sex since Alice was born'.

'Tell me about the delivery', I said and perched more firmly on the couch. The atmosphere became very intense as she described a chain of unpleasant medical events. She had been induced for high blood pressure and the labour had been quick and very painful. They had attempted a vacuum extraction that had failed and Alice was delivered by forceps. Then she had a post-partum haemorrhage requiring a blood transfusion. On her return home, the episiotomy had become infected and broken down. She had needed antibiotics and numerous examinations by the midwife.

I now felt confident once again that I had 'diagnosed' the cause of her problems. Who would feel like sex after this catalogue of disasters and trauma? I did not say anything however, as I sensed she had not finished. I allowed an awkward silence. She still made no move from the couch.

Finally she told me her real pain. Both her partner's parents and her parents lived in her own street. It was about 30 minutes drive from the hospital. She was to give birth to the first grandchild on both sides of the family. Both sets of prospective grandparents had given strict instructions that they were to be phoned for the delivery so that they could be present in the hospital, if not actually in the labour ward. Her partner had phoned his parents who promptly arrived. Before he had time to phone Barbara's parents, the chain of medical events began and he was called back to the labour ward. Barbara's parents, led I suspected by her powerful mother, had taken umbrage at this and their street was now a battle zone. They had not been able to arrange a Christening and the joy associated with this birth had been marred.

I said, 'It must be very difficult to make love to someone when your families are at war'. She became thoughtful, put on her clothes and left without many words. I ran behind her with her prescription for the 'thrush'. The repeat pill prescription was forgotten.

When I saw her again in the baby clinic, I asked how things were and she briskly said that everything was fine now thank you. I felt as if I was being told to mind my own business.

Comment

I have used this case as a demonstration that one can never generalize about the cause of sexual problems. The traumatic delivery may have led me down the wrong path, but I sensed at each stage that she had more to say. I enabled her to gain insight into the reason for her loss of libido. This did not take long. She had already made several attempts to talk to doctors about this and finally presented in the baby clinic with the 'calling card' of Alice's eczema. Even then she had said that she was sore instead of saying that she had lost her libido. Once she was better, their sex life became the property of the couple, it was no longer a medical difficulty and further enquiry seemed prurient. Barbara will need to see me in the future with her own and her daughter's problems and will not want to discuss healthy sexual activity.

I have seen many women whose sexual functioning has been affected by the physical events and traumas of the delivery, leaving them with sore areas, vaginismus and fantasies of damage. Extrapolation from these cases would not have been very useful in this case. Although the problem was not directly related to a physical problem stemming from the delivery or pregnancy, it was disclosed after the genital examination.

AGEING

Although sex in the media is generally associated with the young and beautiful, middle aged and elderly people still have sexual desire and romantic feelings. These feelings into old age are portrayed delightfully in the popular novel, *Captain Correli's Mandolin* (De Berniere, 1998). The lovers, who meet during the Italian occupation of the Greek island of Kephalonia in the Second World War, are not able to consummate their relationship until their old age when they meet again, having maintained a passion for each other throughout an enforced separation. It is often hard for a young doctor or nurse to 'imagine' that elderly or ill people are still having or wanting to have an active sex life, sometimes even with a new partner.

The national survey of sexual behaviour in Britain (Wellings *et al.*, 1994, 137–9) only interviewed men and women up to the age of 59. It did, however, show that the frequency of sexual activity decreases with age. The highest frequency reached is a median of five times per month for women aged 20–29 and men aged 25–34. By the age of 55–59, the median had dropped to twice a month for men. Fifty per cent of women in this age group reported no sex in the last month. The women over 50 were more likely to be widowed, separated or divorced than men of the same age. They commented that some social surveys also showed that the menopause had an effect on sexual frequency.

These statistics are useful, but do not always help us understand the patient or couple in our consulting room who have their own fears, desires, difficulties and expectations. Older people may find it more difficult to ask for help that may be perceived to be more readily available in family planning and sexually transmitted disease clinics that attract a younger

clientele. Particularly in the general practice setting, it is important that sexual health is discussed in the context of physical disease, disability or mental illness.

The menopause

The menopause and the time of change surrounding it known as the climacteric is a life event that means different things to different women. In some cultures it is welcomed as the end of fertility and the onset of old age, which commands respect. In the western world, it is more likely to signify the loss of youth and femininity. The hormone changes may bring about vasomotor and other unpleasant symptoms that can lead to insomnia, stress and possibly depression. The reduction in oestrogen, especially when sudden, as with oophorectomy in a younger woman, can lead to dramatic loss of libido. Studies have shown that it is the menopause and not age that affects libido in women (Hunter *et al.*, 1986). As time progresses, if no hormone replacement therapy (HRT) is given, many women develop vaginal dryness and soreness, leading to dyspareunia. This may cause discomfort during intercourse, leading to secondary loss of libido. Difficulty with penetration can also have an effect on the male partner's ability to sustain an erection. Luckily for the modern woman, many of these symptoms can now be alleviated with HRT. In some women testosterone implants are prescribed for loss of libido, although this is still controversial and more trials are needed.

Any sexual difficulties reported at the time of the menopause must, however, be considered in the context of other changes that may be taking place in a woman's life at that stage. Her partner may be less potent and yet she is presenting with a problem. Children leaving home or grown-up children still in the home may be equally disturbing. A woman may be torn between elderly parents needing increasing care, her own job and her children's problems. Sex may just seem like another chore. Once again no generalization can be made and women may use a discussion about HRT in a specialist menopause clinic or in general practice as a 'calling card' to discuss sexual matters which may not actually be related to the climacteric.

Lifestyle changes

Lifestyle changes can occur at all ages of man, but these are often most dramatic in later years when loss of job, retirement or disability may affect the way men or women view themselves. Major changes can also affect the balance in a relationship. Role reversals may take place when women are able to maintain their job whilst their partner may be made unemployed or become retired either because of ill health or the economic climate.

Case 2

Mr Archer was referred to me by my partner. He was 57 years old, tall and well built for his age. He was losing his hair on top of his head. There was a twinkle in his eye. He told me how he was impotent with his wife. He had very poor early morning erections, but that was all. He said sadly, 'There is nothing there'. I offered to examine him – my partner had checked his blood pressure and other physical parameters. As he started to get undressed, he stopped to show me his arm. 'It was a nasty fracture', he said. It was still swollen and stiff. 'It happened when someone at work had dropped a crate on it. They were very good at the hospital, but I have finished with all the physiotherapy now.'

He spoke wistfully of the doctors and physiotherapists, as if they were comrades or workmates. 'I cannot work any more and I am still waiting for my compensation. Everyone at my old workplace ignores me now.'

I completed the genital examination, which was normal, and he got dressed.

'I cannot play golf any more. I was a good sportsman you know.' I felt he was showing off to the younger woman doctor.

I said, 'You lost everything with that accident'. I remember stressing the word 'everything'. He said, 'Yes, I did. No one has ever said that to me before. I feel I am on the scrap heap now'.

I said, 'It is no wonder your penis will not work when the rest of you has been made to feel so useless'. We sat in silence and stared at his arm. I felt very sad and I related this feeling back to him.

This was just an ordinary general practice appointment and I suggested he came back again. On the second visit he agreed that he understood now why he had become impotent and decided that it was time that he stopped feeling sorry for himself and 'get on with his life'. I asked him about sex with his wife and what they did. It was only then that he started to talk about her breast cancer and recent mastectomy. She had also had a mild stroke and was on a lot of medication for her blood pressure. He said, 'She does not seem that interested at the moment anyway'. Without any formal 'contract' it seemed appropriate that we left it there. He knew he could come back.

I have seen them many times as a couple over the past few years because of his wife's deteriorating health. Sex has never been mentioned. Was this a success or failure? By interpreting the feelings in the room he was able to understand his impotence and accept that it was related to his change in lifestyle. As well as losing a job, which was very physical, he was now unable to play his favourite sport and felt abandoned and let down by his workmates. There was also a role reversal and he adapted very well to becoming his wife's main carer as her health deteriorated.

Comment

The spark of interest in sex, the twinkle in his eye, was still there and was presented to the female doctor. I saw him for himself and looked at his problems and losses before getting involved with his wife's difficulties and their relationship. I had stuck to the 'here and now' of the consultation. Although I subsequently saw them many times together when she had a further stroke, the sexual problem was never discussed and I have never known whether he had even told her that he had been to talk to me about it.

I really had two patients but they did not present as a couple and only one of them, the man, was complaining. His initial problem related to his accident and loss of self-esteem had to be dealt with first before he mentioned his wife. It had been important that I saw him initially as an individual, because it later seemed that the enormity of her problems overshadowed his. It did not seem to be necessary to ask them to attend as a couple to discuss their sexual problem, as they had resolved the issue between them for themselves once he had reached an understanding of his difficulties.

DISABILITY

The practical issues of disability and sexuality have been described elsewhere by specialists working in this field. It is relatively easy to learn about the mechanical ways that lovemaking can be adapted to accommodate a deformed or disabled body. Useful tips, such as the use of analgesics before lovemaking, the employment of extra cushions or the management of a paralysed limb, can be learnt by the professional and the information imparted to the patient. Advice regarding the management of intercourse with a urinary catheter in situ and physical treatment for organic erectile dysfunction can easily be obtained. These subjects are discussed by Cooper and Guillebaud (1999) in their book, *Sexuality and Disability: A Guide for Everyday Practice.*

It is much harder, however, to deal with the feelings and emotions of an individual who may have sexual urges and desires inside what is seen to be by them, and the outside world, as a deformed and ugly body. A disabled person's ability to achieve sexual expression is not only restricted by their physical limitations, but also by their sense of worth and attractiveness. If they feel deformed and unlovable, they will not be able to enjoy their bodies or allow another to do so. A physical relationship may bring a sense of exposure that may be mirrored in the doctor–patient relationship, especially during a physical examination. It is important that the doctor or nurse tries to see the 'person' beyond the disability that may have defined them all their lives. Even a small degree of deformity or disability may leave an individual feeling that they have been 'marked out' and different from the rest of society.

Coulson (2000), in her paper about body image, describes three women in whom their picture of themselves disturbed their sexual function. She defines 'body image' as a 'mental picture of the flesh, as opposed to the spirit, produced by the imagination'. She also poses the question: body image – is it body shape, body function, body health or body strength? It is complex and there may be additional fantasies about ostensibly 'normal' parts of their anatomy in a person who has a deformity or disability, as in Case 3 where the patient felt that she was flawed.

Case 3

Tamsin came to see me in my general practice surgery. It was an emergency appointment and she was seen as a temporary resident. I was not sure why she had come then. She was a 23-year-old art student home on holiday from a northern university. She wore usual student garb, jeans and a dark sweater. Her blond curly hair was dishevelled and unkempt. She had moderately severe acne for which she had not sought any treatment. She hung her head and said nothing. In the ensuing silence I looked on her computer notes, which were available because she was a patient of our practice before leaving for university. I noted a comment that she had repeatedly failed to attend as requested for a cervical smear.

'Well', I said, feeling a little irritated by all this. I was very busy and running late.

'I keep getting these pains', she said, looking at her abdomen.

I was not going to beat around the bush. 'We had better take a look.'

She lay on the couch fully clothed. Reluctantly and slowly she pulled up her sweater and underlying tee-shirt. The atmosphere in the consulting room was very tense. As I went to put my hand on her abdomen she visibly flinched and went to push me away. 'You don't seem to like anyone to touch you', I said. 'Is that why you didn't come for your smear?' She looked terrified and tentatively nodded. 'I could not let anyone do that to me', stressing the word 'that'.

I said, 'Sex must be difficult if you cannot let anyone touch you'. I felt as if I was attacking her. She wept and described how she felt that she was not 'normal' 'down there', pointing towards her genital area, and that she felt that she would never be able to have sex. She could not use a tampon and never had been able to do so. There seemed to be some sort of 'blockage'.

I asked her to get dressed. I felt as if we had gone far enough for that consultation. She got dressed and sat on the chair beside the desk with that type of shudder that follows a bout of tears. She looked me directly in the eye, accusingly, and said, 'You looked straight inside me. How did this happen? I only came to discuss my irritable bowel syndrome'. I said nothing, but the atmosphere had lightened. 'Perhaps we could work on this together', I said. 'If you would like to come back again I could take a look "down there" and we could work the problem out together.' She willingly agreed and the appointment was made.

I saw her for a couple of 15-minute appointments, all that was available, and was gradually able to examine her vagina with one finger. She was able to examine herself and used small tampons tentatively at her next period. She had no boyfriend, but there was a fellow student at university whom she fancied and they had been out together a few times. (Perhaps that is why she had come at that time). She would like to have sex. I even sorted out the contraceptive pill for her – suggesting something that would help her acne. I thought a clear skin might help her feel better about herself. Although she was improving in as much as I could examine her, I still had no idea why she had had this problem and I felt there was a lot more work to be done. Because of the time limitations and the fact that she would be leaving soon, I did not have time to arrange any long appointments. The 'test' would be when she returned to university and was with her 'boyfriend'.

She came a final time to say goodbye before she went back to the North. I fussed around, like an anxious mother, giving her advice about seeing a doctor there if things did not work out or coming to see me in the next holiday if there were any problems. As she got up to leave she said, 'Oh by the way, I have an appointment at the local orthopaedic hospital about my back. Will it be all right if I defer it to the next holidays or do I need to come home especially?'

'Your back', I exclaimed. 'What is wrong with your back?'

She looked really surprised. 'Didn't you know I had a scoliosis. I thought everyone could tell that I was deformed.'

'Is that why you thought you might be different down below?' I said. I was puzzled and concerned that I had missed all this. Should I have scanned her old notes more carefully?

'Maybe', she said, 'But I feel better now'. With a very quick thank you she left and I have never seen her again.

Comment

Maybe it was because I did not know about her deformity that I was able to work with her in this way. I had treated her as a 'normal' sexual being with concerns about the anatomy of her vagina and a fear of being touched. I had discussed the fact that her acne could be treated and that it was fine for her to be sexual and even suggested that she went on the pill. I had shown no aversion or pity when I had examined her. This may have helped her to feel more normal. I had not seen her as a patient with a medical condition. I had kept to the 'here and now' and used the feelings between us in the consultation without exploring the past history. Perhaps this has helped her to feel 'whole'. She may need more help when she embarks on a sexual relationship, but she may now know how to help herself, having achieved a measure of insight.

TERMINAL ILLNESS

When a person is terminally ill the last thing on the doctor or nurse's mind will be sex. Other aspects of a person's comfort and wellbeing usually take priority. This may not be the patient's or their partner's agenda. As 'time runs out', sexual expression may be very important for the couple or an individual and loss of function or desire may be very distressing. There are often physical discomforts and difficulties that can be overcome, but a partner may feel that it is wrong of him or her to expect sex at this stage. There may be fear of causing damage or pain or a sense that it is not appropriate to make love any more. Privacy becomes limited as carers invade the home or a patient is admitted to hospital or a hospice.

There may be feelings of guilt, especially if the disease could possibly be seen to be caused by sexual activity, as with carcinoma of the cervix, and it is important that these issues are aired before death. There may simply be guilt that they are thinking about sex at this time. There may also be feelings of guilt associated with previous affairs, indiscretions or arguments, and the doctor or nurse may find his or herself cast in the roll of priest or confessor.

A couple may seek 'permission' from the medical attendant that it is 'safe' to continue with sexual activity. Practical advice regarding the use of analgesia prior to intercourse may be helpful. Sometimes erectile enhancement drugs for men can be introduced at this stage, even if it is not the man who is dying. The importance of being able to make the best use of the small amount of time remaining cannot be stressed. Women may have been 'castrated' by their chemotherapy or radiotherapy, leaving them with sudden extreme menopausal symptoms. Practical advice such as the use of vaginal moisturizers or vaginal oestrogens that will not affect a hormone-dependent tumour can be helpful.

I recall one young woman with secondary breast cancer who had a new husband of six months standing. I saw her in a local hospital menopause clinic where I worked. Since her chemotherapy and the subsequent acute menopause, they had been unable to make love. She had severe vaginal soreness and dryness preventing penetra[...] She had been [...] gorically by the on[...] [*Holy Shit... something shorten "guilty using something like to have sex"*] [...]ave HRT as her tu[...] [...]ant. I prescribed some low potency vaginal oestrogen which I assured her would have no 'end organ effects'. She came back not having used it as the data sheet in the pack said that it should not be used in women with breast cancer. She felt guilty at using something that might shorten her life, in order to have sexual pleasure, when she had to think about other members of her family, including her young children. We were able to discuss this, but despite my reassurance she would not use the hormone cream. Finally she agreed to use a vaginal moisturizer. The impact of this woman's distress was so great on me that we subsequently started a joint clinic with the oncologists in order to try and alleviate some of the suffering experienced by women with cancer who were experiencing oestrogen-deficient symptoms.

Whilst it is important for the attending medical professional to be aware that there may be sexual difficulties, it is extremely important that the intimacy and privacy of these very precious moments are maintained for the couple. Professionals working within the hospice movement are trained to deal with all physical, psychological and spiritual needs of the terminally ill, but those in the community may find it more difficult. Gilley (1988) describes four cases of terminal care in the community. In each case a terminally ill patient was being nursed by his or her marriage partner. Dr Gilley's role as General Practitioner was very different in each scenario. The level of intimacy before the onset of the illness was reflected in the ability of the partner to care for or receive care from their partner. In one situation a woman considered it an extreme 'liberty' that her husband had asked her to brush his hair, whilst at the other end of the spectrum a man was able to make a sexual innuendo when his wife adjusted his urinary catheter. Gilley concluded that the level of intimacy between the couples and the quality of their previous sexual relationships also influenced the choice of terminal care environment. The man who could not even receive the comfort from his wife when asking for his hair to be brushed needed to be admitted to a hospice before his physical condition dictated this. Other patients with a good relationship were nursed at home until death.

BEREAVEMENT

The loss of a partner has many aspects and one of them is the loss of sex and intimacy. A patient may find it difficult to discuss their loss with their doctor as it may seem selfish and they may feel guilty about exhibiting such feel-ings. There may also be feelings of guilt regarding the cause of death and difficulties with the relationship. Bereavement may have an effect on future sexual relationships which may be sought relatively soon after a partner's death in a society where mourning traditions have on the whole been abandoned and dating agencies are increasingly prevalent. Whilst the new relationship may have been formed in order to overcome loneliness, progression to sexual activity may be too rapid and be influenced by the past.

I remember the oldest person that I ever saw in a family planning clinic. The clerk thought he had come to the wrong place. He was 79 years old, tall, thin and distinguished. He had a new lady friend who was only 74. She had been widowed many years and seemed to want the relationship to quickly progress to a physical one. His wife had died from heart disease about six months ago – she was never as fit as he was. When he tried to make love to his lady friend he was impotent. This, despite his age, had never been a problem with his wife, he proudly told me. I examined him and told him nothing was wrong physically. He then shed a tear and told me how much he missed his wife and we understood, together, the effect that that was having on his penis.

I have also seen a woman who developed a persistent vaginal discharge when faced with having sex with a new partner when deep down she felt that it was too soon after her husband's death. It is our job as medical professionals to enable our patients to gain insight into their behaviour and feelings. To do this we need to be brave enough to go with them into this area which may seem taboo when discussing death and dying.

CONCLUSION

The general practice team in particular has a role that involves caring for the patient from 'the cradle to the grave'. Sexual health of both the body and the mind is part of this. Members of the team may have the benefit of a great deal of background knowledge about an individual and their family that can be an advantage in many situations. It can also be a disadvantage if it creates preconceived ideas about the cause of a problem. With each individual patient in each consultation we must stick with the 'here and now' if we are to help with their sexual difficulty, ignoring our 'good ideas' or theories about the cause of the problem. We can use the feelings that are present in the room and reflect these back to the patient. We are in a privileged position to be present and involved in so many patients' significant life events.

KEY POINTS

- It is important to see an individual with sexual feelings and not a patient defined by their illness, age or disability.
- Every patient's sexual problem is different and extrapolation from one person to another may be misleading.
- Stick with the 'here and now' in the consultation, despite previous history that may be known about the patient.
- Concentrate on the relationship between the patient and yourself. Remain aware that people, whatever their stage in life and whatever their degree of disease or disability, will have sexual feelings.

REFERENCES

Cooper, E. and Guillebaud, J. 1999: *Sexuality and disability: a guide for everyday practice.* Oxford: Radcliffe Medical Press.

Coulson, C. 2000: Body image and sexual problems. *Institute of Psychosexual Medicine Journal* 24, 3–8.

De Berniere, L. 1998: *Captain Corelli's Mandolin.* London: Vintage.

Dixon, M., Booth, N. and Powell, R. 2000: Sex and relationships following childbirth: a first report from general practice of 131 couples. *British Journal of General Practice* 50(452), 223–4.

Gilley, J. 1988: Intimacy and terminal care. *Journal of the Royal College of General Practitioners* 38, 121–2.

Hunter, M.S., Battersby, R. and Whitehead, M. 1986: Relationship between psychological symptoms, somatic complaints and menopausal status. *Maturitas* 8, 217–8.

Wellings, K., Field, J., Johnson, A.M. and Wadsworth, J. 1994: *Sexual behaviour in Britain.* London: Penguin.

Wight, D., Henderson, M., Raab, G., Abraham, C., Buston, K., Scott, S. and Hart, G. 2000: Extent of regretted sexual intercourse among young teenagers in Scotland: a cross sectional survey. *British Medical Journal* 320, 1243–4.

Part Two
Psychosexual Problems

9 Vaginismus and non-consummation

Josephine Woolf

Presentation in a clinic

Reasons for vaginismus

Difficulties working with vaginismus patients

The examination

The term vaginismus is still sometimes used as a diagnosis, as if it were itself a disease. I prefer to think of it as a symptom that can result from physical or psychological causes, or a combination of the two. The phrase 'non-consummation' merely means the absence of penetration, either by choice or from whatever cause. Physical abnormalities, for example a vaginal septum, may result in non-consummation of a relationship, as may psychological causes, such as a fear of pain.

The textbooks define vaginismus as an involuntary spasm of the muscles surrounding the outer third of the vagina that occurs when any kind of penetration is attempted. The strongest of these muscles is the levator ani, whose fibres form a U-shaped sling at the junction of the lower and middle third of the vagina. When it is really severe, the spasm can extend to the thigh adductors, preventing anyone getting near the external genitalia. The woman may be seen to retreat up the examination couch, arching her back and clamping her knees together, without even having undressed.

When the vaginal muscles are in spasm, any attempt at penetration will inevitably be painful, so on the next attempt the woman will anticipate pain and will subconsciously contract her vaginal muscles as a protective reflex to prevent further pain. Mild degrees of vaginismus cause uncomfortable or painful intercourse. Severe degrees are likely to make penetration impossible. Primary vaginismus means the muscle spasm has been present since the first ever attempt at penetration. When the vaginismus is secondary, there has been successful intercourse in the past, but after some emotionally or physically traumatic event the spasm has developed.

Most commonly vaginismus is a bodily reaction to a psycho-emotional upset. A first attempt at penetration proves painful, and the fear that this will happen again leads to an automatic protective reflex, a closing up of the vagina to prevent a recurrence of the pain. This involuntary contraction may also develop as a result of disease or an anatomical abnormality that causes pain on attempted penetration, or because the woman has a fantasy that her vagina is too small, too fragile or too rigid to be able to accept a penis.

Thankfully it seems rare these days for a terrified woman on an examination couch awaiting a smear to be told by an impatient doctor to 'Just open your legs and relax!' or even to 'Stop being so silly!' These sorts of comments indicate a belief that vaginismus is a voluntary condition, implying that the patient could relax if she chose to. Now that we understand that vaginismus is involuntary, it becomes much easier to say, 'There seems to be a problem here – let's try to understand it'. Or, 'I wonder if something like this happens when you try to make love'.

As with so many sexual problems, vaginismus is a condition concerning the mind and the body, and so a mind–body approach is needed in its management. As will be seen below, the consultation, and in particular the examination, is much more than just the exclusion or identification of a physical problem. It can allow patient and doctor access to feelings previously hidden, enabling the patient to 'open up' with her mind as well as her body.

PRESENTATION IN A CLINIC

Recognition by a woman that she has a sexual problem and needs help for it is not easy. Harder still is admitting this to another person in a clinic or surgery, whether a stranger or a GP who knows her and her family well. A health care professional giving out signals that he or she is interested and concerned to hear about a sexual problem is more likely to create an atmosphere in which such intimate matters can be discussed. Sometimes the patient needs to test the doctor's attitude before sticking her neck out. She may bring a 'calling card' of a physical or an emotional symptom, perhaps taking several appointments before she gets to the real problem. The 'hand on the door' syn-

drome is familiar to many. It allows a quick escape route if the woman feels her problem has not been well received, or has been dismissed with a 'reassuring' remark, which indicates to her that the doctor is not interested in her problem.

The presentation may be overt or covert, but there are usually plenty of clues to alert the professional to the underlying problem.

Overt presentation

Many women, with or without their partner, go to their GP or family planning clinic to complain directly that they cannot consummate their relationship, or that sex has become painful. Some present early, but there are those who wait years before summoning up enough courage to face a doctor. The longer they wait, the harder it becomes to disclose this seemingly shameful truth. With secondary vaginismus there is usually some event or circumstance which has triggered the change, and these women are likely to seek help sooner rather than later. Painful sex is a frequent complaint in the gynaecology clinic, and in family planning clinics.

Covert presentation

Sometimes a woman feels too ashamed or too frightened to tell someone directly that her partner cannot penetrate her. She may believe (or may want to believe) that there is some physical reason for this. Certainly she knows that something is wrong 'down there' which needs to be looked at, though she may be reluctant to be examined.

Repeated non-attendance at a smear clinic should lead the practice nurse to wonder whether the patient is reluctant to attend, and why. The woman who does manage to reach the clinic, but who does not take her pants off or is in a state of hunched up terror at the top end of the bed is similarly giving a signal of her need for help. In the family planning clinic, it is noticed that a young girl has been unable to settle on any particular method of contraception and always manages to avoid being examined. It emerges that she has not actually been able to make love with her boyfriend so far. The gynaecologist is consulted for a pain 'down below' or a persistent discharge with negative swabs; are these perhaps signals that this woman wants her genitalia to be looked at because she fears there is something terribly wrong there? Couples not infrequently present at infertility clinics requesting IVF, and are discovered never to have had penetrative sex. The GUM clinic is a place where a worried woman can see a doctor without prior referral from a GP. She will almost certainly be examined and no one else need know she has been there.

These are just a few examples, but they illustrate the importance of being alert for signs of a sexual problem. The atmosphere in these clinics should be such that patients feel that it is safe to reveal their real difficulty; that the doctor or nurse will be receptive and interested in their problem and that they will not be wasting his or her time.

REASONS FOR VAGINISMUS

Physical reasons

Physical reasons for vaginismus will usually be discovered fairly promptly in general practice or in a family planning, gynaecology or GUM clinic, when the patient's story followed by an examination and appropriate tests reveals the situation. Occasionally, patients find their way to a specialist psychosexual clinic, if examination has previously been overlooked. I recently discovered a vertical septum in a patient referred for non-consummation; surgery solved the problem.

A vertical or horizontal septum or a congenital short vagina is likely to result in non-consummation. A thick, tough or rigid hymen may prevent penetration and sometimes surgical removal is justified. Penetration does not always follow hymenectomy, however (Tunnadine, 1970). The vicious cycle of pain causing vaginismus causing more pain on the next attempt needs more than an operation under anaesthetic to break it; it needs a fully conscious understanding of why the muscles are tight and help in learning to loosen them (see below).

Any condition causing pain in the vulva or vagina can similarly cause vaginismus. These include vulval infections such as Bartholinitis and herpes, vaginal infections such as monilia and trichomonas and other causes of vaginitis, for example due to spermicides or lubricants. Perfumed sprays, soaps and detergents can also cause chemical irritation or allergy. Vaginismus may follow episiotomy repair or a vaginal repair for prolapse, because of the painful scar. Vulvo-vestibulitis, an inflammatory condition of uncertain origin, can cause severe pain and tenderness and vaginismus may follow.

Vaginal atrophy following radiation treatment or at the menopause will cause soreness and dryness with a thin, less elastic mucosa, making intercourse painful. Inadequate lubrication for any reason will have the same effect. This can include a lack of arousal, possibly due to inadequate stimulation by the partner, loss of sex drive, fatigue and, of course, the fear of pain itself. Certain medical conditions such as multiple sclerosis can also cause inadequate lubrication, as can drugs such as antihistamines, alcohol and amphetamines.

Deeper pain may arise from infection, for example pelvic inflammatory disease, or from endometriosis. A vault scar after vaginal hysterectomy, adhesions from other pelvic surgery, or a shortened vagina in Turner's syndrome or testicular feminization may also cause problems. These causes of pain are perhaps less likely to result in vaginismus than those lower in the vagina.

Although most of these physical conditions are relatively easy to diagnose, treating them may not instantly cure the vaginismus. The feelings must be dealt with too and the vicious cycle broken.

Psychological reasons

Why is it that some women develop vaginismus whilst others do not, despite apparently similar circumstances? There are women who anticipate their first time with an inner certainty that there will be pain. Maybe they have friends or sisters who have told them it is always painful. They may have been brought up in a family where sex was not discussed, where periods were definitely not something to be proud of, where they were given no encouragement to try tampons. They become afraid. Their vaginal muscles go into protective spasm and any attempt at penetration is painful, confirming their fears and setting up the conditioned response for the next attempt. Other women with similar backgrounds do not develop vaginismus even if they have experienced pain in the past. For them, at the important moment the sexual feelings overcome the apprehension, and they can permit penetration.

This is a complex question, and the answer must lie in the fact that every woman is unique. Their background and circumstances may be similar, but their reactions to them and their feelings about them will not be. Although information is easily available to almost everyone, there are those who choose not to read or to ask, and even avoid television programmes which might be informative. They are choosing to ignore that aspect of themselves completely, perhaps afraid of what they might discover. Values handed down by a mother to her daughter are likely to influence her sexual development. A girl who has been brought up to associate sex with guilt and anxiety may feel that her sexual organs are shameful, dirty or disgusting and must not be touched.

How fascinating it would be to know how and why fantasies about the vagina develop. What remark was made? When did that seed of fear take root? How did it come to be so far removed from reality? Ideas about what the vagina is like inside are very varied. Descriptions I have heard include a narrow rigid tube; a long tunnel; a pin-hole entrance; a thin fragile wall which might split or tear. Some women believe the top of their vagina opens directly into the abdomen, others believe the top narrows down. One woman thought it was like the liver or the lungs, another described it as raw meat, like the inside of the body. The hymen is imagined as a thick solid structure that must bleed painfully when it is ruptured. One woman with vaginismus was afraid to touch herself because she believed there were horrible things inside her vagina that would come out if it was opened. Her vagina was a Pandora's Box of horrors. Another was afraid that her boyfriend's penis might touch her abdominal organs and do damage. A 30-year-old woman, who was still a virgin and ashamed of it, feared that her vagina had become blocked up or stiffened because she had not had sex for so long.

Very common indeed is the fantasy that the vagina is too small to accommodate an erect penis. Sometimes the feeling that she is too small may also indicate that the girl still feels like a child, small emotionally as well as physically, not ready yet for grown-up sex. Part of being a child is that your mother is still responsible for you, and it has been said that a daughter's vagina is the last part the mother lets go. The girl is still attached to her mother and wants to be 'good'. She is not yet in full possession of her vagina, not yet free to allow sex, though she may think she wants it. The mother or other family members are sometimes felt to be 'present' in the bedroom, watching critically, and this inhibits sexual response.

Case 1

Usha had been married for a year. Although she was very clever and had a university degree and a career, her father had never valued her and he disapproved of the marriage. She was pretty and petite, almost childlike, and the doctor felt quite protective.

When she was younger she had tried tampons but they had hurt. Attempts at penetration also hurt and after her wedding she had got 'honeymoon' cystitis. She enjoyed foreplay and oral sex, but she had not had an orgasm and didn't know where her clitoris was.

On examination, Usha allowed the doctor to insert one finger into her vagina with no difficulty. She put her own finger in afterwards and the doctor showed her how to relax her vaginal muscles. She made good progress, but after one more appointment she dropped out of follow up. After 15 months she reappeared, and reported that although she could now get three fingers in easily, with her husband she was dry and sore and he could not penetrate fully. The doctor listened with quiet interest and she went on to say that she felt as though her mother-in-law was always in the bedroom, telling her it was high time she had a baby. She felt she was being rushed. Her husband was very close to his mother and she thought they talked together about her. Other family members seemed to be analysing her too. 'I feel as if they are all trying to get inside me and I want to keep them out!' she blurted out. 'And your body reacts by keeping your husband out of your vagina', the doctor commented.

Usha had only returned to the clinic when she felt ready; she was *not* going to be rushed any more. The atmosphere was unhurried and unpressurized. With the doctor Usha felt valued, respected and understood, and was able to reveal her angry and uncomfortable feelings. Having made the connection between her mind and her body, she began to make steady, solid progress. Once expressed, her anger dissolved, and within two sessions she was enjoying full penetration. She was certainly not childlike now, but potently in control.

The vagina that is too small may be a metaphor for feeling emotionally too small, perhaps not ready to take the huge step that seems to be expected. And conversely there are women who fear that if they open their vagina they might unleash too much sexuality, which might be uncontrollable and unbounded; safer to keep it firmly reined in.

Fantasies of damage may arise following gynaecological procedures and operations, particularly in a woman whose sexuality is insecure. After hysterectomy or even cone biopsy of the cervix, a woman may feel that part of her essential femininity has been removed and she is therefore unable to enjoy sex to the full. Breast cancer patients and others, for example colostomy patients, may also have an altered body image that inhibits them sexually. Scarring after anterior or posterior vaginal repair may indeed cause pain and subsequent vaginismus, but may in addition leave the woman with a fantasy that her vagina is completely altered.

Any traumatic sexual encounter is likely to produce a sexual problem at some time. In particular, rape and sexual abuse may result in a need to keep men out, to ensure protection from further harm. Childbirth may also have this effect, if a woman has felt degraded or invaded in a hospital environment where insufficient attention has been paid to her feelings. The birth over, she is left in lithotomy position awaiting suturing, feeling vulnerable, exposed and uncomfortable. She may deal with this by shutting herself off from all feelings 'down there', including sexual feelings, or by developing vaginismus (unconsciously) to protect herself.

Very rarely, vaginismus highly resistant to treatment may be associated with serious underlying psychopathology. Either the vaginismus has developed as a deep defence against psychosis or there is dysmorphophobia, a persistent, almost delusional, belief that abnormality exists. Continuing to try to break down such a defence could lead to disintegration and the development of an overt psychosis. In these rare cases vaginismus should probably be allowed to continue its protective function and the equilibrium left undisturbed. Long-term psychoanalysis may be an option if the patient wants it.

Cultural and religious reasons

A brief mention should be made of these influences. Although not often a direct cause of vaginismus, they may indirectly contribute to its development through feelings of fear or guilt. The tradition of needing to see blood on the sheets as proof of virginity on the wedding night may fuel a woman's fear that penetration will be painful. An arranged marriage may find a woman on her wedding night being penetrated by a man she has only seen once and has not yet learned to love. Not surprisingly, she may be unable to relax her vagina enough to let her husband in, and intercourse will be painful.

Women who have undergone circumcision often carry with them terrible memories of pain and fear which are reawakened when the time comes to make love. In some cultures the women are brought up to be afraid of the men, who are considered to be more important and more powerful.

Guilt about sex and masturbation before marriage may also cause problems later on. Where there has been a cultural taboo on talking about sex there is likely to be ignorance about anatomy and function.

Religious belief and practice is sometimes used as an excuse or a defence for underlying psychosexual problems. Obligatory abstinence from sex for part of the month may create problems, but may also be a good excuse for those women – or their husbands – who are reluctant to have sex.

DIFFICULTIES WORKING WITH VAGINISMIC PATIENTS

Vaginismus is a very rewarding condition to treat, but it can sometimes take a very long time to get better. This is because the patient's defences are strong and the doctor is denied access to her feelings. She has shut them up along with her vagina to protect herself from pain. She may be angry with her partner, and this anger will reveal itself in the room with the doctor. Sometimes she has a need to be in control, to prevent the feeling of helplessness that was felt at the time of the abuse or rape or traumatic childbirth. The doctor is not going to be allowed to take charge and make her feel helpless again!

All sorts of ploys are used to prevent the doctor doing an examination, which the woman fears will be painful and will make her feel vulnerable and exposed. Excuses such as having a period, not having washed or a straight refusal are common. Telling the doctor about other things, serious things, even death or tragedy or illness, will, she hopes, distract the doctor from the task in hand and divert on to 'safer' ground. It often works! Several appointments may go by before the doctor realizes how powerfully the patient has prevented the examination taking place.

This kind of defensive behaviour is not a deliberate attempt to sabotage the doctor's efforts to help. The patient is there, after all, and keeps coming back, wanting help but too terrified to allow the doctor to get close. The professional who does not recognize this may become frustrated and irritated at the inability to make progress. This in turn can lead to their own defensive behaviour. When information is not forthcoming, what do we do? We ask questions. What does that give us? It gives us answers to our questions. But those answers may not give us the information that we really need. We doctors are used to *doing* things for our patients. If they prevent us helping them, we may at least feel useful if we arrange a test, or prescribe some treatment. We may give advice, teach them about their anatomy, show them pictures of female genitalia, or reassure them, all of which strategies can be useful at an appropriate time. Sending for the partner is another option sometimes used by a doctor desperate to find a way forward. All of these actions may be valid and appropriate. However, it is important to be aware of those occasions when they help the doctor more than they help the patient. A doctor who is stuck may well be tempted to adopt a course of action that amounts to flight from the 'no-win' situation he or she is faced with.

Doctors in training groups have often expressed a fear of 'opening a can of worms' if they touch on sensitive areas. They are afraid the patient's distress will be overwhelming and they will be unable to contain it, or will not have time to allow it to take its course. Yet allowing the patient to release her feelings, giving her permission to divulge the awfulness of how she feels, can be extremely helpful and is itself therapeutic. The doctor who has very little time to listen to a long story may at least have time to let the patient know that he or she recognizes and understands her distress, and wants to set aside special time for her at a later date to hear more. Doctors do indeed feel overwhelmed at times by their patients' distress (Crowley, 1995), and it is all too easy to avoid it and pass on to safer areas. But by acknowledging it, containing it, sharing an understanding of it and giving support and empathy, the patient can obtain relief. The burden of pain is shared, and therefore easier to bear.

The patient who is reluctant to be examined may make the doctor feel invasive, as if forcing her to submit to something horrible. The doctor, of course, does not wish to be put in such a position and might easily agree that examination isn't really necessary. Such collusion may not be in the patient's best interest. An understanding that the doctor feels this way because the patient herself feels as if she is being invaded may lead the doctor perhaps to enquire whether she has felt similar feelings at other times of her life. Our feelings when we are with a patient give us insight into what the patient is feeling, and we can share this insight with the patient, helping her to understand her difficulties and hence overcome them.

Case 2

Janet could not allow her boyfriend to penetrate her. He could put his finger inside, but when he tried with his penis it was extremely painful and he had to withdraw. Despite this she enjoyed an active sex life and reached orgasm with clitoral stimulation. Lately she had become so tense that she could not let go and was no longer orgasmic.

Five years ago, things were very different. Then she was head over heels in love with another man, to whom she had lost her virginity at the age of 30. For two months she had been blissfully happy, and enjoying sex to the full. Then one day she discovered that he had lied to her and was still seeing an old girlfriend. This girl became pregnant and Janet was 'dumped'. She was devastated, shocked and deeply hurt. She could not bring herself to go out with a man for five years. Her relationship with John began as a good friendship, and only became sexual after a year. It was deepening now, and she was desperate for things to 'come right'.

In the psychosexual clinic Janet was apologetic and seemed vulnerable, always close to (or in) tears. She agreed readily to be examined, and the doctor inserted one finger into her vagina easily, with almost no vaginismus. With two fingers there was slight vaginismus, which seemed to reproduce the pain she had felt. The doctor observed that it must have been very hard for her to have waited so long for her first sexual relationship, then to have given herself so totally to someone, only to find herself cruelly betrayed, her joy snatched away so soon. No wonder she needed to hold back now, afraid to be hurt again.

With such an obvious reason and so little vaginismus, the doctor had high hopes of an early 'cure'. But this was not to be! Her anxiety and insecurity was almost overwhelming. She would cry copiously on each visit, and then apologize, saying she never did this at home with John. 'Isn't it interesting that you let go emotionally so easily with me here, yet not with John?' the doctor remarked. 'Yes', she sobbed, 'I am so afraid that if I open up completely he will reject me'.

Janet came to the clinic regularly over the next 18 months, progressing very slowly. The doctor examined her again and she was completely relaxed, yet still experiencing pain with John. But her relationship was deepening and she began to trust him more with her emotions and, in parallel, with her vagina. They moved in together and Janet began to get orgasms again. The pain steadily improved and eventually they achieved penetration.

Janet's very tentative sexual beginnings coupled with a very shaky self-esteem had taken such a hard knock that her secondary vaginismus took a very long time to resolve. With a supportive and caring boyfriend and a patient and encouraging doctor able to contain her distress and 'hold' her through it, she was at last able to move on.

THE EXAMINATION

Why examine?

Traditionally doctors are trained to take a history, examine, make a diagnosis and prescribe treatment as appropriate. The examination is done to detect pathology or to confirm normality. In psychosexual medicine there is more. As doctors we have a duty to examine our patients if they complain of pain. But if their pain stems from a psychological or emotional cause, our examination would be incomplete if we only used it to exclude physical abnormality. A woman who is convinced that her vagina is abnormal will not change her opinion merely because, following examination by a doctor, she has been reassured that it is normal. Our examination must also explore the woman's feelings about herself and her partner. We must explore fully her fantasies about her body before helping her to see and feel for herself the reality of what her vagina is like.

The word 'psychosomatic' is equated in many people's minds with their condition being 'all in the mind'. Of course, this is not true. Vaginismus is a very physical condition. The muscles are in spasm and the pain of penetration is real and may be severe. It helps to explain that the body and the mind are inextricably linked and what affects the one is bound to affect the other. In vaginismus the body has reacted physically to some cause or other, or perhaps a combination of causes, and the doctor's duty is to find all of them, be they physical, psychological or both. So vaginismus is truly psychosomatic – in the mind *and* in the body.

In vaginismus, the examination plays a crucial role. Why? Because at this time the patient's defences are lowered, she feels vulnerable and hidden feelings may surface. This is so often the 'moment of truth' in the consultation (Tunnadine, 1970). From the moment the doctor suggests examination to the end, much information may be gained. The very suggestion of an examination fills some patients with horror, and their reaction to it is of clinical interest to the doctor.

Imagine the dilemma of a doctor faced with a patient who refuses to be examined. Should the doctor agree not to do it and make another appointment? If so, is he or she failing in a duty to examine her pain? Or should the doctor insist on it, thereby running the risk of making the patient feel violated, never to return for follow up, and the doctor feel like an abuser? There is a third possibility. The doctor hears and sees that the patient is distressed at the thought of being examined. This is a clinical sign and should be further investigated before anything else happens. Why is she distressed? Is she anxious that it will hurt? Is she embarrassed and if so, why? Is it something to do with feelings of shame she has about herself? Is it because she has never been able to admit that she cannot allow penetration? Or is she afraid that something terrible will be revealed, some awful abnormality that she believes exists 'down there'? Perhaps she wants to avoid revealing her fear that she might have damaged herself through masturbation, or a sexually transmitted disease.

A comment such as, 'You seem upset at the suggestion of being looked at. Can we try to understand why?' or, 'I wonder if you are having similar difficulties when your boyfriend tries to make love', may facilitate further discussion without withdrawal or retreat.

When to examine

It can be seen that the examination begins well before the patient is on the couch. It begins when the doctor calls her in from the waiting room! From this moment, her behaviour, attitudes and reactions can all be observed and therefore examined, and give important clues about her feelings. In the room, the doctor may be aware of feelings of discomfort, embarrassment, shame, anxiety, anger, reluctance or distress. The woman sitting on the edge of her chair, clothes buttoned to the neck, handbag clutched in front of her, is signalling her anxiety and her need to protect herself. Such feelings should be addressed, not brushed off, since failing to address them is tantamount to failing to examine pain, and our job is to examine the feelings, not to belittle them.

Even if the physical examination is not actually done on that occasion, an exploration of why the woman is unwilling to permit it is still valuable. We must be careful to distinguish our own feelings from those of the patient, and recognize that our own discomfort or embarrassment is nearly always a reflection of the patient's feelings. Feelings belonging to the doctor alone, related to his or her personal life, are not relevant to this professional situation and must not be allowed to confuse the atmosphere.

Case 3

A young woman in her mid twenties was referred to the psychosexual clinic for non-consummation after three years of marriage. Sara was the only daughter in a strict Muslim family, and her mother had brought her up to believe that sex should be regarded as a duty, never a pleasure. She grew up with the feeling that not only was it wrong, but it was dirty, and she did not have any right to enjoy it. On her wedding night she was very tense and her husband could not penetrate her. Later, however, she was easily aroused with her husband's foreplay and could reach orgasm with clitoral stimulation, although deep inside her she felt it was wrong.

The doctor noticed that Sara seemed embarrassed and a little reluctant to tell her about her difficulties, and in response to the doctor's comments she admitted she felt ashamed of her complaint. She spoke also of a painful gynaecological examination in the past and unsatisfactory experiences with counsellors. The doctor remarked that she must be feeling angry and fed up about it all. With some trepidation in this climate of suspicion and anger, the doctor asked how Sara would feel about an examination now. Politely but very firmly Sara declined, leaving the doctor feeling distinctly pushed away. The doctor did not try to persuade her, but noted that she seemed to need to be in control, and interpreted her need for a barrier to protect herself. The doctor explained what would happen during an examination, stressing that Sara would be in control all the time and would not experience any pain. After some thought, she agreed to go for it at the start of the next appointment.

To the doctor's surprise, when she returned she willingly undressed and lay on the bed. The doctor encouraged her to put her finger inside her vagina, but Sara felt unsure of where it should go. However, she allowed the doctor to insert one finger very slowly, moving further only when instructed. It went in easily, with no resistance and plenty of room to spare. 'You try this time', the doctor suggested. This time Sara easily put two fingers inside, and went away very encouraged. By the next appointment she was making love with no problems.

Sara needed to take control for herself. She was mature in her sexuality, but her vagina still belonged to her powerful mother and so she could not give herself fully to her husband. Once she had decided for herself that examination was the right way forward, she was able to take responsibility for her vagina. Self-examination helped her to accept it as her own, along with the sexual pleasures it contained. She may have seen this doctor as another powerful female influence, but one with a different message, which she was ready to accept.

There are no rules about when the physical examination should be done. It may be early on in the consultation, much later or not at all on the first occasion. It will differ depending on the setting, and on the doctor–patient relationship. Each case is unique, and the doctor or nurse must judge when and if it is appropriate for that particular patient. The important issue is that the health professional should always try to understand what is going on in the room. If it is not done, why not? Is the patient preventing the doctor from getting close? Or is the doctor reluctant to do an examination? If so, what is it about this patient that has caused the reluctance? Is the doctor suggesting examination because he or she is at a loss as to what else to do?

The setting

The examination room must be suitably equipped to provide the basic requirements of privacy, dignity and comfort. Ideally the bed should have a sheet, a pillow and a thin blanket. Screens are useful, even when the room is private. The patient can undress in privacy, and if her partner is with her she can choose whether she wants him with her inside the screen or outside of it, though still in the room.

The decision whether or not to have a chaperone is not easy. Some male doctors would argue that a chaperone should always be present when examining a female patient. This must be balanced against the fact that the presence of another person in the room will affect the doctor–patient relationship, making it harder for the patient to reveal painful feelings. A compromise may be to have the chaperone outside the screen, unseen by the patient, although she is aware of her presence. The patient's own partner may be the most suitable chaperone.

Whether or not the partner should stay during the examination depends very much on the patient's wishes. It is important to respect these, but the doctor should be aware of unspoken feelings. She may be trying to indicate that she would really like him to go out, that she would feel uncomfortable revealing shameful feelings or angry ones in his presence but is reluctant to voice this. Sometimes the woman very much wants to include her partner and, indeed, he may participate in the examination, to the great benefit of both of them. She may want him there but outside the screen, where he can share in what is going on whilst still allowing her privacy. There are no rules; alertness and sensitivity will dictate what feels right in each case.

On the bed

How does the patient undress? Quickly – or slowly and reluctantly? What is her position on the couch? Is she hunched up at the pillow end, legs drawn up, pants on and the blanket up to her chin, a look of terror on her face? Or is she lying exposed with her legs apart and looking up at the ceiling, detached from what is going on? Her behaviour should be observed and interpreted. 'You seem very afraid about this' or, 'I have a sense that you are somehow detached from what is happening down here. Does it feel a bit like this with your boyfriend too?' Detachment, terror, anxiety, embarrassment/shame or disgust may all be recognized.

Comments such as 'Ugh! This must be horrible for you, doctor!' or, 'I don't envy you your job!' reveal that this woman thinks there is something horrible about her genitalia. Replying, 'No problem, I do it all the time!' is rather dismissive of her anxiety. Better perhaps to say, 'It seems you feel that that part of your body is not very nice'. Then it may be possible for her to reveal her real feelings about herself.

This moment, with the patient on the couch, vulnerable and with her defences lowered, is a very powerful one. Handled sensitively, by a doctor or nurse listening, watching and interpreting when appropriate, it can be the key to helping that patient confront her fears and fantasies in the safe presence of someone she can trust with these intimate secrets.

It is important to discuss a patient's feelings about her body before being examined. Until these feelings have been brought into the open, any reassurance will be premature and useless; the woman cannot feel reassured if her real worries have not been addressed. Only when she has been able to put these into words can the doctor help her to compare them with reality and so finally lay them to rest.

During the examination the patient needs to feel that the doctor is always 'on her side'. She should never feel rushed, must never be allowed to feel that she is wasting the doctor's time. The doctor must be extra alert, watching and listening for clues to feelings and how she is reacting to what is going on. Nothing should ever be forced, but the doctor should try to give the patient responsibility as well as control.

A small mirror may occasionally be useful. Some women have never looked at their vulva and are afraid to do so. Some may have developed a fantasy about damage after childbirth or a gynaecological operation and be afraid that they are deformed. The doctor offers the woman an opportunity to have a look at herself, and if she agrees gently encourages her to bend her knees, put her heels together and let her knees flop out, relaxing the adductor muscles. The doctor helps her to identify her labia majora. Then, without the doctor touching, she is encouraged to part her labia, identifying the labia minora and the vaginal entrance. She can part them even more and stretch upwards to identify her clitoris. With encouragement it may then be possible for her simply to place her finger between the labia, at the vaginal entrance. If she can do this, she may then be able to try gently to insert her finger a little way inside.

Some women feel unable to look at or touch themselves at this early stage of the examination, and must never be pressured to do so, though it may be very helpful to explore why they feel they cannot. Others who feel comfortable with the clitoral area and may be orgasmic with clitoral stimulation still cannot bring themselves to approach the vaginal entrance with their finger. 'Would you like me to go first then?' the doctor might suggest. Examination should never be rushed. The patient must feel in control – indeed, it is in this way that she is able to regain a sense of control that she has lost in the past. In my clinic the patient sometimes actually holds my finger and moves it herself. This gives her full control without her touching herself. She must be allowed to proceed at a pace that she feels comfortable with, with a promise from the doctor to stop immediately she asks, and not to cause her any pain. The doctor should tell her what is happening throughout the examination. Much patience is required – any 'cheating' by the doctor will lose all trust!

With a finger inside the vagina, the doctor can then show her how to squeeze and then relax the vaginal muscles, thus converting an involuntary movement into a voluntary one. I explain the movement like this: 'Imagine you are sitting on the loo, midway through passing urine. Now stop the flow midstream. This movement makes your vaginal muscles contract, just as they do when you try to make love. Now reverse the movement, as if you are restarting the flow of urine. This is the movement that relaxes the vaginal muscles. Contracting the muscles first makes the relaxation movement more definite, and helps you to be aware of both these muscle actions'. It is useful to practise this at home when actually passing urine. The movement is, of course, just a pelvic floor exercise. Some women learn the movement easily, whilst others have more difficulty.

Doing this exercise with the doctor's finger inside, the woman will be able to feel for herself the difference between the 'squeeze' and the 'relax' modes. On each 'relax' phase, it may be possible to move the finger in a little bit further, until it is completely inside. She must now feel this for herself, and the next step is to encourage her to put her own finger in, and to feel again the difference between squeezing and relaxing her muscles.

With her own finger inside, she may be surprised and delighted to find that what she feels is very unlike what she imagined. The examination serves not only to lay her fantasies to rest and to put her back in touch with her vagina, but also to give her back a feeling of control of her body. She can now accept that her vagina belongs not to the doctors, or to her mother, but to her alone.

Case 4

> Vicky and Sam had not achieved penetration during their six months of married life. After several painful attempts they had given up. Vicky was convinced her vagina would rip and her hymen would tear painfully. Sam could excite her by touching her vulva, and he could put his finger inside her vagina, but she had never tried with her own.
>
> In the clinic Vicky sat anxiously on the edge of the chair, and when the doctor suggested examination she was terrified. She was sure it would be painful and the hymen would split. After the doctor explained in detail what would happen, she nervously undressed and sat on the bed. With encouragement Vicky was able to part her labia and identify her clitoris and her vaginal opening. The doctor then asked her to put her finger gently in between the labia at the vaginal opening, but she was too afraid. It was easier for her to allow the doctor to insert a finger, which was done very slowly. The doctor promised Vicky the finger would only move on her instruction, assuring her there was plenty of time and no need to rush. When she indicated she was ready, the doctor would move a bit more, and would stop – but not withdraw – if it hurt. The doctor's finger went in with ease. The hymen was a very soft thin frill, and there was almost no vaginismus. The doctor was able to move the finger easily from side to side, showing Vicky that there was plenty of room.
>
> With the finger still inside, the doctor asked Vicky to squeeze on it, by pretending she was stopping a flow of urine mid-stream, and then to relax, imagining she was now resuming the flow. She did this several times, until she was sure she could feel the difference. Then the doctor asked her to lay her finger on top of the doctor's, following the line of the finger exactly to guide her in, then slowly slipped out as Vicky's went in. To Vicky's astonishment she was able to put her finger in easily, without discomfort. Her vagina felt soft and elastic, not at all like her fantasy. She squeezed and relaxed on her own finger, discovering for herself the control she had over the muscles of her vagina.
>
> At the next appointment, she came together with Sam and reported that she felt comfortable inserting her own finger. This time the examination began with Vicky putting her own two fingers in, followed by the doctor's two fingers. They went in without difficulty. Vicky felt much more confident. The next step would be to involve Sam more, encouraging him to put his fingers in before progressing to full penetration.

Afterwards

I believe it is better not to try to achieve too much in one session. In primary care appointments are short and it may be necessary to take small steps each time. Even in clinics where sessions are longer, there is only so much a woman will be able to cope with each time. It is important to let her decide when she has had enough, and to respect her wishes. However, the doctor should be aware of avoidance tactics and should not collude in putting things off indefinitely.

The examination may be repeated, or rather continued, on subsequent occasions. Little by little, progress is made. Each time something else is achieved. First, one finger, then two, then her partner's one finger, then two. It may be possible to get this far without the doctor touching the patient. It is more important that the woman experiences it for herself than that the doctor should be able to examine her. Eventually her confidence should be great enough for her to allow medical examinations, smears and so on.

Progress is not always smooth and straightforward. Much support and encouragement is needed. Praise for progress, however slight, is better than disappointment that more has not been achieved. The faith, support and positive attitude of the doctor is of great importance in the treatment of vaginismus. It may take a long time, but the doctor must contain the frustration, disappointment and despair and stick with it. There may come a point when progress seems to have halted, and a judgement must be made as to whether sessions should be discontinued. Treatment cannot go on forever! Sometimes the issuing of an ultimatum serves to 'kick start' the patient into taking responsibility and progress can be made. Other reasons may also hinder progress. One patient with severe vaginismus overcame it completely, only to find that her husband, unable to cope with her new found sexuality, lost his erection.

Between appointments the woman is encouraged to find a time when she can feel relaxed enough to slip her own or her partner's finger into her vagina. I am trying not to use words like 'exercises' and 'practising' and 'homework' in this context, because it is all too easy for this to become a chore or a duty, and to become separated from the joy of lovemaking. Doing it at home helps to increase confidence and familiarity with her body, but it is much better if done as a part of sexual activity. Sometimes patients need to be reminded to stop 'working' on their exercises and go back to having fun in their sexual play. Digital penetration will in any case be easier when the woman is aroused or post-orgasmic.

CONCLUSION

I have not included a separate section on treatment, because the examination is also the treatment, as we have seen. There are, of course, other approaches to the management of vaginismus. Vaginal trainers (dilators) are frequently prescribed, particularly by gynaecologists, and some patients feel they can gain confidence and control using these. My personal viewpoint is that the vagina needs not stretching but relaxing. Putting a mechanical instrument inside may keep the vagina remote or detached. However, if the patient is well in touch with her body and her feelings, there is no reason why she should not have trainers if she so wishes. They may also be useful for a woman who has a fear of vaginal speculae and has been unable to have a smear. Once or twice I have lent a small speculum to a patient to get used to it at home, and this certainly did help to reduce the fear of the instrument.

Behavioural techniques such as those described by Masters and Johnson are also sometimes used. The danger with these is that treatment programmes and timetables may be set up before the underlying reasons for the vaginismus have been understood. Patients then return having failed to do their 'homework'. If this failure is then explored and the reasons for the difficulty are understood, then the technique will have been of some value. I maintain that the vaginal examination, together with an understanding of the doctor–patient relationship, is a much more powerful tool, focusing as it does more directly on the area of difficulty. This approach has been shown to be of value (Bramley *et al.*, 1983), even helping couples who have not responded to other treatments.

There are no hard and fast rules as to what is the 'right' treatment. What is certain is that every woman is a unique individual, who has reached this moment of her life with a complex of experiences and attitudes different from those of every other human being on earth. Management must be tailored to fit her needs and personality exactly. Vaginismus is a very common problem. The sooner it comes to light, the easier it will be to treat. Even so, many women who wait years before seeking help can sometimes be rid of their problem within a few sessions, once their fears and their fantasies have been brought out into the open and laid to rest.

KEY POINTS

- Vaginismus is a symptom, not a disease.
- We should always examine pain, be it emotional, physical or both.
- Feelings should be addressed, not ignored or avoided.
- Fears and fantasies should be explored, verbalized and understood.

- Reassurance will be of no value if the real worry has not been understood.
- Patients can be given responsibility as well as control.
- Self-examination allows the patient to compare her fantasy with reality.
- The examination is a vital part of the therapy.

REFERENCES

Bramley, H.M., Brown, J., Draper, K.C. and Kilvington, J. 1983: Non-consummation of marriage treated by members of the Institute of Psychosexual Medicine: a prospective study. *British Journal of Obstetrics and Gynaecology* 90, 908–13.

Crowley, T. 1995: Seminar training and the development of boundaries. *Institute of Psychosexual Medicine Journal* 9, 6–8.

Tunnadine P. 1970: *Contraception and sexual life.* London: Tavistock Publications.

FURTHER READING

Lincoln, R. (ed.) 1992: *Psychosexual medicine: a study of underlying themes.* London: Chapman & Hall.

Tunnadine, P. 1992: *Insights into troubled sexuality.* London: Chapman & Hall.

Skrine, R. 1997: *Blocks and freedoms in sexual life.* Oxford: Radcliffe Medical Press.

10 Lack of sexual desire

Jane Botell

Some patients have never had one and many more have had one and have lost it. What? A sexual desire – a libido.

Certainly, 28 per cent of the patients (25 per cent male and 75 per cent female) attending my referral psychosexual clinic seem intent on finding one.

I am reminded of one such man who came into the consulting room, sat down arms akimbo and legs wide apart, saying, 'I want a libido'! To this doctor it felt somewhere between being asked for an item in a grocery store much like a John Cleese sketch and being asked for a lifeline in ER.

WHAT IS LIBIDO?

What exactly is this elusive libido, what does it mean to us, and do patients and doctors mean the same thing when they use the word? Chamber's dictionary defines it as: a vital urge, generally or sexually. 'Vital' implies essential for life, a manifestation of life, hence 'vital organs' and 'vital signs'. No wonder patients use expressions such as 'dead' or 'lost' when they find it missing.

The clinically depressed patient can demonstrate the antithesis of this living urge, both in general and sexual life, as if the vital signs are dying or indeed dead. This deadness can be felt in the consulting room in the doctor–patient relationship. So it comes as little surprise to the clinician that the patient complains of loss of libido among the list of other depressed symptoms. We know from our work in psychosexual medicine that genital behaviour reflects general behaviour and vice versa. However, even for the depressed patient this desire might not be completely lost, seeds still being found even though deeply buried.

Sexual desire has been described as consisting of three stages: libido, willingness and arousal (Cutler, 1996). Many patients I see have not in fact lost their libido at all. It remains very much alive in their minds in thoughts and fantasies, often emerging through self-masturbation. They keep it to themselves. What they have lost or perhaps never had is a willingness to share their sexual life with another. For libido is the vital urge for what? If I listen to patients, it is to Make Love. This is the goal of their search, to share themselves with a partner through sexual intercourse.

'MAKING LOVE'

Making love implies letting go of oneself on all levels. It is a moment of intimacy between two people, a moment of vulnerability, even one of exposure. To be mutually satisfying, each partner needs to be in touch and at peace with all aspects of his or herself, emotionally and physically, those perceived as strengths and weaknesses. Each needs to accommodate those of their sexual partner and each needs to trust the relationship.

Does lack of desire or unwillingness to share this desire always mean no sexual intercourse? Apparently not, according to patients. The expression 'making love' appears to be distinct from 'having sex', a term commonly used by the media and also by patients. It can be critically applied by one member of a partnership to the sexual behaviour of the other. 'She just wants sex, I want to make love!' So our patients make a distinction between these two actions,

despite their both resulting in sexual intercourse.

'Sex' does not require intimacy. It can be a means to an end. Sex to secure a pregnancy and a much-wanted child. Sex through fear, to diffuse the anger of a demanding partner. Suppressed and denied feelings can remain safely hidden in the presence of a prostitute, or a casual relationship, but making love in an ongoing, intimate relationship could expose unbearable vulnerability.

One patient told me, 'I can't say I love him and I pull back from compliments and hugs even though he has given me all I have ever dreamed of in life. It's as if, if I made love, you might as well hang me in the street naked for all to see'. That is what intimacy meant to her; it is no wonder she had withdrawn from it.

WHY CAN WE LOSE IT?

To block such pain, defences are required and reference has been made to these elsewhere in this book. Play safe, masturbate alone, have sex with somebody you will not wake up with tomorrow, lie back and think of England, anything but touch feelings. It is easier and less painful to disconnect.

However, the human subconscious can create even more subtle defences. The man attempts to penetrate the vagina of his partner but he meets a barrier, the vagina hurts, the vaginal muscles respond and contract down on his penis. He is obviously unwelcome in his partner's inner world. Her psyche has been somatized. Her vagina has said 'No' for her.

The woman makes sexual advances to the man and his penis says 'No' for him in a more public way. He does not get an erection or loses it, ejaculates too early or not at all. He will not or cannot share his inner self with this female, but it is his physical body that has told the story.

So patients concentrate on the physical organ and its dysfunction, as it takes on the responsibility and blame for the sexual problems, and professionals to whom they turn for help are encouraged to follow. Physical symptoms or problems are presented, as have been illustrated in other chapters. Both doctor and patient lose sight of the suppressed feelings.

A man struggled, searching for the words to describe how he felt at the moment when he could not sustain his erection. 'My partner said, "cut it off", and then we would be all right'. That is what he had done with his feelings, cut them off and buried them. However, it is physically painful to have dyspareunia, it is not imagined. It is emotionally painful to watch one's penis shrivel away. The same patient said 'it (the penis) feels hollow, as if the inside has been scooped out'. So the penis still held feelings even if in a dismembered form.

THE ULTIMATE DEFENCE

The subconscious has something else up its sleeve to help us to run even further away from this intimate confrontation. Let's not be interested in sex at all, make such a state a diagnosis in itself and give it a fancy name, loss of libido.

The patient can now be totally free of responsibility and pain, leaving his feelings with the diagnosis or projecting them elsewhere, perhaps on the partner. The partner can feel hurt, abandoned, rejected, angry, exasperated, frustrated and even guilty, carrying the feelings by proxy.

So back to my original patient, sitting in his chair, arms folded, waiting for the doctor to deliver the goods. In the face of the patient's inactivity, the doctor can become super active searching for the culprit. Sexual abuse, diabetes, the menopause, the new baby. Surely one of these will fit and if all else fails there are always hormones to blame, the repository of loss of libido of unknown origin.

PHYSICAL CAUSES

Although the purpose of this book is to address the psychosexual origins of sexual symptoms, this is not to deny that we are also physical doctors and that physical science underpins our work in psychosexual medicine. As part of our search facility, we need to pay tribute to the possible physical aetiologies of the symptom of loss of desire.

Sex hormones

Males need oestrogen and females need androgen. High levels of oestrogens in the male brain in early life seem necessary for male sexual imprinting and oestrogen has a role in spermatogenesis and maintenance of bone mineralization in men (Davis, 1999). Conversely, androgens play a role in the female physiology.

Androgens are worthy of closer attention, for in some circles they have impacted on therapy for loss of sexual desire, particularly in the female.

In the male, testosterone is produced in the Leydig cells of the testis through the hypothalamic–pituitary axis via gonadotrophin releasing hormone (GnRH) and luteinizing hormone (LH). About 2 per cent of testosterone is not bound to sex hormone binding globulin (SHBG) and is free to enter cells and bind to intracellular androgen receptors. Although various disease processes and aging may alter the levels of SHBG, the level of free testosterone tends to remain within the normal range because of a negative feedback adjustment of GnRH secretion (*Drug and Therapeutics Bulletin*, 1999).

In the female in the reproductive years, androgens are produced by the adrenal glands and ovaries. They act directly via androgen receptors on bone, skin, sebaceous glands and hair follicles and as precursors for oestrogen biosynthesis in ovaries and at extragonadal sites including bone, brain, the cardiovascular system and adipose tissue.

What is the significance of androgen deficiency in females and of lower levels of free testosterone in either gender? Is there a direct link between low testosterone and low libido? We still do not know the answers to these questions. There is a dearth of prospective controlled trials in this area compounded by the insensitivity of most testosterone assays at the lower end of the normal range, particularly in the female reproductive years.

Endocrine disease and loss of sexual desire

The effects of endocrine disease on libido are summarized in Table 10.1.

Drugs and loss of sexual desire

It has been observed that certain prescribed drugs can produce an adverse effect on sexual desire.

- **Antidepressants.** Tricyclics, SSRIs.
- **Antihypertensives.** Alpha agonists, e.g. methyl dopa and beta blockers, e.g. propranolol.
- **Phenothiazines.** Chlorpromazine and thioridazine.
- **Diuretics.** Spironolactone.
- **Hormones.** Corticosteroids.
            Oestrogen in men.
- **Hypnotics.** Benzodiazepines.

Depression and loss of sexual desire

Although the relationship between depression and sexual dysfunction has already been addressed in other chapters, I will take this opportunity to look briefly at it with reference to loss of sexual desire.

Sexual dysfunction may be an early symptom of depression with drug therapy contributing to the problem, or can arise from the impact of the illness on the patient or the relationship. The sexual problem can lead to the depression or even predate it, and I have certainly seen patients treated with antidepressants where the patient and physician are living in the expectation of the libido's being re-found as the mood lifts, only to find it is not. The depression seems to have suppressed the feelings that led to the loss of libido in the first place. Now with the covers off, other defences have to be found and the libido remains the same.

Existing studies report wide discrepancies with regard to the association between depression and loss of desire, ranging between 31 per cent and 77 per cent in untreated patients, with some contradictory views on gender difference and uni- and bi-polar depression (Bartlick *et al.*, 1999). Perhaps more studies will emerge as more questions are asked.

The list above of possible physical- and drug-induced causes of loss of libido is not exhaustive and more detail can be found in other texts. To the list could have been added any debilitating disease producing general fatigue and lack of well-being.

PSYCHOLOGICAL CAUSES

Why is it that disease and medication produce sexual dysfunction in some patients and not in others? What is the missing link? The individual patient.

Our frustration in the consulting room can reach impotence levels when we have run out of physical search engines and yet the symptom persists. We can flounder like the patient. We need to look elsewhere for the answers.

Our only hope of understanding the universal symptom in the individual patient is to understand the patient in front of us in the here and now. Everybody is unique, everybody writes his own textbook. The patient has the solution there among the pages, but for some reason he can not or will not read it. So he comes to us to crack the code, to try and put the body and mind together. The doctor struggles alongside him, also in ignorance. Of course, in the end it is the patient who does the cracking. It is the patient who is the expert in his own case.

VARIATIONS IN LOSS OF DESIRE

The meaning of loss of desire will be different for each patient, and the details need to be understood. Is it lost altogether and for everything? Is it lost for just one partner, or for everyone? Just at this time or always, under

Table 10.1 Endocrine disease (Hawton, 1991)

Organ	Activity	Effect on libido	
		Men	**Women**
Adrenal gland	INCREASED (Cushing's Disease)	Can be decreased	Variable
	DECREASED (Addison's Disease)	Can be impaired	Can be impaired
Pituitary gland	INCREASED e.g. Pituitary Adenoma producing hyperprolactinaemia	Can lead to erectile dysfunction and consequent loss of libido	
	DECREASED	Can be impaired	Can be decreased
Thyroid	INCREASED	Variable	Variable
	DECREASED	Usually decreased through general debility and through testosterone synthesis and androgen and oestrogen metabolism	
Pancreas	DECREASED (diabetes mellitus)	Can lead to erectile dysfunction and consequent loss of libido	
Gonads	DECREASED		
Female	Congenital, e.g. Turner's Syndrome		Can be decreased
	Acquired, e.g. Post bilateral oophorectomy, chemotherapy and irradiation		Can be decreased
	Post-menopause		Variable
Gonads	DECREASED		
Male	Primary hypogonadism:		
	Congenital, e.g. Klinefelter's Syndrome	Can be decreased	
	Acquired, post orchidectomy, infection eg: mumps, trauma, irradiation or chemotherapy	Can be decreased	
	Secondary hypogonadism*:		
	Hypergonadotrophic hypogonadism (*Drug and Therapeutics Bulletin*, 1999)	Can be altered	
	Congenital, e.g. Kallman's Syndrome	Can be decreased	
	Acquired, e.g. Pituitary tumour**	Can be decreased	
	Systemic illnesses, e.g. end stage renal and respiratory disease, obesity, poor nutrition, long term over exercise, supra physiological doses of steroids, marihuana, ketaconazole and spironolactone		

*The symptoms of altered sex drive, decreased secondary hair, and reduced shaving without changes to the voice, body proportions or penis size would alert the doctor to the possibility of secondary hypogonadism. A single measurement of the morning basal total testosterone, luteinizing hormone, follicle stimulating hormone (FSH) and prolactin could confirm it.
**Headaches, impaired visual fields, polydipsia and an elevated serum prolactin would indicate a hypothalamic or pituitary tumour.

every circumstance? Does the interest return if new interest is expressed in them? Have they moved the interest elsewhere, onto somebody else, in an affair, or have they withdrawn it into a fantasy world?

The cherished, romantic heroine of a Mills and Boon novel, the shared cigarette and crashing waves on the shore of the old black and white films can seem preferable to a real world of responsibility, drudgery and conflict. In the fantasy the patient can be in charge of feelings, people and events.

There are patients who say 'I am not interested but if he starts I do get aroused'. It is worth wondering if such patients will only work with the doctor as long as he continues to express interest in them? Are they unable to hold the desire for themselves? Finally there are the patients who say 'I am only interested when I have had a drink, or am asleep or at certain times of the month', when they do not have to own their sexual feelings for themselves.

WHY DO PATIENTS COME?

What motivates a patient whose complaint is disinterest to be interested enough to present to a doctor, or particularly a psychosexual medicine clinic and all that that could entail? I am not surprised that 17 per cent of 154 patients referred to me with this complaint did not attend their first appointment. As with intercourse, their motivation had disappeared at the first hurdle. However, the remainder did attend; there was interest in something. What?

To understand the disinterest

For some patients just to understand the origin of the loss of interest is the key to resolving the problem. One man 'did not want medication, only to understand'. In fact he already knew the origin, but needed to speak it aloud in the safety of the surgery. They were considered to be the perfect couple, recently married in their sixties with high expectation of good lovemaking. Failed erections, a dry menopausal vagina and a mother in law permanently installed in their new marital home dashed their hopes. 'It's not conducive to spontaneously use my quick erections. It's a bit irritating but much easier to give up.'

Another man also wanted to understand his sexual withdrawal. Ten years of abortive IVF treatment had ended in failure, except for one success that had resulted in a miscarriage. He silently cried for the loss of 'his child'. The couple were about to embark on their final IVF attempt. He felt it was pointless. They had last made love two years before. 'I don't want to share my feelings with my wife. I want to disconnect', and he had. Despite understanding his feelings in the consulting room, he was not able to use the insight at home.

To collude with the disinterest?

If a patient without a sexual desire marries a partner who is happy with the situation, is there a problem? Not if the relationship is balanced. However, it could be that both partners have problems and their collusion provides a shared defence. One seeks help and the other can be exposed.

Case 1

Mrs E had presented with dyspareunia. She was a strange mix of 1990s city slicker and 1950s frizzy pony tail. She wore a mask of makeup, thick powder and bright red matt lipstick. A psychosomatic genital examination revealed a complete absence of pain and vaginismus, and self-examination was also painless. She was able to admit that she knew it was not a physical problem, she just did not want sex. She had come because she thought she must be missing out on something. She must be some sort of freak; all these young teenagers getting pregnant did not seem to have a problem! She obviously had feelings about this and the doctor felt led to ask 'What if you became pregnant?' 'I would be suicidal. I have never wanted children, never interested in them, don't know what to do with them. My father was not interested in us and left us and my mother told us she would have been happier without children. With those genes it's unlikely I would make a very good job of it. . . . So it's fortunate I am not interested in sex and my husband (of ten years) says he loves me with or without it.' Here was collusion. Could the doctor call her bluff and break the shared defence? She suggested they leave it there and said she could always return should she want to work further. The patient hesitated as if on a cliff edge. Should she jump? The doctor used the moment to draw the distinction between sex and making love, where intimate feelings could be shared. Was that a tear in those eyes, interestingly the only part of her face that was not made up? The doctor risked drawing attention to them and the tears welled over. She could not cope; she looked away, even turned her body away. Rivulets formed down her white mask exposing pink bare flesh underneath. She smudged the tears away, covered by a torrent of apologies. 'I came today expecting nothing but this is great.'

To rekindle lost interest

If something enjoyable in life dies it can be devastating; no wonder patients try and resurrect it. Some reclaim it for themselves, some for the partner or the relationship and others for all three. Psychosexual medicine offers help by struggling with the patient, in joint ignorance, to seek the truth. It is not about generalizations.

Mrs F and Mrs G were approximately the same age, both married, both post-menopausal, and both complaining of loss of libido. The difference lay in their individuality and that is where their solution was to be found.

Case 2

Mrs F had been referred to the psychosexual clinic by her general practitioner. Her referral letter had given the doctor an abundance of physical pathology to work on. Mrs F was in her late fifties and married. She had a history of cardiac disease, resulting in a mitral valve replacement a few years before, and she was being treated with HRT for menopausal symptoms. An ongoing anxiety state had many years ago resulted in alcohol abuse and suicidal thoughts, culminating in a psychiatric admission. Currently, she had a raised serum prolactin level. With all these contributing factors, why look further for the origin of her loss of libido? A non-motivated patient would have more than enough to blame, but Mrs F insisted the origin was psychological. It was obvious that the GP thought otherwise and the psychosexual doctor caught the mood of pessimism, but Mrs F was motivated to come and that was encouraging.

She looked much younger than her years. She was dressed casually, her make-up well applied; she took an interest in herself. Her affect and facial expression were flat, but when she smiled, she lit up, she was beautiful.

Mrs F came to the point with little prompting. She had lost her libido 18 months ago and she wanted life to be back the way it was when she and her husband had mutually enjoyed making love. That was it, she gave no more just as in her sexual life. The doctor tried to find an opening and wondered whether her husband did the same. Could she help? It had just gone one day, no reason. The doctor kept trying and commented that she seemed to have enough interest to come to the clinic. Her husband was a good man, he would like it back, she responded. In the silence that followed she added she wanted it for herself.

The atmosphere in the consulting room felt aimless. Where to begin, how to begin? This feeling was coming from Mrs F. Is this how it was in sex? The doctor was 'up a gum tree' and so became very active searching for some history that might help. As with all good ideas it bore little useful fruit, just a story, a list of events. It was the pain revealed associated with her father's death in her mid teens that seemed important. She was the eldest of seven children. She had upheld the family and it was not until two years later that she allowed herself to grieve. This appeared to be relevant to Mrs F. Was she showing she could only reveal feelings when there was time, did she put the needs of others before herself or was it a red herring? She had developed panic attacks and had contemplated suicide to rid herself of these feelings, they were so painful. The talk of her childhood connected her with her own child, a son in his late twenties. Three years ago, having left home some years before, he had returned to live with her and her husband. Her face lit up and caught the doctor's attention. She recounted the great times they had together, the things they did, 'we have a wonderful relationship'. She looked a different woman, alive and even younger. Here there was very obvious interest. Was this the key? There was certainly less interest surrounding the description of life with her husband. 'That's when it all started, three years ago not 18 months'. She had always found it embarrassing when her son had returned home for a short while as an adult and 'I went to the bathroom after making love', she confided with much blushing. The time had to be right to release messy feelings, the doctor was reminded. Initially, Mrs F had noticed she was no longer orgasmic, but the loss of desire soon followed. Her husband was very patient and believed it would return. 'I have told him straight that I am no longer interested'.

Her son had now left home, was this the 'why now'? He had made her feel young and told her he loved her. Her husband told her the same, but there was no life in it. 'We do talk about everything though', as if she needed to show the doctor the relationship was all right or perhaps remind herself. 'I wonder whether I should just reach out and succumb'. The doctor mused on the word. 'That is how it feels, dare I risk it'. She could offer no further explanation. Then she added 'I do have sexual dreams and wake in the night in the middle of an orgasm, no particular person involved'. She was full of surprises. She could not tell her husband, she was ashamed and embarrassed. She was a good Catholic girl, she thought she was abnormal. There was much of the confessional about this consultation.

The doctor felt optimistic. They shared the fact that she did still have a libido but was keeping it under wraps, unwilling to share it with her husband but had done so with the doctor. Mrs F left that first session with a firm handshake and the intention of telling her husband.

The second session brought a beautiful smile, some anxiety and an averting of the eyes away from the doctor. She awkwardly blurted out that things were going really well. She had started to have sexual thoughts toward her husband during the day: 'wasn't that awful', said the good Catholic girl. However, she had reached out to him in bed that night. 'I wanted to go all the way but I feared I would not get an orgasm and would go backwards'. The doctor could feel the joy and optimism, yet the fear of disappointment. Would it live up to her memories or the displaced fun with her son? Mrs F reflected in silence as if in a state of disbelief. She had told her husband it would all take time. Was it going too fast for her? Maybe her talk of HRT and breast disease at this point slowed everything down.

In the third and final consultation, Mrs F did not stay long. She kept her coat on, but the beaming smile filled the room. They had made love once, 'well actually five times but no organism'. She laughed at giving the wrong word. 'That would be the icing on the cake'.

The doctor pondered with the patient as to the origin of her loss of sexual interest. Mrs F had no explanation but was sure of its affect, death and consequent grief. It was everything and then it became nothing.

She and her husband were thrilled with the outcome. It had happened quicker than she had thought possible. Her husband had thought the doctor would discharge her now. He wanted it to be over, he wanted her back for himself. She was happy, but kept an insurance policy by taking the clinic number. Her revitalized libido had spilled over into her general life. 'I am so happy', was her parting shot and it was obviously true.

Despite copious medical history, Mrs F knew the origin of her problem was psychological, even if she never clarified it for herself. She was motivated to work even if embarrassed and it was a bit fast. She had risked showing her feelings to this doctor without attaching medical jargon to it. She had used the work she had done with the doctor when she was at home. She had re-found what she had lost.

Case 3

Was Mrs G motivated? She came late to her first appointment, actually one hour late. She had been held up in traffic. Her husband was in hospital; she was on the way to visit him. Another appointment was negotiated.

Removing her coat, she revealed the frame of a fragile bird with pretty eyes that seemed dulled. Her body was still and expectant, yet her hands, with carefully manicured nails, were constantly gesticulating, somehow speaking for her. She and her husband were not having a sexual relationship, well not with Mrs G anyway. Her husband was having an affair. She covered her mouth as tears mounted in her eyes. 'I mustn't cry'. The doctor's surprised 'why not?' was drowned by confusion, lots of words and a long convoluted story, including mention of her father, boarding school and not liking to be touched. Was there a connection with the now? It was the 'not touching'.

Mr G had been working away recently. Mrs G had noticed a distancing on the phone. She had never mentioned her feelings to her husband; they were 'private' people. However, his miserable mood, when home at the weekend, had prompted her to voice her fears. They were instantly confirmed. Within hours he had made an appointment with Relate.

The doctor was mildly irritated: was this really a psychosexual problem or more a relationship one? They were splitting the work between two agencies. Mr G saw the problem as to do with the relationship, Mrs G as sexual. She remained impassive. Did she have feelings about the affair? She supposed she was angry, but could not express it; she might lose everything. She had a 'nice' home, 'nice' child and a 'nice' marriage. Friends would be amazed to know they had a problem. She excused his behaviour as out of sight, out of mind. However, if he did leave her, then she would let out her anger. Currently it was all displaced onto his model railway, which took up her full spleen and his full time when he was with her.

The doctor could not feel sad for this lady, although her situation was sad, only irritated. This must be coming from the patient; why was the doctor having to carry it by proxy? 'What about sex?' Everything was fine sexually until four years into the marriage. She had recently given birth to their son and her husband, again working away, rang to admit to his first affair. She really could not remember how she felt; angry, she supposed. She did remember buying sexy underwear as a response, although what she had was not frumpy, she complained. Her memory lapsed, but with more prompting from the doctor about her sexual symptoms, she admitted to superficial vaginal pain at that time and no interest in sex since, even recoiling from his touch. That was 13 years ago. The doctor felt hostile to this man she had never met.

'I don't feel sexy. Look at me. I am all bony and B says he does not even fancy me'. The doctor's heart sank and she spluttered, 'How does that feel?' Mrs G felt she would never match his recent partner in sex, but was more cross he had not used a condom with her 'after all, he isn't a child'. She was talking more easily about her feelings now, and the description of her own bed attire, of long nightdress and underwear, in contrast to her husband's nakedness, highlighted the gap between them.

Even after this long session, the doctor did not really know what the patient's needs and expectations were. The idea of examination had passed through her mind, but she was not sure why she would be doing it, or for whom. The patient had complained of dyspareunia, but the doctor felt the genital pain was associated with a denied emotional pain. However, these thoughts remained in the doctor's head. Mrs G kept the doctor away, just as she kept her husband away.

Mrs G was half an hour late for her next appointment; traffic was again the reason. 'It is as if I am not meant to be here'. Everything was fine, she told the doctor, and she looked unburdened. The doctor felt the change was a bit too quick and easy. The source of her relief appeared to be the fact she now had her husband safely at home. He was recuperating from an injury to his leg and was unable, temporarily, to go back to work away from home.

Mrs G still complained of not feeling sexy, adding she needed a pill or a hypnotist. An external force was required. The doctor was becoming exasperated. Was this how it was with her husband? Did she make him exasperated too? The doctor reflected aloud that she seemed to deal with situations on a superficial level; surely the reason she felt happy was that she had her husband caged up at home. 'You have put it exactly', she said and smiled. Other people saw her as scatty, but she knew she was not. It was an act. In the presence of others she becomes a frightened mouse, others seem to know so much. Was she trying to make the doctor the expert in the consulting room? The doctor suggested that Mrs G was the expert on her self; she knew there was more to her. The patient recognized she wore different masks for different situations. At work she said that she was so happy and smiling that her customers asked her what she was on.

What had to be hidden so effectively? The doctor went back to the pain in the vagina 13 years ago. Mrs G repeated she could remember it had hurt at penetration. No mention of making love there.

This was the doctor's cue to offer a genital examination. Mrs G had stuck with the superficial penetrative pain and was locked into it. Could she and the doctor together reach beneath it? The doctor felt rather silly suggesting the examination and covered her self-consciousness with psychosexual explanations. This was not the doctor's usual custom. This was coming from the patient. Mrs G delayed the examination further by explaining she had already been examined by her GP and it had hurt. A warning to the doctor! There was a battle in the room, albeit a 'nice' one.

Mrs G slowly undressed, taking off her lower clothes. She lay impassively on the couch, yet her true feelings were expressed by the clenching of her arms and hands. Her body was still expressing her feelings for her. She wore a fixed smile and stared at the ceiling. She appeared cut off from the waist down. Surprisingly, the examination was very easy, the vagina was relaxed and moist. There was no vaginismus. The doctor asked how it felt and Mrs G replied, 'There's no pain'. She was surprised. The doctor pushed deeper, metaphorically, by questioning the source of the pain if it was not to be found in the vagina? The patient was confused. It was then that the doctor became aware of her semi-nakedness as she lay there, yet Mrs G appeared relaxed. 'You seem to want to reach out to your husband, what is in the way, what is the pain?' Mrs G broke through her barriers. She feared the relationship was still going on, although her husband denied it. She admitted she did have feelings and she remembered the days of crying when she had heard of the first affair. She had thought their marriage was as wonderful as was their sexual life; it came as such a shock. She had cried a couple of days ago with her husband, but he had not wanted to hear it and preferred to go out on his own and sort himself out. Also she did not want to upset her son. The doctor suggested she was good at hiding her feelings and wondered where they went. 'They are inside bursting to get out', she said. 'And ending up as pain in your vagina', the doctor added. It was then Mrs G became aware of herself on the couch. She felt rather self-conscious and wanted to dress. She had exposed enough, the doctor thought. 'If I get in touch with these feelings, will I be different?' What did she think? She was not sure, but it felt scary.

The third session found Mrs G bereft. There was no eye contact, no smile and her head hung down. A favourite pet had died! It was as if she was pouring all her grief from life onto this event. She no longer apologized for her tears. She had found a justified outlet for her feelings. No prompting from the doctor this time. She did want a sexual relationship for herself, but she feared what might be released. She could not selectively reveal feelings. Her husband had gone back to work. If she was angry, she could push him further away. If he did leave, then she would let it out. She had used the doctor's wondering of the previous session of why her husband did not leave her permanently, but he had responded by stating he did not want to do so.

This couple appeared to collude and give the illusion that everything was 'nice'. Mrs G picked up the thread and described how her son had looked on at his mother's distress over the death of the family pet and had wondered why it was so excessive. Was this 'nice' family becoming more real?

'I want him back home', Mrs G screamed.

Time was up in the consultation. The patient was amazed. She wanted to claim another as soon as possible. However, when that day came she cancelled the appointment, asking for the file to remain open.

So the doctor had to remain in ignorance. She had used her psychosexual skills to help Mrs G release her own feelings and the genital examination had provided a catalyst, but the outcome for the patient was unknown.

Comment

Love-making requires a triad of two people and a relationship. Mrs F had two parts of this triad in place, her husband and the relationship ready for her to join. Mrs G had none. She was hiding, her husband appeared to be doing the same and the relationship could not be trusted. It was not surprising that she was ambivalent about attending. Mrs F knew she had something missing that she wanted back for herself as well as for her husband. Mrs G wanted to save a marriage with a veiled interest in a sexual life for herself.

Two women with an apparently similar presentation. It is only by walking around in the individual patient's shoes that the difference can be felt and used by the doctor to whom the patient comes for help.

PHYSICAL TREATMENT

For a sense of completeness, it is worth addressing the use of testosterone in the treatment of loss of libido if all other possible reasons for the problem have been explored. It is generally agreed that testosterone is of little use in men with normal serum testosterone, but there are mixed views about its use in those with low levels. Severe mood swings can be a side effect.

In women where testosterone in the form of implants and patches is used, the dose must be titrated to maintain physiological levels to avoid masculinizing side effects. In the postmenopausal woman, it must only be used in conjunction with oestrogens. There are ethical dilemmas with androgen therapy in the older woman in competitive sport.

- There are no methodologically sound studies to support the use of ginkgo or yohimbe, although the latter stimulates the libido in male rats (Clarke *et al.*, 1984).
- We are now in the era of sildenafil (Viagra). It has given welcome hope for many men with sexual dysfunction and it may soon be licensed for women and give them hope too. But Viagra is ineffective for patients without a libido. Nitric oxide is the major neurotransmitter involved in the production of an erection. It stimulates the production of cGMP, which is then broken down by the enzyme phosphodiesterase 5, which Viagra inhibits. Nitric oxide is only formed on demand following sexual arousal. No libido, no nitric oxide, nothing with which Viagra can work.

CONCLUSION

No libido is the ultimate defence for patients unwilling or unable to share their intimate feelings with a sexual partner. Doctors grounded in physical medicine can use the skill of body–mind doctoring, with motivated patients, to reach behind the dimly lit mirror and see face to face what lies there. The patient is then free to choose what happens next.

KEY POINTS

- Genital behaviour reflects general behaviour and vice versa.
- 'Making love' and 'having sex' are different.
- Loss of libido is the ultimate defence.
- The effectiveness of androgens in the treatment of low sexual desire is yet to be proved.
- We need to walk around in the patient's shoes.
- Each patient is unique.
- We are all physical doctors; we could be psychosexual ones also.

REFERENCES

Bartlick Barbara *et al.* 1999: Sexual dysfunction secondary to depressive disorders. *The Journal of Gender-Specific Medicine* 2(2), 52–60.

Clark, J.T., Smith, E.R. and Davidson, J.M. 1984: Enhancement of sexual motivation in male rats by Yohimbine. *Science* 225, 847–9.

Cutler, W.B. 1996: *Love cycles: the science of intimacy.* Chester Springs, PA: Athena Institute Press, 172–211.

Davis, Susan R. 1999: Androgen treatment in women. *The Medical Journal of Australia* 170, 545–9.

Drug and Therapeutics Bulletin 37(1) 1999: Replacing testosterone in men.

Hawton, K. 1991: *Sex therapy. A practical guide.* Oxford University Press.

11 Erectile dysfunction

Andrew Stainer-Smith

Physical causes

Physical treatment for impotence

Psychological factors

I write as a doctor, both a specialist in sexual dysfunction and also a General Practitioner. But I am very conscious of the fact that nurses, counsellors and a range of therapists are presented with exactly the same spectrum of humanity. Rarely does a doctor hold any special expertise that can solve this problem. More commonly, a doctor finds that he or she can learn from those skilled in counselling and other therapies. Workers who are not doctors more often possess the attributes needed to form therapeutic relationships of the sort that enable a patient to express real fears. An attitude of listening from a position of ignorance is needed to allow a patient to feel empowered to offer his expertise. When there seems no solution, we are tempted to explain, to teach, to reassure and impose our framework over a sea of helplessness. But if we are prepared to give of ourselves and see our patient as an expert in managing his life, we can listen and hear what he has to say.

The pressure is on in all fields of state-funded healthcare. We have to work quickly. We must prioritize. We must be cost efficient, evidence based, perceptive to clinical governance, team and cell responsible or whichever politically correct description holds sway. We are acutely aware that impotent men need time over and above that which they have already been given. A man who feels helpless to help himself can quickly make others feel helpless. One may have to swallow hard to begin the process of trying to understand his feelings. This is commonly referred to as the heartsink scenario. Without doubt we all try to avoid losing heart, and the quickest way with a patient is to refer him on to another agency. As workers in the field of impotence we have to bear the brunt of this. We take on men where others have given up, or not begun to try.

We are a strange breed, having chosen to try to offer help where others have failed. This may not be an attractive field of healthcare. From the outset we are dealing with people who have acknowledged that they carry a negative label. It is difficult for our patients to reach us for help. We hear time and again that men have asked for help in the past, being given a reassurance that things will improve when they are less stressed. Men have been advised to have a holiday, to engineer protected time with their partner, to cut their smoking and alcohol, but still they have a problem. They may have been advised to ban penetrative sex and graduate physical intimacy in the hope that relieving a pressure to perform will work a certain magic. They may have been discovered to have type 2 diabetes, to need antihypertensives, thiazides, analgesics for a back injury, be getting over depression and so on. Their problem may have appeared after a heart attack, a transurethral resection of prostate, a change of partner and so the playing field is presented to the doctor or therapist. I continue this narrative referring to doctors' working with patients, but meaning to include all others in the field.

How do we react when we have a man where there are several sources of difficulty? The traditional answer is to ask questions and take a detailed history. But we must question the very nature of this process. As a basic mark of respect for a man's autonomy and integrity, we must accept that he will already have agonized over what could be wrong. He will already have questioned of himself whether his difficulty coincides with his diabetes, is consistent from day to day and whether he is together with the right partner. Men have usually made a judgement as to whether they could be vulner-able to psychological impotence. The doctor's first role is silently to be open to what is being presented.

There may be a phone call in advance from the partner warning the doctor that our man has something special to talk about. There may be a missed appointment. He may have changed doctors or be asking for a second opinion. There may be a referral letter expressing an opinion about the nature of the problem. Letters often contain warnings from the referrer not to question areas of the patient's life.

Pause for a moment and think. If the referrer emphasizes a supportive partner, what is going on? This is usually a feeling coming from the patient via the referrer. The patient has already let you know that he has travelled that road and discounted relationship difficulties as being relevant. Question that early, and you are in for a difficult consultation. Share with him that he has put effort in to trying to see if his relationship is at fault and he may reward you with his interpretation of what may be the most likely cause.

> A caring GP wrote 'Please would you see this man who is impotent. I feel sure his problem is physical in origin as I also know his wife who agrees that they have no marital problems.' They first came together. At a later consultation, on his own, he told how hurt he was on retirement to learn that his wife did not want him to work freelance in the media. He had tried to suppress the feelings, but they were still there and affecting his prowess with her.

PHYSICAL CAUSES

Age

Patients often ask whether 'at my age, do I have to say goodbye to sex?' Yet we know that men often father children at great age. So how do we respond to the question? The temptation is there to agree, and the patient has offered an easy way out with perhaps a swift end to the consultation and time to catch up on another case. It takes courage to say 'No', and to explore what he is really asking. It may be that his partner has told him that it is time to down tools, or that he himself is looking for permission to return to her saying that the doctor says that this form of intimacy should be over. It is a dangerous scenario in which doctors are at risk of collusion. If a patient has got as far as a consultation on the matter, it is likely that he will appreciate all the possibilities being explored.

> An elderly man asked if his time was over. Yet he described a wife whom he remembered in her prime and fondly described their earlier romance. He spoke of an abusive experience as an adolescent, as if offering it as an excuse for his failure now. But listening to the narrative, the doctor heard that the sex went wrong some years ago, when

there was a family row over how to cope with their daughter who was in an anorexic state. He and his wife, for a while, moved into separate beds. Apparently reconciled, the conflict was far from resolved. He cried as he described his pain in agreeing with his wife to estrange their son who had criticized what they had done. The doctor listened, feeling sure that when this man went home he would talk there about the past. The doctor did not need to direct or give instructions about what he and his wife should discuss. A second consultation revealed that they had managed successful intercourse and the patient brought down the curtain of privacy, saying that 'all along, I knew that there were no problems in our marriage'. This was now not a time for intrusive history taking, teaching, explanation or the doctor needing to be acknowledged as the specialist expert.

Epidemiological studies reveal decreasing coital frequency and increasing prevalence of erectile dysfunction with age. A large Veterans study from the US quantifies this (Mulligan and Moss, 1991).

It is easy to say to an older man that at his age he should be thinking of mechanical or chemical means of boosting his erection. If he is set on wanting an artificial treatment, one may have to offer sildenafil or another means of help. But this can be considered as a path to be walked with him. Follow things up; ask how he feels with this as an answer. Often you will hear that medication or devices are not used, having been put away in the cupboard at home. Having been listened to and granted the respect of the doctor in giving that for which he initially asked, he may want to talk about other things.

A man tried sildenafil, which worked for him. His wife, however, was not happy and didn't like him using it, asking for the old, real erection that they used to enjoy. The doctor sensed that his patient was holding back in accounting for his relationship at home. Why had this man become frightened of the assertiveness of his wife when he spoke of how useful it was that she kept her good health? It transpired that he had become unsafe driving and he had had to relinquish this to her. He needed to grieve for the loss of his independence.

Grieving requires that anger and frustration be given vent. In this case, sex fell foul of this. He had not linked the two and the doctor could only wonder if there was a connection. It is the sort of area where again it is tempting to guess and have a good idea to suggest to him that there could be a link. But he went away with an open agenda and returned to tell the doctor that he felt his driving ban was the cause of his loss of potency.

We cannot assume that older men will be less bothered by their loss of potency than their younger counterparts. An evaluation of sexual dysfunction in men with benign prostatic hypertrophy showed no correlation between age and problem assessment scores (Namasivayam et al., 1998).

Arterial disease and diabetes

These are the commonest physical causes of impotence.

In insulin-dependent diabetes, the prevalence has been shown to range from 1.1 per cent at age 21–30 to 47.1 per cent in those 43 years or older (Klein et al., 1996). The danger is to make an assumption that in the presence of diabetes, we know the answer.

So often we hear men talk of a mixed pattern of sexual response. They say that they cannot maintain an erection long or hard enough for sex, yet they can occasionally wake with a hard one. If a man can sometimes be hard, is it not likely that the cause of his impotence is psychological?

In the presence of proven arterial disease or diabetes, there is pressure to assume a physical cause. One may feel drawn to first offer a physical answer to the problem. Intracavernosal injections, sildenafil and apomorphine work well. We can be fairly certain that offering these will lead to a man returning with the report that he can get a better erection.

I suggest that we need to listen very carefully to what is reported back. And the doctor has to be honest with himself as to the dynamic revealed. If it all sounds successful, is the doctor truly sharing the delight of the patient? Or could the doctor be rewarding himself as having been a successful expert? Is the happiness of the patient tinged with any regret at being told that his days of independent unassisted sex are over?

Patients deserve a second look at the situation. Patients appreciate a second look at their new-found potency. Is it really what they want? Of course, it may be correctly left at that. But I have already described a man where, after sildenafil, a second look revealed unhappiness that he wanted to address.

Venous insufficiency

This is a difficult area. During erection, the cavernosal blood is held in the chambers of the penis. This has been described as a process of pinching off the venous return through the tissue of the cavernosal sheath (tunica albuginea) by a pressure effect. This is called the 'veno-occlusive mechanism' and is akin to how blood flow is clamped off from the placental bed by uterine pressure after delivery. But anatomically there are no discrete veins to be pinched. Under electron microscopy, there are holes in the tunica large enough to allow red cells to pass. It may be that the size and openness of these holes determines why some men retain better erectile capability. Research is being directed to look at how the structure of the tunica may change with age and disease.

Hormonal problems

Testosterone is needed to fuel the libido. But young boys, and indeed the foetus in utero, have erections. Eunuchs can be potent. The singer and eunuch Bagoas, who serviced both Darius III and Alexander the Great, was reported to be potent.

Men with very low testosterone levels do not feel the urgent need for sexual release. It is likely that they lean away from consulting doctors. At times a man is found with a low testosterone level. In rats after orchidectomy, there is a reduction in nitric oxide synthetase activity. However, the main action of testosterone is thought to be on the higher centres of the brain, particularly the limbic system.

Testosterone levels do not fall significantly with age.

It is surprising to see the range of testosterone levels in potent men. Indeed, the standard ranges have been scaled down in recent years, so that we now regard as normal levels of the hormone that would earlier have prompted intervention. A double-blind trial of replacement in men with low levels is needed. Surely, the placebo effect of an injected treatment would be profound. If the colour of tablets can affect the placebo response, then one would expect an injected mode of delivery to do so.

An unblinded trial from Coventry of the usefulness of testosterone in erectile dysfunction found improvement in potency in only 10 per cent of the low testosterone group. The authors concluded that 'Measuring testosterone was not helpful in assessing potency or libido' (Fahmy et al., 1999). Patients expect to have their hormones considered. One must be careful to be honest in one's prediction as to whether or not increasing a level will help.

This lack of correlation is associated with a burgeoning of treatment in the private field. If random testosterone levels do not correlate with treatment results, then patients may be drawn in to treatment on the grounds that their early morning levels are low, or that their free to bound testosterone ratio is low. Wearing an evidence-based hat, there is a need for doctors to challenge this practice.

Hyperprolactinaemia is quoted as a cause of impotence. The mechanism is unclear. Excess prolactin secretion is a feature of a reduction in dopaminergic control from the limbic system and hypothalamus via the posterior pituitary. It is interesting that other conditions associated with a reduction in dopamine production (depression, Parkinson's disease) are associated with impotence. It may be that hyperprolactinaemia is more ordinarily a secondary association of a state of cerebral function causing impotence.

Hormone therapy in the form of oestrogen, antiandrogens and gonadorelin analogues profoundly reduce libido. As these are used more and more in treating prostatic cancer, we are seeing more impotent men. Terminal care nurses are asking for guidance in how to help men and couples in distress. Yet there is a dichotomy. We have evidence that obliterating androgens may improve symptomatology and PSA blood results. But the evidence that it improves longevity or the end result is lacking.

Should we withhold testosterone on this evidence? It is an area where doctors may feel uncomfortable with patient empowerment. Doctors need to learn from other workers how listening needs to be active. Listening may reveal that a patient is happy to risk his disease becoming active in return for sexual activity.

Adverse drugs

Textbooks and the *British National Formulary* will indicate whether particular drugs have been reported to cause impotence. We need to know about a few important ones.

Thiazides are bad for sex. It can be worthwhile modifying antihypertensive treatment to eliminate them. Vasodilators cause less problem and indeed nitrates are recreational drugs used to enhance the sensation of orgasm.

Betablockers do not consistently cause impotence. Reducing the effect of sympathetic tone may be expected to reduce the detumescent effect of the sympathetic system. Patients and doctors frequently blame these drugs. Stopping them rarely helps.

A man was impotent from the day of his 5-vessel coronary artery bypass graft. On the face of it, he expressed gratitude and asked what I could do to adjust his medication to help sex. I asked to examine him, not expecting to discover anything that I did not already know. But I learnt from him. He hated his scar, and his persistently swollen leg below the vein donor site was an assault on his body image. As he told me more about the operation, he admitted that he was gutted by its only partial success and his need for continuing medication. The doctors blamed his drugs. But he had not been impotent the night before surgery, and his medication with his betablocker was essentially unchanged. On the internet he had read that the occlusion rates of several grafts was over 50 per cent in 2 years. He had also discovered that he could not expect an improvement in his life expectancy. He was angry and felt deceived. He made the link between this and his impotence.

Tranquillizers and antidepressants can spoil sex. It is useful to consider the pattern of response when there is a problem. Both can make erections sluggish. Tricyclic antidepressants in particular make orgasm difficult. It can be useful to reduce the dose to restore sexual function once the required antidepressant effect is achieved. Trazodone has been reported to cause priapism. It has a weaker anticholinergic (antimuscarinic) effect than other tricyclics and would be expected to have a less inhibiting effect on the parasympathetic pathways essential to erection.

In a placebo-controlled trial of clomipramine in men with premature ejaculation, both they and the controls showed a significant reduction in nocturnal penile tumescence and delayed ejaculation. Even 25 mg has a significant effect (Haensel *et al.*, 1996).

Some drugs are known to have an effect on the hormone environment. Drugs that can cause gynaecomastia (digoxin, cimetidine, chlorpromazine) are in the list of those that can cause impotence.

Antiparkinsonian drugs increase the availability of dopamine. They can cause a state of increased sexuality. This neurotransmitter is central to the function of the limbic system, pleasure appreciation and mood. As with trazodone, we again begin to see links as to how drugs work. Sympathomimetic drugs can be expected to increase sympathetic tone and facilitate detumescence. Dopaminergic drugs increase parasympathetic outflow and tend not to spoil erections.

Peyronie's disease

The plaques of this are associated with radiologically demonstrable blood leakage from the corpora cavernosa. Excising a stable plaque can restore potency. The problem is that the operation results in a loss of penile length and requires circumcision. Both these results can affect how a man feels about his penis. Urologists know the scenario of a man who after surgery complains that the operation has caused a worsening of his impotence. This is an area where a psychosexual consultation beforehand may prevent misunderstandings and it is sensible to offer help later if problems ensue.

Radical prostatectomy and transurethral resection (TURP)

Radical prostatectomy is a cause of impotence. It is tempting to lump together the operation in one's mind with TURP for benign hyperplasia. However, the two should not be expected to have the same effect.

There is no anatomical reason to expect simple TURP to cause impotence. The nerves are not damaged. Nor is the blood flow to and from the penis affected. So why is it that studies of TURP show it to be related to impotence? Perhaps this association is similar to studies that show the contraceptive pill to reduce libido. There may be something special about the type of man who suffers in this way. Unfortunately, it is not possible to do a blinded trial of TURP to discover any real effect.

We need to consider in a holistic fashion what happens when a man has an operation on his prostate.

> A man was devastated to find himself impotent after TURP. He agreed that the operation was essential. What hurt him was that he suffered a readmission with clot retention and a second catheter for several days. When a nurse joked with him that he was going to be 'out of action for a while', he replied that he was 'relieved, because otherwise it may get up and bite her!' In fact, he was far from relieved, in truth mortified that his manhood should have to be exposed for a second time.

We know that sexual dysfunction in women is related to obstetric events and unfavourable gynaecological experiences (Skrine, 1997). Similarly, we should expect that a man's sexuality is sensitive to things that go on in hospital.

It is too easy to suggest to a man in a vulnerable position that he should take a macho stance and not let things bother him.

This fronts up the matter of whether it is ever right for a health worker to reassure a patient. It used to be thought an important role of doctors and nurses to give reassurance to relieve anxiety. But this is a minefield, full of areas of partial doubt and temptation to bluff. If evidence is concrete and unshakeable that, for example, yes, the prostate histology is benign, then the information can be given. Patients are always intelligent enough to understand this. They must then feel their own assurance if it is real. Whenever a worker feels the need to reassure, he must ask himself what is going on. How can a worker reassure a man that his potency will return? The days have passed when we would reassure a woman that she would get over a miscarriage because it was 'only a blob of jelly'. I heard that said in my earlier professional life. Likewise, when a man loses his prostate, he deserves to have someone understand exactly what he has lost.

Pelvic surgery, injuries and radical radiotherapy

A study from Edinburgh quantified the effect of radical pelvic radiotherapy for bladder cancer over more than 4 years. The effect is variable. Seventeen per cent could not achieve any erections. Of the 71 per cent who reported deteriorated function, 44 per cent of these reported that they were not concerned by it (Little and Howard, 1998). It is interesting that several epidemiological studies report the sporadic prevalence of impotence to be in excess of 17 per cent. We must question what is going on here.

Pelvic fracture with urethral injury leads to long-term impotence in a large number of cases, 62 per cent in one long-term study (Mark et al., 1995). This erectile failure has the features of neurological damage, suggesting that the cavernosal nerves lateral to the postmembraneous urethra behind the symphysis pubis are particularly vulnerable.

Neurological problems

It is helpful to consider damage to the nervous system in terms of whether it represents a closed episode or ongoing disease.

Once the initial phase of brain injury, spinal cord injury, pelvic fracture and other things damaging nerves is over, we are left with a condition that should stabilize. There are patterns of cerebral and high spinal injuries that can leave erectile function sensitive to the point of being overactive. Without higher modulation, the erectile response can be triggered by afferent stimulation through the spinal cord up to the L1 level. Men in this position can be gratified to see erections useful for intercourse. Ejaculation can still occur, though the sensation may be poor. Low lesions usually result in complete anaesthesia and cause frustration to the patient and doctor.

The most important caution is that denervation sensitivity leaves the penis very sensitive to chemical agents. Injected intracavernosal agents should be started at very low dosage (2.5 mcg alprostadil). Similarly, sildenafil can be expected to have an exaggerated effect.

As ever, one has to consider the whole man. Certainly, consider accurately what the consequences will be of the anatomical lesion. But also think hard what you know about how this injury has affected this man as a unique individual. What is it about him that may make him react differently from the last man you saw with a spinal cord injury? What clues are there in how he treats you? How is he special?

Low back problems present particular difficulties. A vertebral body fracture or spinal disc decompression do not usually affect the parasympathetic supply to the penis. But when litigation is in the air, complaints abound. Working with unhappy patients requires the helper to listen at length to what has gone on. The man may still be in a state of grieving for the loss of his abilities to live a normal life. A doctor may be drawn in to being asked to criticize the actions of a surgeon or another specialist. One may have to tackle overt depression with drugs that are known to affect erections. One may have to plan to tackle one problem first, such as the pain, agreeing to look at the impotence later.

It is unusual to be able to give a solicitor a clear answer as to whether an injury or other assault on the back fully explains a man's sexual state.

Ongoing neurological disease has to be considered in terms of exactly what the nerve damage is.

In diabetes, the lesion is basement membrane damage of the fine blood supply of the vasa nervorum. This affects sensory, motor and autonomic fibres. Similarly, multiple sclerosis can affect all types of nerves, though primarily with an upper motor neurone pattern. Again, use of erection enhancing drugs should start with low doses to avoid priapism.

Motor neurone disease, cerebellar degenerative diseases and muscular dystrophies should not primarily affect erection and ejaculation. The psychological consequences, however, can be appalling and are often brought to a psychosexual doctor.

PHYSICAL TREATMENT FOR IMPOTENCE

Vacuum devices

These have an old-fashioned image, derived from sex toys. Modern devices have been modified to an extent that involves irrelevant extra considerations. It does not ordinarily matter whether the pump is hand operated or battery. Having a flexible tube connection between the pump and the chamber is of no particular advantage, and the design of constriction rings with a ventral sparing notch is more a gimmick than an improvement. It is important not to use petroleum jelly on the rubber parts of the o-ring or flange, as they will stretch. Otherwise, a simple device marketing at around £120 fits most needs.

A constriction ring on its own will help many men. If a man can get a partial erection on his own, it will be boosted as the penis tightens inside a band alone. Men frequently buy the whole device and end up using only the rings.

Intracavernosal injection therapy

Originally papaverine, now alprostadil, is the drug of choice. It has a lower priapism rate than papaverine. There are at least three styles of syringe and needle. The patient literature contains instructions about what to do if an erection lasts more than four hours.

The technique needs to be demonstrated. Graduated doses can be accounted for by giving an incremental dose in a clinic into the opposite corpus. Bruising is often worrying, more noticeably in those on aspirin, and although warfarin is not an absolute contraindication it does usually lead to too much bruising to continue. The worry is also that repeated bruising

and reabsorption may cause fibrotic Peyronie-like plaques.

It is sensible to obtain written consent to treatment. Accident and emergency departments must be happy with arrangements to call a urologist or other with experience in dealing with priapism should this happen. Reduction of priapism requires a large (23G+) butterfly needle and rapid aspiration of blood with a firm suction on the syringe. The needle should be left in place for half an hour or so afterwards in case tumescence recurs. Failing this, 200 mcg phenylephrine can be injected and repeated under blood pressure monitoring. Shunt procedures involve opening a channel between the glans and the corpora.

Intraurethral alprostadil

The UK marketed product has been disappointing. Although insertion of the pellet should be pain free, later discomfort is fairly frequent. It is less effective than by the intracavernosal route, though withdrawal rates from studies are lower. A head to head study of alprostadil reported intercourse rates as 55 per cent for intraurethral and 85 per cent for intracavernosal routes (Shokeir et al., 1999).

Specific vasodilators

Intense interest surrounded sildenafil and apomorphine when they first became available. Both facilitate erection, but by action at very different sites – sildenafil peripheral and apomorphine central.

Sildenafil acts as a phosphodiesterase type 5 inhibitor in the chemical cascade that leads to vasodilation of the penile arterioles. Prevention of the breakdown of cyclic GMP within the arteriolar smooth muscle cell stimulates an enzyme protein kinase G (PKG). Rising levels of PKG close the calcium inflow channel, leading to a fall in calcium levels within the smooth muscle cell and resultant relaxation of arteriolar muscle. This allows blood flow to the penis to increase and consequently, erection (see Fig. 11.1).

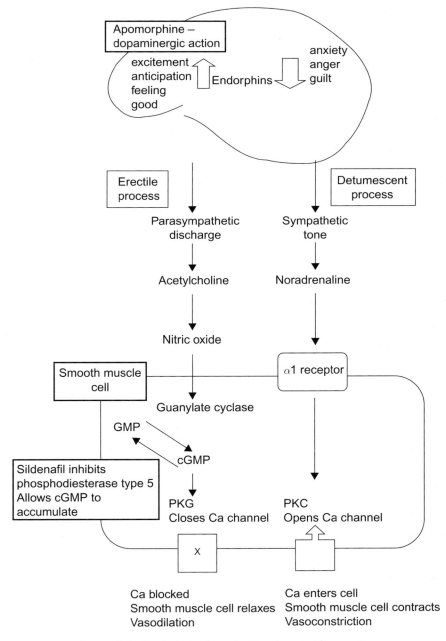

Figure 11.1   The brain to the penis. How drugs improve erection

Apomorphine is a centrally acting dopaminergic drug. From the brain it increases parasympathetic activity that, via acetylcholine as the neurotransmitter, stimulates production of nitric oxide outside the smooth muscle cell surface. Nitric oxide enters the cell, stimulating guanylate cyclase to catalyse cyclic GMP production and leads to erection through the same mechanism described in the previous paragraph. Apomorphine has an unusual side-effect profile of yawning, somnolence, nausea, vomiting and sweating – all features of parasympathetic activity. The US manufacturer's submission data to the Food and Drug Administration showed a 60 per cent drop-out rate due to side effects. This may affect its value as a drug, though the quickly acting sublingual route of delivery is attractive.

These drugs again point to the importance of the parasympathetic system in leading to erection.

Additionally, it is well known how the sympathetic system releases noradrenaline. Noradrenaline, through the $\alpha 1$ receptor, activates a series of enzymes leading to the production of protein kinase C (PKC). PKC opens the calcium channel, allowing calcium into the smooth muscle cell, contraction and a cut off of blood flow to the penis.

Surgical procedures

Penile lengthening involves freeing the penis from its attachment under the pubic arch. It does not interfere with the parasympathetic supply, but leads to a drooping of the angle of erection.

Dorsal vein ligation is now rarely performed. The rationale is suspect, as the critical point of blood flow from the penis is not the large veins, but within the cavernosal sheath.

Frenulum release can be useful to prevent repeated tearing that can result in alarming, though rarely serious, blood loss.

Implants, rods and more complex reservoir devices may be the only solution where all else has failed.

Testosterone therapy is a difficult area. Blood levels do not correlate well with potency. Some preparations are not detected in laboratory assays. Commonly, testosterone proprionate is detected. Mesterolone is not. Assays may include a measure of free to bound hormone, but this is not of practical use.

Acupuncture, as with all forms of complementary medicine, has been used in erectile dysfunction. It has been shown to help (Kho *et al.*, 1999).

PSYCHOLOGICAL FACTORS

Psychological factors may be consciously acknowledged or subconsciously hidden.

A man may speak openly and sadly about a failed marriage and his difficulty in giving of himself in a new relationship. He often knows what his problem is. So how do we help him tackle it?

This is the crux of psychosexual medicine. We cannot assume that his difficulty is the same as that of the last patient we saw who was impotent in apparently the same circumstances. Our guide has to be the relationship that we form with him as an individual. The doctor–patient relationship.

A man appeared to have missed an appointment. When he came for his next he explained that as he was in the car park, 15 minutes late, he gave up and went home. He thought that the doctor would be annoyed and not want to see him. So the doctor asked what this was about. How could he know what the doctor felt? The pattern of his marriage had been that he repeatedly felt to blame for not picking up the clues when his wife wanted sex, and being too slow for her. At times he faked his orgasm. Now he was in a new relationship and, from all descriptions, she cared for him greatly. So the doctor reflected that as he had misunderstood the doctor's reaction, he may be misunderstanding other people. Next time, he returned thrilled that she didn't mind if he didn't come quickly and still wanted to be with him when he didn't feel like sex.

A doctor may find that his relationship with the patient is being driven to emphasize that what the patient thinks is necessarily right.

A man kept telling the doctor how he had had many girlfriends, had studied sexual techniques and done a counselling course. But he was impotent with the woman he really wanted. The doctor felt uncomfortable with all the intimate details disclosed and reflected to the patient that too much talk of a perfect technique was off-putting. The doctor felt put off. The doctor had to leave this with the patient to see what he made of it. Later he returned, explaining that his girlfriend had also said that she wanted more privacy and he realized that she was entitled to it.

Through a patient, a doctor may feel grief, sadness, a longing for missed opportunities, anger, guilt, paranoia: indeed the whole gamut of human feelings. Psychosexual medicine asks the doctor to think with a clear head, be certain that what he is picking up is real, based on the evidence presented and to try to reflect those feelings in a way that the patient can use.

When dealing with impotence it is a particularly difficult path to tread. It would be so easy if one could use a checklist or a standard sexual history format of enquiry. But real men deserve real personal consideration.

Observe, and seek clues without asking questions.

Men coming for help with sexual problems are particularly nervous. Where else is there such a wealth of non-verbal body language to observe? He may creep in hoping that nobody has recognized him. He may have a confident swagger, announcing that nothing you can say will surprise him. Again, think. Here are two very different men who came my way.

One man crept in wearing a grey raincoat with a hand deep in his pocket. He dutifully produced a urine specimen for testing in a jar bound in duck tape and double wrapped in polythene, which he put at a distance on the window ledge. It transpired that this man had powerful unexpressed feelings about what penetration and ejaculation could do to his partner. He blamed his intercourse for his partner's precipitate delivery years ago. Ever since, his penis had let him down.

Another man strode in explaining how his confidence from working in the media left him able to solve his own problems. Being made redundant had been an opportunity to spend more time at home. So why had he failed in bed? Rather than reassure him that all he needed was time to find a new career, the doctor struggled to understand the incongruence of his confident entry when he was in such distress. Later he told the doctor that his wife could not talk about the fact that he needed regular checks for bladder tumours. Indeed, he had defaulted follow up to show her how little he worried. But between them they were both very worried. Being unable to tell each other about their real fears, they could no longer share sex as a form of communication.

As doctors we are required to examine men. Indeed, we are licensed to do so. All workers who touch patients hold a special brief. Be they nurses, physiotherapists, midwives or others, workers who touch patients should be conscious that they share a particularly close link with their patient. It requires a special degree of respect and can also enable a patient to open the door to talk about things that would otherwise go unsaid.

For investigating impotence, there is no standard examination format, though one may like to look for evidence of arterial disease, diabetes and hypogonadism. When we examine, we are best to use our senses to understand how a man feels about his body and sexuality. We are likely to be going over old ground where doctors have examined before. We may want to examine his prostate – and in older men this is often essential. At those times we must listen carefully.

> A man with advanced neurological disease vigorously refused to allow the doctor to examine his prostate. His wife was next door and had indicated that if the doctor needed help she could give it. The patient explained that, not unreasonably, he was worried that his condition could lead to incontinence. This real fear was making him shut off thoughts of his lower body. His wife expressed her worries, but with a reasonable certainty that she could cope. The doctor acknowledged how dreadful the patient's predicament must feel. And as the doctor agreed that a prostate examination was unlikely to affect management, the patient changed his mind and said that really he wanted it done to check that there were no signs of cancer. The atmosphere in the room lifted and he went on to talk openly about his fears of losing his sexual function altogether.

CONCLUSION

We who examine are in a special privileged position. We share this responsibility with biomedical technicians, osteopaths and many other complementary therapists. The effect of touch in relationships has been noticed in several spheres. Aromatherapists, beauticians and hairdressers touch. John Steinbeck wrote: 'People tell a hairdresser things they wouldn't dare confess to a priest: and they are open about matters they'd try to conceal from a doctor'.

Those who touch facilitate communication. We know that when we are physically close to a patient he is particularly likely to talk of the things closest to his heart. It is a serious responsibility, to be acknowledged and respected. If we can be aware of it and attune to those moments of revelation, we can extend our antennae and listen.

It can feel daunting to sit down with an impotent man, not knowing how the talking will go. It is difficult to hold back from barraging him with questions. When we lose sense of direction it is tempting to be diverted to wondering whether his partner has difficulties of her own. But stick with him. Why is he here now? What atmosphere has he generated here and now in the room with you?

When you feel sure that you have identified something special about him and how he feels, try to reflect it back as an observation. If it strikes a chord with him, he may there and then be able to move on, seeing connections with his sexual function. Or he may take the thought home to ponder.

Do not expect to be rewarded or thanked. Psychosexual medicine is strewn with uncertainty and not knowing. We have to tolerate this. Show your patient true respect, exposing your ignorance that you cannot know what he really feels. His mind and body do not work together in the same way as the last impotent man you saw.

From time to time you will hear that things are better. And when that happens you are entitled to share your patient's delight.

KEY POINTS

- Never generalize about the cause of sexual dysfunction.
- Men deserve to be listened to by a doctor who can start from a point of ignorance.
- The doctor must be prepared to form a relationship with the patient.
- The doctor must regard the patient as the expert.
- There can be value in examining when one does not expect to find any abnormality.

REFERENCES

Fahmy, A.K., Mitra, S., Blacklock, A.R. and Desai, K.M. 1999: Is the measurement of serum testosterone routinely indicated in men with erectile dysfunction? *British Journal of Urology* 84, 482–4.

Haensel, S.M., Rowland, D.L. and Kallan, K.T. 1996: Clomipramine and sexual function in men with premature ejaculation and controls. *Journal of Urology* 156, 1310–5.

Kho, H.G., Sweep, C.G., Chen, X., Rabsztyn, P.R. and Meuleman, E.J. 1999: The use of acupuncture in the treatment of erectile dysfunction. *International Journal of Impotence Research* 11, 41–6.

Klein, R., Klein, B.E., Lee, K.E., Moss, S.E. and Cruikshanks, K.J. 1996: Prevalence of self-reported erectile dysfunction in people with long-term IDDM. *Diabetes Care* 19, 135–41.

Little, F.A. and Howard, G.C. 1998: Sexual function following radical radiotherapy for bladder cancer. *Radiotherapy and Oncology* 49, 157–61.

Mark, S.D., Keane, T.E., Vandemark, R.M. and Webster, G.D. 1995: Impotence following pelvic fracture urethral injury: incidence, aetiology and management. *British Journal of Urology* 75, 62–4.

Mulligan, T. and Moss, C.R. 1991: Sexuality and aging in male veterans: a cross-sectional study of interest, ability and activity. *Archives of Sexual Behavior* 20(1), 17–25.

Namasivayam, S., Minhas, S., Brooke, J., Joyce, A.D., Prescott, S. and Eardley, I. 1998: The evaluation of sexual function in men presenting with symptomatic benign prostatic hyperplasia. *British Journal of Urology* 82, 842–6.

Shokeir, A.A., Alserafi, M.A. and Mutabagani, H. 1999: Intracavernosal versus intraurethral alprostadil: a prospective randomized study. *British Journal of Urology* 83, 812–5.

Skrine, R. 1997: *Blocks and freedoms in sexual life*. Oxford: Radcliffe Medical Press, 90–101.

12 Problems with ejaculation

Jane Whitmore

Therapeutic approaches

Premature ejaculation

Retarded or absent ejaculation

Painful ejaculation

Factors affecting outcome

Ejaculation can be defined as the ejection of semen from the body at the moment of sexual climax. It is often thought of as the visible manifestation of orgasm, although the two events are distinct neurologically. Ejaculation, as a marker of orgasm, is usually the climax of sexual excitement, and results in a sense of fulfilment and relaxation. This is the case both during masturbation and during sexual intercourse with a partner and, as with female orgasm, is associated with a letting go of control and abandonment. Men may have difficulty with such abandonment, which may have its roots in the fear of letting go of emotions, particularly anger. It is no coincidence that orgasm is regularly defined as an explosive event. This emotional difficulty can result in ejaculatory problems that may occur in all situations. With a sexual partner there is the added requirement of feeling safe enough to allow such abandonment and loss of control in the presence of another. If difficulties with the development of intimate relationships exist, then the ejaculatory disturbance may only be significant when a partner is present. This has obvious implications in fathering children, and in the development and maintenance of satisfactory long-term sexual relationships.

To understand how and why ejaculatory problems develop at any stage in life, it is use-ful to consider the natural history of ejaculation from infancy to old age.

Male infants enjoy having a penis, are proud of their erections, and experience genital pleasure from an early age. They become aware of adults' attitudes towards their interest in their genitals, and if their pleasure is perceived to provoke adult disapproval, they may feel ashamed or guilty, and become secretive. Seminal emissions, which like erections are difficult to hide, can occur in childhood, but become noticeable with more forceful ejaculation as nocturnal emissions, or wet dreams, at puberty. With a healthy acceptance of sexual awareness and experimentation, and increasing experience with and without partners in adult life, most men should achieve orgasm and ejaculation that is pleasurable and fulfilling, and not experienced as threatening in any way.

There are many ways in which this normal development from infantile genital pleasure, through nocturnal emissions and awakening adolescent sexuality at puberty, to a rewarding, orgasmic adult sexual life can be disrupted. A child's experience of his family's attitudes towards sexuality and personal relationships is likely to have a profound effect on later psychosexual development. If sex is never discussed in a family, because it is a taboo subject for whatever reason, a child might develop a sense that normal sexual responses are wrong or shameful. The mortification or guilt provoked by the messy bedsheets of pubertal nocturnal emissions can result in powerful inhibitory responses on ejaculation in later sexual life. The ability to develop intimate relationships with others is also laid down by early experience, usually with parents and other family members. How children experience their parents' relationship, and their own relationship with each parent, is likely to be important in determining vulnerability to later sexual and other interpersonal difficulties. Furthermore, religious beliefs may compound this vulnerability, particularly when strong, uncontrollable sexual urges and responses appear to conflict with religious ideals.

Many men are fortunate enough to receive 'good enough' experiences of parenting and sexual development, and enter adult sexual relationships with a 'good enough' ejaculatory ability. As with all other sexual dysfunctions, there will then be the potential for life events to act as precipitants for the later emergence of ejaculatory disturbance, which may include:

- Discord in general relationship.
- Infidelity.
- Childbirth.
- Bereavement.
- Unemployment.
- Sexual dysfunction in partner.
- Reaction to physical and mental illness.
- Traumatic sexual experiences.
- Unreasonable expectations.

When such ejaculatory disturbance occurs, spontaneous resolution without recourse to professional help may be possible, particularly if the developmental groundwork has been satisfactory. For some men, however, resolution of these problems may not be easy and they may present to their GP for help, with or without their partner.

With increasing age, levels of sexual arousability in men decline, with noticeable effects on both erections and ejaculation. More stimulation for a longer period of time may be required for ejaculation to occur – 'having to work so much harder for it' is not an uncommon comment. The forcefulness of the ejaculation can diminish, and the amount of seminal fluid produced can decrease in volume and change in consistency and sometimes colour. The refractory period may lengthen considerably, and the frequency of desire or need to ejaculate can decrease. An awareness and understanding that these somatic changes can be a normal effect of ageing can allow a man to accept them without experiencing them as a threat to his manhood. If they are viewed as inadequacy, secondary ejaculatory and erectile disturbances can occur. This might be in the context of a longstanding relationship, or particularly relevant given today's divorce statistics, in new casual and long-term relationships in middle age and later.

Problems of ejaculation of psychological aetiology are mainly related to timing. Thus men will seek help if their sexual satisfaction is significantly impaired by experiencing orgasm and ejaculation much sooner than they or their partner would like – so-called premature ejaculation. Conversely, sexual satisfaction can be impaired by delayed or retarded ejaculation, or by the complete inability to ejaculate – absent ejaculation. It is important to ascertain whose sexual dissatisfaction is being presented, i.e. a man might be sent for help with his inability to ejaculate in the vagina by the female partner who wishes to conceive.

Rarely, the ejaculatory dysfunction is experienced as pain. It is common for men with this symptom to be seen in urological or genito-urinary clinics, to exclude prostatic or seminal vesicle pathology. They find themselves being referred to psychosexual services only when investigations reveal no evidence of organic pathology, or physical treatments have been ineffective.

THERAPEUTIC APPROACHES

Often the initial presentation of ejaculatory problems is made to a doctor or nurse in primary care, and occasionally in genito-urinary, urology, psychiatric and other hospital clinics. The first health professional to whom the disclosure is made will probably have had little or no training in psychosexual medicine, and the initial response may be a feeling of dismay and inadequacy. There are no easy answers to psychogenic ejaculatory problems, nor any prescribable effective treatments. But a surprising amount can be achieved using everyday communication skills in such a consultation. The patient needs time and space to put his symptom into words, and then the health professional and the patient can puzzle together over the history. How long has the symptom been present? Why seek help now? In what circumstances does the problem occur? To whom is it a problem? In what way? How has the patient managed his problem so far? What is his motivation for seeking help, his expectations? Is his partner present – does he wish his partner to be present? By observing and listening to the story of the patient's symptom, some factors, emotions or feelings hitherto not recognized by the patient may become apparent. The attentive health professional may observe this, and wonder with the patient what it is about. After all, the answer to the patient's problem lies with the patient, not in the health professional's head, or in a textbook.

Often when the problem is presented to a doctor, a physical genital examination is required. This may be to ascertain the absence of organic pathology, perhaps to reassure, or to provide the opportunity for any anxieties or fantasies the man may have about his genitals to be explored. This is the psychosomatic genital examination – paying attention to the examination findings in relation both to the psyche and the soma.

These consultations and examinations may feel unsatisfactory to the doctor, because no tangible result may be evident. But the experience may have put the patient in touch with hidden or unconscious factors, which may provide him with more insight as to the nature of his problem. This may only be realized after he has left the consulting room, and he then may

be able to use such insight in improving the problems in his sexual relationship.

Some men will request and require referral on to specialist psychosexual services for further help. Specialists trained in psychosexual medicine will employ a variety of therapeutic models depending on the nature of their training and experience. However, the previous sharp division between behavioural and psychodynamic theories is becoming less evident in practice as a more eclectic view prevails. Behavioural techniques of sex therapy, such as sensate focus, and the stop-start and squeeze techniques for premature ejaculation, well described elsewhere (Bancroft, 1995), require both members of a couple to be involved in therapy. The success of sex therapy may depend on subtle changes in the unconscious interpersonal power balance in the relationship brought about by embarking on a behavioural programme. The unconscious factors may not need to be understood for this type of therapy to be successful.

Psychodynamic interpretative therapy is much more dependent on the exploration of unconscious factors, which can be highlighted by focusing on the experience of the here and now of the consulting room. The development of the doctor–patient relationship and the understanding of the interactions between the doctor and patient provide living evidence about that patient and his relationship with others. In the words of Tom Main, the psychoanalyst who founded the Institute of Psychosexual Medicine, 'If you examine what the patient is doing with you, you can see him in action elsewhere'. These observations and insights can be interpreted and shared with the patient, and he may begin to react differently in his sexual relationships. In this way it is possible for therapy to be successful despite the absence of a partner.

PREMATURE EJACULATION

There have been many attempts to define premature ejaculation. Masters and Johnson (1970) defined it in terms of the extent to which a man could delay ejaculation long enough for his partner to reach orgasm. Other definitions have been based on the amount of time in the vagina following penetration, and whether this was viewed as normal compared to other men. Interestingly, a large study (Kinsey *et al.*, 1948) found that two out of three married men interviewed would like to last longer. The same study revealed that 75 per cent of the men interviewed estimated that they ejaculated within 2 minutes of vaginal penetration. There would probably be agreement that ejaculation that occurs before vaginal penetration, or immediately after penetration is premature. Rapid ejaculation is common in young men in their first sexual experiences, and an occasional lack of control over speed of ejaculation during sexual intercourse may occur in many men without becoming a persistent problem.

In the absence of a satisfactory definition, it is the extent to which the perceived prematurity of ejaculation by the patient affects him and his partner's sexual satisfaction that is important. A man who regularly ejaculates prior to penetration may be delighted to be able to last 1–2 minutes of vaginal penetration, whereas another man might view 1–2 minutes as premature.

The problem of premature ejaculation is often compounded by the partner's response. If the partner's sexual pleasure is disturbed by the rapid ejaculation, the resultant frustration and sometimes anger, can increase the man's guilt and sense of inadequacy, and may in turn engender resentment. Men who have not attained some control over their speed of ejaculation during earlier sexual development have to feel safe enough to gain this control in the presence of a partner. Unconscious fears of the vagina or the power of women may threaten this safety. Additionally, the partner may have his or her own problems in allowing another to take control.

Premature ejaculation is often a primary problem, i.e. it has been experienced continuously by a person since sexual activity first began. Rapid ejaculation during masturbation and initial sexual encounters in adolescence is not uncommon, but some men fail to develop control over their speed of ejaculation later. Guilt, associated with sexual activity of any sort, because of a child's experience of negative adult attitudes to sex, might predispose to a failure to develop ejaculatory control. There may be an unconscious hostility towards women, a hangover from earlier relationships. Anger can be a frightening emotion, especially to a child and especially when the object of the anger is a close and loved person. At the time it is felt safer to suppress the anger, which can cause problems in later relationships.

Premature ejaculation sometimes develops as a secondary problem, i.e. one that arises after a period of satisfactory sexual functioning. Life events such as those listed earlier, which provoke guilt or a loss of confidence, can result in loss of control of ejaculation. Many men with premature ejaculation express serious fears of inadequacy in their failure to control their ejaculation, even if the partner is uncomplaining or attempting to be reassuring. The interactions in the consulting room that expose this inadequacy might be useful in enabling the man to regain a sense of being good enough, reducing the anxiety and increasing confidence enough for the symptom to improve.

Case 1

Mr A was referred to the psychosexual clinic by his GP because of his premature ejaculation, which had developed after the birth of his first child, a son, 18 months ago. He ejaculated immediately after penetration and was certain this had never been a problem previously. He reported that he always tried to make sure his wife was satisfied, but over the last 6 months intercourse had become very infrequent, as she seemed to be losing interest. They had not had intercourse at all for 2 months. Prior to the birth of their son, his wife was very enthusiastic sexually, but she now often complained she was too tired. 'I know I'm no longer satisfying her', he said. During the 18 months he'd tried everything to solve the problem – having a drink before sex, trying to distract himself with other thoughts during sex. He'd even looked it up on the Internet, but had decided not to order the various creams advertised as certain cures. The doctor commented that the patient seemed to be working very hard to solve the problem himself. 'Oh I'm like that in every way', he said. 'I've always managed to solve any problems I've had in the past by working at it. I've had to – my two brothers were much brighter than me and went to university. I knew I couldn't do that, but I've made a success out of my electrical business by sticking at it and working hard.'

At this first appointment the doctor noticed how polite and eager to please the patient was, and how outwardly confident he appeared to be. A second appointment was arranged, but before leaving the patient asked if there was anything he should be doing in the meantime. The doctor had a vision of him working hard at his homework, and just suggested they should talk again at the next appointment.

The second consultation started with the patient apologizing that he had nothing to report. After some questioning from the doctor, it transpired he'd tried to have sex once, but it had been a dismal failure again – he'd ejaculated immediately after penetration. 'Well that isn't exactly nothing to report', said the doctor. 'Perhaps you feel there is nothing good to report. Are things only worth talking about if they are a good report?' The patient thought carefully about this before remarking that only success had ever counted in his family. He spent some time describing what a failure he felt he must have been to his father, a university professor, that he wasn't clever enough to get to university himself. To be good enough, he'd felt he'd had to work doubly hard in his training as an electrician – failure wasn't an option. He'd built up his own business, which was very successful, and said that he'd always felt he'd had to work very hard to be good enough for his father.

The doctor observed that it was interesting that he had become, in his own eyes, not good enough in his sexual relationship after the birth of his own son. 'Yes', the patient agreed, 'before Sam was born I would have said that I had developed such self-confidence, but since this sexual problem started that's all changed. Sometimes I feel pretty useless.' They discussed the possibility that the birth of his own son had reawakened in him his own fears of inadequacy.

At the third consultation, the patient reported that the symptom was improving – he had instigated intercourse a few times and was lasting longer.

In this doctor–patient relationship, the patient had needed to impress upon the doctor how hard he was working at trying to succeed. His fears of inadequacy were exposed and faced – they had been well hidden by his success as an electrician and in his business. It was the birth of his own son that reawakened in him a fear of his inadequacy in his father's eyes, which manifested itself as sexual inadequacy with his wife. The consultations had provided him with a safe space to recognize this, and being accepted as good enough in that situation had allowed him to begin to feel good enough for his wife again.

RETARDED OR ABSENT EJACULATION

Retarded or absent ejaculation may perhaps best be considered as inhibited ejaculation, the inhibition being total or partial. Total ejaculatory inhibition, i.e. the inability to ejaculate under any circumstances, is less common than partial inhibition, i.e. able to ejaculate with masturbation, but not in the presence of a partner or in the vagina. Men will often delay presenting this problem until pushed to it by a partner who may desire to conceive, or who has become intolerably dissatisfied with the lack of ejaculation. Occasionally, men will seek help in order to obtain greater sexual pleasure for themselves. There is some evidence (Lincoln and Thexton, 1983) that men who are actively seeking pleasure for themselves have a better prognosis than men who are pushed into seeking help by dissatisfied partners.

Once again the symptom of inhibited ejaculation may be primary or secondary and, as it often originates in the unconscious, can respond to a psychodynamic approach. Inhibitions in the release of sexual feelings in adult life may be because of a restrictive upbringing, or dysfunctional relationship with either parent, which has interfered with the normal sexual development during childhood and adolescence. Not uncommonly non-ejaculating men, being able to maintain their erections for long periods, are much appreciated initially by their partners, but the inequality in sexual satisfaction may create tensions, which make the sexual relationship unsustainable. Unconscious hostility can often be found in these men who are allowing their partners to be orgasmic, but in not giving of themselves are denying their partners any joy in sharing and reciprocity.

During successful intercourse, each partner shares closely with the other. Each is aroused and responsive. One partner does not give the other an orgasm – they both have to feel safe enough in the vulnerability of letting their feelings show. Boys learn to relate to women through interaction with the important women in their early lives. Ejaculatory problems can occur when their unconscious feelings about women, causing anxiety and hostility, persist from those earlier experiences. The unconscious

feelings can prevent a man from enjoying his sexuality by spilling his semen too soon, as in premature ejaculation, or withholding it, frustrating the partner and being destructive of his own joy of sharing. Thus similar unconscious factors may operate in premature and inhibited ejaculation.

There is one situation where the unconscious factors are more likely to produce inhibited, rather than premature, ejaculation – the desire or threat of fatherhood. Men who have had unsatisfactory relationships with their own fathers may have a distaste for fatherhood. They may lack a satisfactory father model with which to identify. Men who feel uncertain of their own value in a relationship may fear the rivalry the presence of a baby may provoke. Interestingly, in the study of 22 men with inhibited ejaculation previously mentioned (Lincoln and Thexton, 1983) seven of the 22 men had been born a twin (13 times the national incidence) and many others talked about siblings of whom they had been very jealous.

Some men have learned to view childbirth as a painful and negative experience, and may have fears of inflicting such damage on their partner.

Men who have difficulty ejaculating often have difficulty letting go of other emotions, and forming intimate relationships. They often come from families where the showing of emotion of any sort was not encouraged. They may appear rigid in consultations, displaying little spontaneous emotional reactions or lively behaviour. Consultations with these men can feel flat, emotionless and hard work.

Case 2

Mr B, aged 40, attended the psychosexual clinic with Pauline, his girlfriend of 2 years, because of his inability to ejaculate in her vagina. Ejaculation was very rarely possible with masturbation in her presence, but fairly easy when alone. He had experienced this problem with the few short relationships he'd had in the past, usually ending the relationship himself rather than confront the problem. 'But with Pauline it's different', he said 'because she's very important to me and I don't want this relationship to go the same way. And besides, I'm 40 now – surely I should be able to have a better sex life.' The doctor suggested an examination to which Mr B easily agreed. The examination was unremarkable, with Mr B showing no embarrassment or uncertainty, and no anxieties about his genitals were revealed. The doctor noticed that Mr B seemed very matter of fact about the whole thing, unlike Pauline who appeared nervous and on edge and occasionally looked tearful. He commented on this fact. 'Pauline says I have difficulty showing my emotions', Mr B responded. 'She's always asking me how I'm feeling. When she does that I try to let it out, but I feel the shutters come down and I just tell her to shut up.' The doctor commented that it sounded like an angry comment, and Mr B agreed that he did get irritated when Pauline grilled him like that. The doctor wondered where this fear of letting his emotions show came from, and Mr B went on to describe his mother, who appeared to be a cold, strict and dominating women who rarely showed any emotion. There were no memories of displays of affection, and discipline was maintained with icy stares and an air of disapproval which filled the house. Mr B said he didn't want his house to feel like that. The father appeared timid and shadowy, completely dominated by his mother. He rarely saw his parents now.

Another appointment was made for 2 weeks and the doctor was left wondering if Mr B was a hopeless case – the story of his cold childhood and the longstanding nature of his problem seemed overwhelming and hopeless. It was a big surprise then when Mr B attended his second appointment with a smile on his face. It transpired that following the previous consultation he and Pauline had had a blazing row, something they had never done before. Apparently Pauline had, in Mr B's words, 'pestered me and pestered me about how I was feeling following the appointment and I got more and more irritated until finally I blew my top and told her to shut up and go away!' There followed a brief shouting match in which some angry and hateful comments were exchanged before the anger blew itself out, leaving both of them a bit surprised. Mr B had immediately felt panic that this would end the relationship, but instead he found they were both upset, in need of comfort, and wanting to comfort each other. They ended up in bed and he had ejaculated inside her.

In that and a third appointment, Mr B discussed his fear of expressing his anger and how it felt safer to bottle things up, rather than risk mayhem by letting them out. He felt that he had bottled up a lot of powerful feelings for a very long time, and realized that the fear of showing his feelings dated back to his childhood. He remembered that talking about his mother in the first consultation had made him feel angry, and when Pauline made emotional demands on him that afternoon, he allowed some of that anger to escape. The link between the fear of letting go of his feelings and letting go with ejaculation was made. Mr B felt after the third consultation that Pauline and he could manage on their own.

After many years of bottling up his emotions, Mr B was ready for change. The hopelessness the doctor had originally felt was perhaps indicative of the enormity of Mr B's fear that to let go would involve huge risk. The doctor, by drawing attention to the lack of emotion, had allowed Mr B to focus on the reasons for this. The consulting room and the certainty of a return visit provided enough of a sense of safety for Mr B to dare to let out some emotion with Pauline, and subsequently ejaculate with her.

PAINFUL EJACULATION

Compared with inhibited or premature ejaculation, the symptom of painful ejaculation is rare. Not unreasonably perhaps, the doctor's initial concern will be to exclude an organic cause, and thus these men will often be referred to departments of genito-urinary medicine and urology. Local infection (involving the urethra, seminal vesicles, prostate gland or bladder), abnormalities of the foreskin, and urethral and prostatic pathology may be confirmed or excluded.

Some healthy men experience hyperaesthesia of the glans penis after ejaculation so the glans is painful if touched. Kaplan (1979) has also suggested that painful ejaculation and post-ejaculatory pain could be caused by spasm of the perineal muscles because of a man's anxiety about ejaculation. This interesting hypothesis could be seen in psychodynamic terms as analogous to the superficial dyspareunia with the muscle spasm of vaginismus in women, and might be amenable to a psychodynamic therapeutic approach. Whatever the aetiology, the symptom will be affecting a man's sexual life, and a thoughtful, listening doctor may be able to hear and interpret evidence of emotional pain during the consultation, which may be relevant to the presenting symptom.

Case 3

Mr C was seen by a psychosexual doctor following several appointments at the urology clinic, because of his complaint of pain on ejaculation. Infection screening, examination and investigation of his urinary tract had failed to reveal any physical pathology. The history, already elicited, was that the pain had started approximately 3 years ago. In response to the doctor's query as to how this was affecting Mr C's sexual life, Mr C, who was 52 years old, reported that it had been over a year since he and his wife had made love. The doctor was silent for a short time before asking gently what problems that caused in the marriage. Mr C was on the verge of tears as he blurted out – 'well, she'll never get pregnant now, will she?' It transpired that Mr C and his wife had undergone extensive infertility investigations 12 years previously. No cause for the infertility had been identified, but Mrs C had never managed to conceive. Three years ago Mrs C had celebrated her 40th birthday. Whilst Mr C thought they had both accepted their childless state, he knew that after the age of 40 a woman's fertility declined precipitously. The pain of being able to give his semen to his wife, but not the longed for baby, expressed itself with every ejaculation. Once this pain was acknowledged, the grief, disappointment and sense of inadequacy could be explored and tolerated, and Mr C and his wife started to make love again, painlessly.

Because painful ejaculation is such a physical symptom, it is easy for the man behind the symptom to get lost in the activity of tests, examinations and the hunt for a physical diagnosis. As in Mr C's case, exclusion of pathology is essential, but examination of the emotions and feelings provoked by the symptom can give the clue as to the real cause.

FACTORS AFFECTING OUTCOME

Motivation

The importance of motivation has already been discussed with regard to men with inhibited ejaculation presenting for help because a partner wishes to conceive. It would seem likely that for many psychosexual problems a favourable outcome would be more common in those whose motivation was to increase their own sexual satisfaction. Ejaculatory problems, originating in the unconscious, depend for their resolution to a greater or lesser degree on confronting the repressive forces which inhibit the ability to freely enjoy ones own sexuality. Experiencing these repressive forces, usually of fear – fear of loss of control that may lead to an intolerable intensity of feeling, fear of vulnerability, exposure or loss of dignity – in response to demands of another may be too much to ask. Understanding the 'why now' with the patient and exploring the true feelings evoked by a partner's demands may provide useful insights.

Cultural differences

Interpersonal and intrapersonal difficulties lie at the root of most psychogenic ejaculatory problems. Effective therapy is aimed at understanding these factors for each individual in order for change to occur. When the patient and the doctor are from different cultures, there can be additional barriers to understanding the consultation and the meaning of the symptoms. This may be due in part to subtle differences in use of language, and in part to a variance in the sexual values of different cultures. For example, men from Asian cultures have a very different view of the concept of female partners having equal opportunity to initiate sexual activity than men from white Caucasian cultures. Additionally, fear and guilt that masturbation may have been 'weakening' seems stronger in Asian cultures. There may also be very different expectations about the women's role in the sexual relationship and in the understanding of the effect of arranged marriages.

In such situations, some understanding of the sexual values of the particular culture of the patient is desirable. It becomes even more important than usual for the doctor to listen with an open mind to what the patient says and feels.

Deeper psychopathology

Ever present during consultations with patients with psychosexual problems is an interaction between factors in the current situation and those from the past. Often the feelings and reactions provoked in the patient and the doctor in the here and now mirror those occurring in the sexual relationship, and these clinical findings and other unconscious elements brought to light can result in improvement or resolution of the sexual dysfunction. This is much more likely to happen if the patient's sexual development has been 'good enough', as discussed previously. If it hasn't, therapy offers a chance of making amends for defective sexual development, through re-learning and re-experiencing problematic areas. There will be some patients whose unsatisfactory sexual development may be too disturbed to be amenable to the relatively brief interventions of focused psychosexual therapy. Or the sexual dysfunction may be just one expression of a much broader failure in development with regard to the ability to communicate with others, and the expression and management of intense feelings of anger and intimacy. Some of these patients will require more prolonged, in-depth psychotherapy. In the absence of recognizable psychiatric symptomatology, it can be difficult to predict initially which patients are likely to fall into this category. This is particularly so with men with inhibited ejaculation, as this can often be associated with inhibited experience of feelings generally, and the inability to form intimate relationships with others. Sometimes these men provoke optimism initially in the doctor–patient relationship that therapy will be fruitful, in the same way they initially engage with their sexual partners. With the passage of time, the difficulty with the sharing of themselves frustrates and thwarts the doctor, particularly female doctors, much as it does their partner, and the therapy, like the relationship, fails. This initial raising of expectations of success in the doctor can delay the appreciation that the prognosis with brief therapy is poor and that longer psychotherapeutic help will be required, if the patient can accept it.

Case 4

Mr D, aged 48, attended the psychosexual clinic because of a lifelong inability to ejaculate. His only experience of ejaculation had been as a teenager, once during masturbation, and on several occasions with wet dreams. He had had one sexual partner only, marrying her at the age of 25 and separating from her 10 years later. 'She said that I never showed my feelings', was his response to the doctor's enquiry as to why the marriage failed. He was referred to the clinic by the Psychiatry Department, whose care he had been under for depression resulting in two half-hearted suicide attempts during the previous year. He had been taken into care as a young child, and reported a cold unhappy emotionless childhood. During his marriage and adult life he had failed to make any significant friendships, describing himself as 'a loner, with no mates'. In the first consultation the doctor's hopes of some improvement were raised, despite the history, by Mr D's flattery of her as being easy to talk to, and the first person with whom he had been able to discuss his sexual problems freely. This doctor would be better than the psychiatrists, and his wife! An agreement was made for three further appointments, with the possibility of more, if progress indicated they would be beneficial. During the following sessions the doctor found herself working extremely hard to reach any feelings in this patient, and whilst he remained affable and polite, he remained completely in control of himself and the consultations, and no progress was made. On feeding this back to the patient, his response was that he had suspected it would be a waste of time all along.

As with his sexual relationship, after initial engagement, Mr D's difficulty with letting go of his defences and sharing with another resulted in a frustrating, unsatisfying and ultimately fruitless relationship with the doctor. The doctor could only recommend that long-term psychotherapy might help.

CONCLUSION

Ejaculatory problems commonly present as premature ejaculation, delayed or absent ejaculation, and more rarely as painful ejaculation. Ejaculation is a powerful psychosomatic event, whose neurophysiological basis is poorly understood. Doctors and other health professionals, to whom these problems present, often feel inadequate to deal with these symptoms, as there are no clearly effective treatments. The consultation and communication skills used daily by health professionals become powerful tools in helping patients to understand their own symptoms and facilitate changes, resulting in resolution of the symptoms. Active listening, empathy, an ability to puzzle with the patient and tolerate uncertainty and 'not knowing', will enable the patient to feel heard and understood, and perhaps lead to increased self awareness. The more advanced skill of recognizing and using the unconscious material in the interaction with the patient, and relating it sometimes to the patient's past, and always to the presenting symptom, may be achieved with further training.

For doctors, the use of a sensitive genital examination as an examination of the mind – feelings, emotions, fears and fantasies – as well as the body, can be a powerful tool to shed further light on the problem for the patient.

All health professionals need to be aware of the limitations of their abilities and when to refer men with ejaculatory problems on to more appropriate services.

KEY POINTS

- Ejaculatory problems often are caused by emotional and psychological difficulties, rarely by organic disease.
- Clues to the cause of the problem can often be found in the consultation.
- A thoughtful, listening doctor with good communication skills can help the patient to identify emotional factors that might contribute to, or maintain the persistence of, the problem.
- An exploration of the patient's feelings can provide useful insights.
- The genital examination can be helpful in eliciting further insights into the patient's perception of his sexuality, fears and fantasies.

- Whilst a supportive, sharing partner can be important, men without partners can benefit from psychosexual therapy.
- Referral to a specialist psychosexual service should be a joint decision between the doctor and patient.

REFERENCES

Bancroft, J. 1995: *Human sexuality and its problems.* Edinburgh: Churchill Livingstone.

Kaplan, H.S. 1979: *Disorder of sexual desire and other new concepts and techniques in sex therapy.* New York: Bruner/Mazel.

Kinsey, A.C., Pomeroy, W.B. and Martin, C.E. 1948: *Sexual behaviour in the human male.* Philadelphia: Saunders.

Lincoln, R. and Thexton, R. 1983: Retarded ejaculation. In Draper, K. (ed.), *Practice of psychosexual medicine.* London: J. Libbey.

Masters, W.H. and Johnson, V.E. 1970: *Human sexual inadequacy.* Churchill: London.

13 Problems with female orgasm

Gillian Vanhegan

Normal female orgasmic response

Failure to orgasm

Physical reasons for anorgasmia

Psychosocial

Psychosexual

NORMAL FEMALE ORGASMIC RESPONSE

The female orgasm is a natural reflex in response to the right kind of stimulus, associated with the psychological ability to 'let go'. Physiologically, the response is similar in all females, but the stimulus varies considerably between individuals. Each woman has her own particular erogenous area, which when stimulated leads to orgasm. Some believe in one particular spot for stimulation, the so-called 'G spot', but there is conflicting evidence for this, as some women remain orgasmic even after extensive surgery in the genital area.

The physical reactions in the various stages of female arousal are described in chapter 1. The pleasurable physical sensations are accompanied by an exciting altered mental state, which cannot be measured and is described in different ways by women. After orgasm, there is detumescence of all the organs. During the recovery phase, a feeling of well-being persists; often the woman can be brought to orgasm again quite quickly if love-making continues.

FAILURE TO ORGASM

Orgasms can occur in quite young girls due to the right sort of stimulation, usually to the genital area, such as in rocking games when sitting astride an object or riding a horse. Masturbation begins as a part of normal adolescent development and the girl usually finds a way of replicating the pleasurable sensations for herself by pressure or rubbing. In order to reach orgasm with a partner, the sexually active young woman has to experience her particular stimulus that produces orgasm. As the type of stimulus varies between women, communication is needed in the relationship so that the woman can be stimulated in the right way for her.

The woman who can climax when she stimulates herself, or when her partner learns to do so with clitoral stimulation, may wish to appreciate the deeper feelings within the vagina. She may also feel under pressure to do so from her partner, who considers himself a failure if he cannot satisfy her with his penis.

Despite the physiological demonstration by Masters and Johnson (1967) that there is no difference between clitoral orgasm and vaginal orgasm, most women are aware of a difference, and see vaginal orgasm as the ultimate goal.

Primary anorgasmia, in which the woman has never experienced orgasm, although she may or may not have felt sexual excitement, is a not uncommon complaint in the psychosexual clinic and in the pages of women's magazines. This can be due to deep suppression of sexual feelings or to a lack of proficiency by her partner.

Secondary anorgasmia occurs in an individual who has previously been orgasmic but ceases to be so for certain physical, psychosocial or psychosexual reasons, which will be considered below.

PHYSICAL REASONS FOR ANORGASMIA

Endocrine

Conditions leading to hypopituitarism will result in hypogonadism and a failure to achieve orgasm. Secondary hypopituitarism is rare and can be the result of a severe post-partum haemorrhage that leads to Simmond's disease or Sheehan's syndrome (Mackay, 1983). This is an extremely rare occurrence. Careful history-taking and physical examination would ensure that such a patient would be referred to an endocrinologist rather than a psychosexual clinic. Follicle stimulating hormone (FSH), luteinizing hormone (LH) and prolactin levels would be initial investigations leading to diagnosis.

Neurological

An intact lumbosacral pathway appears to be necessary for an orgasm to happen and this can be disrupted by conditions such as multiple sclerosis, which destroy neurological pathways and connections. Advanced stages of diabetes mellitus can also lead to neuropathy and arteriolar damage. Whereas male sexual function as regards erection and ejaculation is affected at a relatively early stage of the condition, diabetes has to be far more advanced before the female orgasm is affected.

Malignant disease

Extensive surgery for cancer of the pelvic organs can lead to failure to orgasm. This failure is probably due to destruction of the neural pathways rather than of the organs themselves. It can be difficult to differentiate between loss of orgasm for physical reasons in such cases, as there will be a degree of psychosexual distress overlying the loss of organs, which are perceived by many women as representing their sexuality. Sometimes there can be feelings of guilt or blame as to the reasons for acquiring a malignancy in the pelvis. If she has feelings that her enjoyment and freedom of feeling in sex have lead to her condition, she often loses the ability to relax and enjoy sexual activity. Her male partner can similarly be impeded in intercourse and have anxieties about causing damage or further harm following surgery.

Cancer of the vulva is treated by disfiguring surgery and this alters the woman's self image as a sexual and attractive person. Psychosexual treatment can address this problem and allow the patient to express her feelings about the different body image.

Dermatological conditions

Sexual activity can be curtailed by dermatological conditions that affect the vulva. As with malignant disease, there is a combination of physical and psychosexual reasons for failure to orgasm. Eczema often becomes particularly weepy and sore at the vulva. The appearance of the area, or dyspareunia, can disturb normal intercourse. This is similar for other fairly common conditions such as psoriasis, vestibulitis and lichen sclerosis.

Drugs

The female sexual response is often dampened down by the use of suppressant medication such as narcotics or antidepressants, although use of these drugs denotes an altered mental state that might lead to a psychosexual reason for anorgasmia. Some antiepileptic drugs reduce the ability to orgasm, but in the consultation the anxiety of the epileptic patient about producing a fit by sexual activity must be addressed.

The reduced ability to have an erection in males who take beta blocker medication as an antihypertensive has been recognized. This medication seems to have a similar effect on some female patients, who lose the ability to have an orgasm when prescribed these drugs.

The most common medication that patients will be taking is the combined oral contraceptive pill and often they will blame it for their failure to orgasm. In rare cases the pill might alter the woman's hormonal state sufficiently to lead to this problem. More commonly, this will be due to a psychosexual difficulty, such as a desire to get pregnant, but circumstances prevail which necessitate her staying on the pill. In this situation the woman would not be able to feel happy in her sexual life and this would lead to orgasmic failure.

Whilst there are few rare physical reasons for female anorgasmia, the vast majority of cases are due to psychosocial and psychosexual causes.

PSYCHOSOCIAL

The male and female orgasm are both of a purely reflex nature. Some men may become stimulated more easily, and the external environment seems to be less important to them. In contrast, a woman may be more aroused by being in a good relationship, with a suitably romantic environment, and the reflex is easily disturbed by situational difficulties such as having to live with her partner's family. The fear of being overheard by parents in an adjacent bedroom is enough to produce anorgasmia in a previously orgasmic woman. In the consultation the woman will admit to an ability to have an orgasm when she is away from home, for example on holidays.

Relationship problems also come into play in inhibiting the orgasmic reflex. The female has to be able to trust her mate and betrayal in the form of an affair, however brief, can sow the seed of doubt that leads to failure to orgasm.

These social and interpersonal difficulties are usually amenable to resolution when brought to a relationship counsellor. In other cases the cause of the anorgasmia is more deep-seated and psychosexual therapy is required.

PSYCHOSEXUAL

Childhood sexual abuse

Abuse in childhood may lead to various psychosexual difficulties. In the Institute of Psychosexual Medicine, research into adults with sexual difficulties who had been abused as children (Vanhegan *et al.*, 1996) found that almost a quarter of the subjects complained of an inability to achieve an orgasm. The child may be disturbed by any feelings of sexual excitement produced by the inappropriate activity of an abuser and thus develop strategies for suppressing these feelings. In adult life, the woman experiences difficulties in allowing herself to be aroused to orgasm and requires psychosexual counselling to be able to cope with the reawakened feelings from her childhood. She needs to work through these feelings and develop adult sexual feelings on her own terms, so that she can use her sexuality for her pleasure and become orgasmic, as illustrated in the case below.

Case 1

Martha came to see me at the psychosexual clinic for young people. She had already seen a counsellor on 10 occasions and they both felt that she was not making any headway with her problem of failing to have an orgasm.

She was a delicate, fragile 20-year-old, with a beautiful oval face and a sad demeanour. At the beginning of the consultation, when I asked her what the problem was, she said 'I don't enjoy sex because I cannot get at all excited'. I wondered aloud what happened when she was making love with her boyfriend. 'When he starts to move inside me I feel my mind falling away so that I'm not really there'. 'It seems as though you do not want to be there', I said. 'I am afraid that he will lose control and hurt me'.

I pointed out that these feelings must come from something inside her and seemed to make her so sad. 'I've bottled it all up', she said. Then, in a distant and unemotional voice, she told me that when she was about 10 years old she had gone to the dancing class that followed her older sister's class, so she had to sit in the car with her grandfather while she waited for her class. He would put his finger inside her little vagina and make her kiss him. 'I hated it', she said 'He always gave me sweets afterwards'.

I wondered how she felt about what had happened and she admitted to being afraid and unable to tell anyone in the family, in case she disrupted the family life. Eventually, the classes changed and with relief she was able to take the bus, instead of having to go in the car with her grandfather. That was the end of her first visit in which I noticed how I had been put in the position of a caring mother figure to this fragile and damaged childlike girl.

At the next visit she was still not having orgasms with her boyfriend and we talked a little about him. He was at college with her, but she found problems in trusting him because of her experience with her grandfather. She felt that she might not be having orgasms because of something not being normal inside, and she wondered if she had been damaged in some way by the abuse. This seemed a good moment for a psychosomatic examination of her genitalia.

She lay on the couch with her legs completely abducted in a very vulnerable looking position and when I started to examine her she seemed totally uninvolved and detached from what was happening. I commented to her that she seemed to have no feelings about what was happening to her and that she seemed to be cut off from her body below the waist. She said 'That was the only way that I could cope with what my grandfather was doing to me'. I suggested to her that that was why she was not having an orgasm, as she was not letting herself feel any sensations. Then she started to take more interest in the examination and to ask questions about herself and seemed very relieved that she was physically normal and no actual physical damage had been done.

By the third visit she was able to express anger at what her grandfather had done to her and was able to see that she had also at times been angry with her partner for taking his pleasure in something which she could not enjoy. In the following visit this childlike young woman began to own the feelings in her own vagina and to move away from the damage that she perceived had been done to her in her youth, and eventually to own her vagina as an adult. As she went through this process she became less childlike. At the end of psychosexual therapy she was enjoying the relationship with her boyfriend and had become orgasmic.

A note of caution in relation to sexual abuse. Women who have been abused may have no problem at the beginning of their sexual lives. The difficulty may start later, perhaps following an important life event. At this stage she and her partner may blame the abuse. The doctor has to try and work out with the patient how much the old feelings have been aroused by recent events, and how much the old abuse is being used as an understandable reason for the difficulty. It may be easier to blame the past than to accept present feelings, for instance of anger or hurt in the on-going relationship.

Rape

Some patients have had happy and fulfilling orgasmic relationships, which have been destroyed by sexual assault. The male partner can be very supportive following a rape, but the woman is unable to trust and lose her inhibitions in intercourse after such a destructive experience, because her faith in all men has been undermined.

Difficult and distressing cases are the ones where the woman is attacked by a partner she has previously rejected. It is particularly distressing if he follows her in anger and assaults her. This patient needs to acknowledge the pain and invasion felt by such an assault and to work through this before she is able to allow herself to lose her fear, and relax with her new partner sufficiently to achieve orgasm.

As doctors we must remain aware of the concept of 'medical rape'. What we see as a normal medical procedure may feel to the woman as an uninvited invasion of her body. For example, the patient who has had a painful catheterization may in fantasy confuse the small urethra with the adequate vagina, and fear that intercourse will also be painful.

Younger patients may be subjected to a rectal examination as part of the investigation of acute abdominal pain. I have seen a non-orgasmic adult who had suffered this indignity as a 12-year-old in casualty in front of a group of medical students. The examining doctor had not asked her permission to do the rectal examination and she saw the experience as a gang rape by him and the students.

Termination of pregnancy

In the UK at the present time there are a large number of unintended and often unwanted pregnancies, not only in teenagers but also in older women. Although in most areas there is reasonable access to termination of pregnancy, it is still a difficult decision for a woman to make. Many women are lucky enough to have the support of partner and friends, but even so the longer-term effects can lead to psychosexual problems. Sex has often been happy and fulfilling until the resultant pregnancy and the trauma of the decision to have a termination. The actual procedure and its aftermath can lead to a loss of sexual drive and a loss of sexual satisfaction.

Case 2

Jeanette was a beautiful thin, fragile looking woman of 26, who was referred by her GP to the psychosexual clinic as she was distressed by her inability to enjoy sex since her termination of pregnancy. She was originally from the continent and there were still hints of her origins when she spoke, although her English was fluent. When I asked her what the problem was she said 'I cannot get any pleasure from sex since I made (sic) an abortion last year. My boyfriend tries to be very understanding'. I wondered what happened between them now and she said 'I can let him kiss me but when it comes to touching me and having sex I want him to . . .' and she pushed her hand forward. 'To stop him', I said, 'you feel like pushing him away'. 'Exactly', she said, and I wondered aloud but quite quietly, in response to her delicacy and vulnerability, why this should have happened after the abortion. She expressed an inability to understand why she needed to reject him.

In the doctor–patient relationship I felt protective towards this fragile little soul. She continued by saying that she had met her boyfriend when he had been studying overseas and they had always used condoms. She had been extremely surprised when she moved to England to find that she was pregnant. She said 'It was very early when I made the abortion, I did not have the big tummy'. I asked 'Is that important to you, that you did not have a big tummy?' She explained about her Catholic upbringing, the religious school and how she felt that abortion was not right, but she said that she thought that it had been the right decision for her. 'But something has changed deep inside you', I said. 'Yes', she agreed 'I have nightmares about killing babies'. I asked if she herself was killing the babies, and she said that it was always somebody else. The dreams had been bad over the previous week and we wondered whether it was because it was exactly a year since the actual abortion had taken place.

She seemed to need to relive the experience in some way, so I acknowledged this and she began to talk about it. 'When I had the abortion I felt I was on a conveyor belt, there were too many of us in the room, and when one came back from the operation another one was moved along. It was not the fault of the staff, they were very kind, but there were too many people'. I sensed that she had wanted to be alone, 'Yes, I had made a very special decision', she said. 'I did not want to be part of this conveyor belt'.

I was still puzzled over exactly what it was in the situation of the abortion that had caused her to stop being able to feel things and to be unable to have an orgasm during sex. She said, 'I just do not feel anything when I have sex'. I felt that the time had come to examine her. She said that she had a heavy period and that she did not want to be examined while she was bleeding. Fortuitously, I had a cancellation for two weeks later. She seemed so relieved at the thought of being examined that she closed the consultation by jumping up and saying, 'Yes, yes I will see you in two weeks time', and she hurried away.

When she returned she had not had any opportunity for sex with her boyfriend, as he had been working abroad. She had missed him dreadfully and was looking forward to him returning home. We covered a little of the old ground about the termination, but I felt that we were both working towards the important genital examination. On the couch she lay in a very rigid way and I said 'You seem to have some problems with relaxing', to which she replied 'It takes some time'. 'Is that the same when you are having sex?' 'Yes it is', she said. When I began to examine her I wondered what it was like for her and she said 'There is no feeling'. 'Just like sex', I said. 'So why should that have happened after the abortion?' I wondered aloud. 'There were so many of us', she said again. 'It was such a conveyor belt'. But then she added 'Perhaps they cut an important nerve'. I said 'Would that be the nerves that give you feelings down there?' She nodded her agreement.

I continued to examine her very thoroughly so that she could see that I was not treating her as if she was on a conveyor belt. As I examined each area I commented that physically it all looked normal and she said 'I think it is probably me, I will not let myself feel any more'. After the examination she talked about how being under the anaesthetic had been very frightening because she was a person who needed to be in control and she still had deep fears about what had happened when she was asleep. She wanted a more thorough explanation of the termination procedure and seemed very relieved that actually no scissors and scalpels had been used near this delicate part of her anatomy, as her fantasy of cut nerves was very real to her.

She was able to work in the consultations to allow herself to feel again, now that she was not anxious about damage to nerves. Later, when she was making love with her boyfriend, she began to feel sensations, and sex became pleasurable once again.

It was important in her case that I had felt her fragility in the doctor–patient relationship and been able to help her to work with her fear of damage that she had been able to reveal at the psychosomatic genital examination.

Homosexuality

Some female patients who complain of an inability to orgasm are in marriages or relationships with men and have never faced up to their homosexual feelings. This puts great stress on the partnership and the woman will not become orgasmic until she breaks away and forms a homosexual relationship. She will have tried to live the type of life which she sees as required by convention, but eventually during psychosexual therapy she will be able to release her true feelings about her sexuality and, although this often leads to the breakdown of her heterosexual relationship, it will free her to live a life in which she can find sexual happiness and become orgasmic.

Sexual problems can arise in homosexual relationships in response to all those emotions that occur in heterosexual relationships, although help appears to be sought less often. Is this because there are less often children for whom the couple want to stay together? When

faced with the ambivalent feelings that arise in any relationship, and that are so often expressed in the form of sexual dysfunction, it may be easier to split and start again if there are no children involved. The other possibility is that it is still less easy for those in homosexual relationships to ask for help.

Childbirth and motherhood

The act of giving birth to another human being and changing to the role of a mother can have an effect on the woman's feelings about her body and how the process of birth has changed it and also about sexual activity, now that she herself is a mother. The post-natal check visit is a good time to sound out the patient on whether she has resumed sexual activity. Often there are comments such as 'My stitches are still too sore' and even when an examination in this case shows a perfectly healed perineum, the examination will give the woman the chance to express her anxieties about damage or change caused by the birth process. In other cases it may take a number of months before the patient is able to ask for help with a psychosexual problem following childbirth, as is illustrated by the following case.

Case 3

Mrs M was a 30-year-old woman who was referred to me by her GP with dissatisfaction in her sex life since the birth of the child. Her daughter was 18 months old. She was a well dressed, pretty woman and I started by asking her what was meant in the referral letter by dissatisfaction. As soon as she began to talk she became very tearful, saying 'Everything has shut down like a door since I had my baby, but she is wonderful'. She seemed to add the end to the sentence to reassure me that she had no regrets about having the child. Then she continued, and told me that since seeing her GP two months earlier she had not had sex at all. Before that, it had started to get painful, and she was only able to do it a few times when they had been on holidays and she had had a few drinks.

She was still crying and sounding exhausted. 'I feel everything weighing on my shoulders. I am trying to do some work and care for my baby and keep the house tidy. Do you have children?' the latter question to ascertain whether she had a sympathetic and understanding doctor. I agreed that I could sense the awfulness of the situation. It would have been easy to diagnose this patient's problems as being due to the fatigue of modern life for a 30-something career woman, but it was a more deep-seated problem. She wanted to tell me about her long, induced labour and the epidural, which had not worked at first, and had to be re-sited correctly. She said that they had needed to do a foetal blood sample, and her legs were so out of control that her husband had to hold them apart for the doctor to take the sample. 'I wonder how that made you feel?' I said. 'I felt invaded and a complete failure'. 'Why did you feel a complete failure?' 'Because I had seen someone on TV having a baby and they put the baby on her tummy, but they gave Emily to David and he held her first; it was not what I planned'.

During pregnancy she had been a regular visitor to the gym and kept really fit. She had planned a natural birth and had wanted to stay at home and relax until the last minute, instead of being in hospital with epidurals and monitors. At first she had trouble breast-feeding. 'Emily screamed every time she tried to feed because I could not give her what she wanted. Everybody said what a marvellous father David was and I resented him.' There was a pause. 'Does that sound awful?' I reiterated how she felt, and said I could see that these feelings were getting in the way of their previously happy relationship.

At the second consultation, she became tearful again and said that they had been away together and they had tried sex once, but it had been too painful. I felt the time had come for a genital examination. She lay on the couch sobbing gently and saying 'I feel abnormal, I should be having sex'. The examination was not painful for her. I was able to use two fingers and a speculum. I said 'The examination was fine, but you are still angry with him, so you are keeping him out'. She came to sit down again and said that she had wanted everything to be perfect after having the baby, but when they had started to make love again she had found that she was no longer having orgasms. It had all become too painful, and in the end they were not having sex at all. I said that I could feel how perfect she had wanted it all to be and how things had gone wrong from the birth onwards. She said 'Yes it is better not to have sex at all than to fail at that as well as everything else'.

The healing process began with her being able to voice her anger and resentment about the birth and how everyone had praised her husband and seen him as marvellous, when she saw herself as such a failure.

CONCLUSION

The ability to achieve an orgasm is an important and integral part of most women's lives, and failure in this basic area of existence is deeply frustrating and depressing to non-orgasmic women. They expect there to be a simple physical explanation for their problem, but the physical causes of anorgasmia are extremely rare and easily excluded in the general practice setting. The psychosexual reasons are as varied as the patients themselves and can occur at all times of life.

The treatment begins in the non-directive patient-led consultation as illustrated in these cases, in which the doctor is aware of the effect that the patient is having on her. The doctor tries to offer an interpretation so that the patient can see how she acts in relationships both inside and outside the consulting room. This helps to free her to talk about her concerns and anxieties about her sex life. The psychosomatic examination of the genitalia can be a moment of truth for the patient and doctor alike, and often allows the woman to reveal her fantasies about her genitals. In the ensuing consultations the psychosexual doctor can help the woman to work through her difficulties and lose her anxieties and inhibitions in order to become orgasmic.

KEY POINTS

- Physical causes of anorgasmia are very rare.
- The cause is usually either psychosocial or psychosexual.

- Secondary anorgasmia can occur at any stage of life.
- Treatment begins with the interpretation of the doctor–patient relationship.
- The psychosomatic examination of the genitalia is an important event.
- The orgasm is a normal reflex that requires adequate physical stimulation and an emotional ability to 'let go'.

REFERENCES

Mackay, E., Beischer, N., Cox, L. and Wood, C. 1983: *Illustrated textbook of gynaecology*. W.B. Saunders.

Masters, W. and Johnson, V. 1967: *An analysis of the human sexual response*. London: Panther.

Vanhegan, G., Tunnadine, P. and Kwantes, P. 1996: Treatment of psychosexual disorders in previously abused patients. *British Journal of Family Planning* 22, 191–3.

14 Painful intercourse

Marian Davis

Physical causes

Pressure to find a physical cause

Psychosomatic factors

Painful intercourse, or dyspareunia, provides a perfect illustration of the desirability of combining the body–mind approach with the patient. It is a symptom that may have a number of physical causes that require straightforward physical treatments. However, a patient may well have feelings about the symptom or the condition that causes it, and it can be helpful to acknowledge these. There is another group of women who have persistent dyspareunia for which no cause can be found in spite of extensive investigations and in whom no treatment is successful. Psychosexual skills may help these women to make links between their physical and their emotional pain.

Dyspareunia may be defined as pain or discomfort that occurs in association with sexual intercourse. It may be superficial or deep and may occur at the start, during or after intercourse. The causes will be considered under the broad headings of physical and psychosomatic, although, as will be evident, there is a significant degree of overlap and so the distinction is to some extent artificial. No attempt will be made to give an exhaustive account of diagnosis and treatment of physical causes of dyspareunia – this is covered in

standard textbooks of gynaecology (e.g. James *et al.*, 1999).

PHYSICAL CAUSES

The physical causes of dyspareunia can be considered as either superficial or deep (see chapter 19). Superficial dyspareunia tends to occur at the start of intercourse and deep dyspareunia on deeper penetration. The pain may just be there at the time or may persist for hours or even days afterwards.

The patient may come complaining of pain or may present with a problem such as thrush, perhaps on a recurrent basis. It may be easier to complain of thrush than to tell the doctor that sex is painful. Alternatively, a sensitive doctor/nurse doing a vaginal examination for a smear, for example, might realize that the examination is uncomfortable or that the woman is not engaged with what is going on, and may then ask if the discomfort occurs at other times.

Diagnosis of dyspareunia is made by taking a careful history, elucidating when the pain occurs in relation to intercourse and the menstrual cycle. It is important to clarify exactly what is meant by painful sex. After taking the history, a thorough examination is performed, looking in particular for signs of systemic upset, obvious ulceration, warts, inflammation, signs of atrophic vaginitis, discharge etc. Sites of tenderness are noted and any masses palpated. Investigations may include swabs, blood tests and ultrasound examination. Referral might be indicated and laparoscopy carried out to establish a diagnosis. For example, laparoscopy is the investigation of choice for suspected endometriosis. During the examination, the psychosexual doctor will be aware that the patient may well have feelings about her symptom. She may need to switch from being a physical doctor to a listening doctor to a teacher in the same consultation. The examination in particular can be an opportunity to 'listen to' the patient's feelings. A listening examination may prevent a future psychosexual problem or treat a co-existing one.

The main physical causes of dyspareunia are listed in Table 14.1. The treatment will vary depending on the cause, but includes hormonal medication, antibiotics or antifungals, steroids, treatment of the underlying condition or surgery.

Even though the patient may have an obvious physical cause for her dyspareunia, she will have feelings about it. There may be fears as to what is happening to her body that make it difficult for her to ask for help. She may fear disease or what has caused it, or what it may mean to her in the future. Such fears may not be fully conscious, and may include fantasies about her body.

Table 14.1 Main causes of dyspareunia

(a) Superficial
Infections: thrush, trichomonas, genital herpes, genital warts or HPV infection, infected Bartholin's gland etc.
Allergies: soap or personal deodorants, creams, pessaries and other irritants.
Interstitial cystitis or urethral syndrome.
Systemic diseases: e.g. lupus, Behcets syndrome, or Reiter's disease.
Skin conditions: skin bridges and fissures, vulvar vestibulitis, psoriasis, lichen sclerosis, lichen planus and lichen simplex; pemphigus, linear IgA disease or dermatitis herpetiformis.
Malignancy: e.g. squamous cell carcinoma, vulvar intraepithelial carcinoma.
Iatrogenic: e.g. on the site of an episiotomy scar.

(b) Deep
Endometriosis.
Infections: salpingitis, appendicitis, chronic pelvic inflammatory disease, urinary tract infection.
Irritable bowel syndrome or constipation.
Inflammatory bowel disease, or diverticulitis.
Rectal or bladder tumours (rare).
Ovarian cyst: benign or malignant; polycystic ovarian disease.
Pelvic vein congestion.
Pelvic adhesions.
Physiological: Mittelschmerz syndrome, pre-menstrual syndrome.
Hip disease.
Ectopic pregnancy.

Case 1

The doctor's surgery was running late. Due to a computer failure a few days previously, there were several double bookings. Each time she went out to the waiting room, several expectant faces would look up. One of them was Mrs A, a pleasant round-faced smiley woman in her mid fifties. Eventually it was her turn. Still smiling and dismissing the apologies for keeping her waiting, she followed the doctor to her room.

The practice nurse had suggested that Mrs A see the doctor only that morning. The doctor asked what she could do to help, silently hoping that it would be something simple so that she could catch up. Mrs A had never spoken to anybody about this before and it was very difficult. Sex had been really painful for a long time. The doctor asked if she had told her husband, noting internally how uncomplaining she had been with the doctor. The smiley face crumpled and Mrs A's eyes filled with tears as the story came tumbling out. She loved her husband very much and had never told him how much it hurt, but it had been getting worse and worse and now it was like salt on an open wound. 'That sounds terrible'... She dissolved into tears and the doctor sat back and waited. The tears subsided and she looked up and continued. She just couldn't bear it any more, but felt so guilty about letting her husband down. Things had come to a head because they were going away on holiday by themselves for a month. It should have been a really special time. The doctor asked a few medical questions – making love had been painful for about five or six years. Mrs A's periods had stopped about six years previously and she was troubled by flushes as well, but had never linked all these things. She had wanted to avoid HRT.

The doctor suggested an examination. Mrs A slipped off her clothes and climbed up on to the couch. The doctor noted that she was very nervous. She held her arm over her face. The vulva showed the changes of atrophic vaginitis with an inflamed and pale mucosa. The doctor explained what she could see and said that topical oestrogens should be helpful in alleviating the symptoms. The woman's relief was palpable. 'You had feared it was something else?' – 'I thought that I was getting smaller and that it was going to close'.

The woman's distress had been because she thought that the sexual part of her marriage was over. The doctor was able to reassure Mrs A that, apart from the atrophic vaginitis, the examination was quite normal.

The atmosphere had changed completely. The doctor explained about the use of topical oestrogens and arranged follow-up after the holiday. The consultation had taken a little over 10 minutes. When Mrs A returned, her symptoms had completely resolved. 'It was better than I ever thought it could be. In fact it was so good that I got honeymoon cystitis at first!!' She had visited a local casualty department and the nurse had grinned when she'd told her about the pessaries. There was a sense of female fellowship, and more than a little excitement. The cystitis had responded to antibiotics and the rest of the holiday had been wonderful. Had Mrs A felt able to share her previous distress with her husband? No, it would have been too upsetting for him – he was just delighted at the change in their relationship. Again there were tears in Mrs A's eyes, but this time they were tears of joy and perhaps a tinge of regret that she hadn't sought help sooner. 'I thought this was just what happened as you got older'.

Comment

There was an obvious physical cause for Mrs A's dyspareunia. There is no way of knowing whether her symptoms would have persisted if her fantasy of her vagina closing up had not been explored, but a listening doctor and a psychosexual examination revealed what that problem meant to her, and with topical oestrogens she was able to move on.

PRESSURE TO FIND A PHYSICAL CAUSE

Pressure to make inappropriate therapeutic decisions can come from the doctor's perceived role. The doctor is supposed to be all-knowing, to make a diagnosis using the history, examination and appropriate investigations and then to 'make it better'. Not to do this can be seen as failure. The patient, or her partner, may put pressure on the doctor for referral to various consultants in the search for a physical explanation for her pain. Sometimes these women are subjected to years of fruitless investigations, including scans, blood tests and laparoscopies.

Occasionally, they can even undergo therapeutic interventions, such as division of adhesions or total pelvic clearance. The pain may persist because, although many doctors are trying to put things right, no one has stopped and asked a different question – why are they wrong?

Case 2

A 28-year-old woman presented with a 6-year history of pelvic pain and dyspareunia. She had been seen by a variety of gynaecologists and had had a laparoscopy and division of adhesions, but this had not helped the pain. The referral letter said that the pain was affecting what had been a very happy marriage. The letter asked for an urgent appointment and was from out of the area – the GP had had to do a bit of research – but the patient said that she couldn't be seen for several months. When she was offered an appointment, she failed to respond and so she wasn't seen until 9 months after the initial referral. So even before she was seen, there was some contradiction in the way that the doctors were under pressure to put the pain right and her ambivalence about attending. At the first meeting, Mrs B gave all the appearances of wanting to address the issues that might be important. She told the doctor that she had had dyspareunia since before she had got married. She readily and emotionally told the doctor about an unloved childhood, a 'promiscuous' adolescence, a traumatic obstetric history and a sexually inexperienced husband. She seemed to be fully engaged with what went on and responded thoughtfully to the doctor's reflections. Mrs B kept the second appointment in spite of feeling very unwell, again giving the impression of being really well-motivated. The doctor thought that she had pyelonephritis and spent the session making an appointment at the patient's own surgery. At the third appointment, Mrs B was sedated from strong painkillers but had still driven herself to keep the appointment. It proved impossible to do any work because of the medication. She failed to keep her next appointment and there was a further exchange of letters before she was seen some 4 months later. Not surprisingly, there had been no change. This time, she wanted to talk about her attempts at weight loss. At last the penny dropped. The doctor reflected that for the last three appointments, Mrs B had kept her from looking at her problem. This freed the situation and the patient was then able to look at her feelings towards her husband. She wondered if she had ever loved him and certainly now did not fancy him or love him in a sexual way. She acknowledged that the pain meant that she had not had to face up to these issues. She did not want a further appointment and said that she would suggest to her husband that they go to Relate. It is not known whether she did so or whether she is still complaining of pain.

The pressure for a treatable physical condition is not only apparent in the individual doctor–patient relationship but in the relationship between women and the profession as a whole. This is illustrated by the profusion of investigations, differential diagnoses and treatments for vulvodynia. This term is used to describe superficial vulvar pain and dyspareunia for which no obvious cause is found. There is a pro-fusion of professional and self-help organizations addressing this issue. Many of them have sites on the Internet. An American web-site, run by the medical profession, entitled 'Vulvodynia and Vulvar Vestibulitis Syndrome' (Cracciolo, 1998), lists a variety of potential *physical* causes for un-diagnosed vulval pain, including a recent delivery of a baby; early use of oral contraceptives or an early age of first intercourse; fibromyalgia; high urinary oxalate levels; impaired killer lymphocyte activity; and increased levels of mast cells. It would seem likely that psychosomatic factors may well be involved in the first four of those.

With respect to high urinary levels of oxalates, researchers measured the urinary oxalate levels in 130 patients with vulvodynia and in 23 controls. There was no significant difference. However, 59 of the vulvodynia group were treated with a low oxalate diet and calcium citrate diet for three months. Only 10 per cent could have sexual intercourse, but the study concluded that some women may still benefit from a low oxalate diet. Other treatments reported include xylocaine gel, often used for intercourse in an effort to numb the pain, steroid creams and baking soda douches. Interferon has been used in women who have signs of HPV infection, but has been found to be of more use in women who don't have signs of HPV infection.

This research is reported here as an illustration of the pressure that the profession is under to come up with an answer for unexplained vulval pain.

PSYCHOSOMATIC FACTORS

There will be a significant group of women in whom no diagnosis is reached. For some patients this will be reassuring and the pain may well resolve; for example, if the woman feared she may have HIV or cancer. However, reassurance that all is normal will not necessarily solve the problem because the doctor is not finding out what that pain means to that patient.

A woman can feel that if no physical cause is found then the pain isn't 'real' or that the doctor thinks the pain isn't real. This may contribute to the pressure on the doctor to find a physical cause or to keep giving repeat prescriptions for 'thrush' etc. If the doctor acknowledges the reality of the pain and then works in ignorance with the patient to try and link the pain to feelings, then progress might be made.

In contrast to the physical causes, the psychosomatic 'causes' of dyspareunia do not easily lend themselves to tabulation. They may be thought of as unresolved feelings about grief, previous abuse or difficult delivery; an expression of anger or sadness in the woman's current relationship or about her current situation; fear of cancer, infection or loss; a calling card for another problem; a means of avoiding sex in a failing relationship etc. However, in psychosexual medicine every patient has a different story, as the following cases illustrate.

Influence of past relationships

Case 3

Miss C was a 25-year-old who had suffered from dyspareunia for three years, in each of her last three relationships. Prior to that there had been no problem. She had been extensively and repeatedly investigated. Tests had ranged from swabs to scans to laparoscopy. All had been normal. When she went to a new GP, again complaining of pain in a new relationship, the GP referred her for psychosexual counselling. She appeared to be much younger than her 25 years. When asked about her problem she began to talk about her father who had warned his three daughters about boyfriends – 'They were all after one thing only'. When they had a boyfriend, he asked about all the details including their shoe size. The doctor asked about this boyfriend – 'No' – she smiled in a sheepish way; she felt guilty about not having told her father at all about this new relationship. The doctor's suggestion that it was OK to have boundaries had not occurred to her. It felt 'naughty'. There were five children and she and her three sisters had endless discussions about how controlling their father was. There was a lot of anger and resentment. The doctor noted that there had been no mention of a fifth child. Miss C talked about her brother who had cut himself off completely from the family – it seemed that there was no middle way.

She described what happened when she and her partner had sex. She had soreness as he entered her and this pain continued afterwards. The doctor suggested an examination. At first, Miss C sat on the couch, arms folded over her legs, which were covered completely by a long skirt. When invited to lie down she did so, but was completely detached from what was going on. The doctor explained that Miss C could stop her at any time if there was pain and gently did a vaginal examination using one finger. As she described the spasm that she found and began to talk about the muscles, Miss C became quite involved; she was able to relax and squeeze the muscles at will. Miss C left that first consultation remarking that she felt quite hopeful, observing that the most helpful thing she had gained was that it could be OK not to tell her father about her boyfriend. The doctor observed that she could take control of her own body as well as her own life.

In the two sessions that followed, Miss C explored her resentment that her boyfriend found her sexy. In previous relationships, she had gone out with boys that she didn't feel overly attracted to just because they fancied her. There had been no emotional commitment on both sides and so the relationship was equal. Dad was right, the boys just wanted sex but that was OK because she just wanted sex as well! In a relationship where she began to realize that she actually cared for somebody, she feared that Dad was still right. This fear was expressed as pain. She hadn't been able to embrace the sexual and caring aspects of a relationship. She didn't feel able to talk this through with Sebastian because it wasn't his problem. Through the sessions, Miss C was able to realize that she could make her own decisions about her relationships and still remain on good terms with her father. She actually brought Sebastian to one of the sessions, but after a social interchange he remained in the waiting room. It was almost as though she had brought the boyfriend to meet the mother. Boundaries were being drawn in all areas of her life. At the fourth session, Miss C reported that the pain had disappeared and that she did not feel the need to come again. She was able to draw a boundary in her relationship with the doctor as well.

Comment

Miss C had been subjected to several years of investigation in the quest to find a cause for her pain. It was only when the doctor took a step back and listened to the patient in a different way that she was able to connect her father's attitude as she was growing up to her persistent pain.

The body or the relationship?

There is a particular intimacy between doctor and patient during an examination. Just as the patient can have an effect on the doctor, and this can be used therapeutically, it is important to be aware that the doctor may have an effect on the patient. Careless observations about a discharge or an episiotomy by a health professional can affect the way a patient feels about an episode. This may contribute to the patient's fantasies and lead to sexual problems subsequently. However, just as a woman with physical causes for her pain will have feelings about it, and the two factors will be intimately related, so there may be more than one cause of her emotional pain.

Case 4

Mrs L, a 30-year-old woman, was referred by her GP, with a 3-year history of dyspareunia that had been much worse since the birth of her child, 7 months previously. Recently she had been unable to have sex at all. The GP had discussed positions, lubricants, inserting fingers and not contemplating intercourse for some time, but all to no avail. When the doctor went out to the waiting room, Mrs L was over-shadowed in a physical sense by an enormous bear of a man – Mr L, an ex-rugby player who was cradling their son in the crook of his arm. They rose as one – a united front. Mrs L started to tell her story. They had been together for four years and married for three. She had worked as a nanny and had always wanted her own children. She had had an ectopic pregnancy about a year after the marriage – she shed tears as she described how this had not been in her life plan, she had expected to get pregnant and have a normal baby. 'Why me?' The question still sounded relevant. After that, she had had a miscarriage, and then Angus – she looked at him. He had been a much-wanted baby. But now she resented him. She couldn't go out. Sometimes she just wanted to shut him up in a room and leave. When the doctor observed that the reality of being a mother had not lived up to the dream, Mr L joined in very assertively. 'He's Number One! I've adjusted to fatherhood 100%' etc. etc. This felt quite angry and targeted at his wife. Most of the consultation revolved around Angus and he was indeed the focus of attention in the room. The doctor pointed out that they had spent most of the time talking about their son. 'Oh we do', said Mrs L, somewhat resignedly. 'Oh we do', said Mr L contentedly.

The doctor noted Mr L's comment about Angus being Number One. 'Yes', said Mr L, 'And that's why we're here. I had expected everything to be back to normal after six weeks and its not...' there was a short pause. 'I need sex and I ask for it, and she says no and I get angry.'

It seemed that Mrs L had feelings about this that she was finding difficult to express in front of her husband and baby. The doctor suggested an appointment with her alone.

Mr L was resistant at first. 'We do everything together'. The doctor again had the sense that they were joined at the hip. Mrs L said that she would like to come alone next time – beginning to lay claim to her individuality perhaps.

At the next appointment, Mrs L reported that they had managed to make love the night before. It had still hurt but she had wept for joy. She went on to talk about how she wasn't 'Number One' any more, and of how her husband expected that everything would be the same as before. 'Of course things have changed – I'm four stone heavier than I was – I don't feel the slightest bit sexy'. There was more than a hint of anger in her voice. The doctor commented that though her husband had certain expectations of a return to 'normality', Mrs L felt that her body was different. There was a silence. Mrs L started to describe one particular midwife who had looked horrified at her episiotomy and said 'Oh my God what a mess!' A look of disgust came on Mrs L's face as she described this. She had never dared look at her vulva since. She described it as raw, bloody, red and gaping. That was all she could think about when her husband made love to her – no wonder it hurt!

The doctor suggested that they might look at this part of her together. She was aware of a feeling of dread as to what she might see – this was how Mrs L felt. Hesitant at first, Mrs L climbed on to the couch and lay there looking at the ceiling. Tentatively, she opened her legs and the doctor described what she saw – a perfectly healthy, normal vulva. 'If I had not known, I would not be able to tell that you had had a baby.' Mrs L immediately became involved and interested. It was a real moment of truth. She had feared that this much-wanted baby had changed her forever. Mrs L phoned to cancel her next appointment, saying that things were completely better, the pain had disappeared.

Comment

Childbirth, hysterectomy, cone biopsy or a loss of fertility can alter the way a woman feels about her sexuality. In this case, careless words by a midwife had a lasting effect on how Mrs L felt about her body. However, she was also feeling rejected by her husband and resentful against the much-wanted baby. It was necessary to provide an opportunity for these feelings to be expressed, as well as exploring the body fantasy. The importance of verbalizing fantasies before confronting the reality has been described (Skrine, 1997). An examination with reassurance in this case, without first finding out how Mrs L felt about her vulva and about her husband, may not have been very helpful.

Pain as a cry for help

Pain can sometimes be a calling card to gain help with another problem. The patient may not even be aware of this. In such a case the pain has to be considered the presenting symptom of something that may be far removed from the genital area of the body (Tunnadine, 1970). Pain may draw the doctor's attention to a troubled part of the self, to a troubled relationship or, as in the following case, a troubled partner.

Case 5

Mrs V was a 54-year-old woman who was referred by the GP with a 4-year history of dyspareunia. This had been so severe that she had been unable to have intercourse for 18 months. She had been treated with seven oral types of HRT and various vaginal creams and pessaries, all without success. She had also been treated with anti-depressants. When she was seen, although she complained of being dry and tight, she was well-oestrogenized on vaginal pessaries. She had been told by a midwife that her vagina was too small when she had a caesarean section in 1977 and when she started getting pain she feared that that was the cause. The doctor noted without voicing it that the pain had started nearly 20 years after the remark – why now? As she was examined, Mrs V said that her husband had told her that she had healed up. Angry tears began to fall as she described how worried she was about her husband. He had been injured in an industrial accident about 5 years ago, and was now unable to work. However, what had really rocked him was the death of his father and mother 2 years previously. She felt that he was still not over that, but he would not admit that there was a problem. She felt too small to cope with this alone. Presenting with pain proved to be a way of exploring how to get help for her husband.

Pain expressing hidden feelings

Pain can be an unconscious way in which a number of different emotions may be felt if they cannot be expressed verbally. In the next case anger with the partner could not be expressed in the relationship where talking about feelings was too difficult.

Case 6

A slim, attractive, beautifully made-up 18-year-old woman presented with dyspareunia. She had recently moved in with her boyfriend, aged 28. As she talked, it became clear that all she wanted in the world was to marry this man and start a family. She loved him very much but was furious that he was so happy with the status quo. After discussion with the doctor she was able to tackle this with the boyfriend, who became her fiancé. She came back to show the doctor her engagement ring and to report that the pain had disappeared. This young woman felt unable to talk to her older boyfriend about her needs. She used the doctor–patient relationship to try out her ideas. When they had been accepted by the doctor, she was able to take them back to her boyfriend and move on.

Comment

In this case the patient was able to use her feelings to strengthen her relationship. However, in some instances, the woman may have an investment in keeping the symptom in a relationship that is failing. The pain may have a subconscious benefit in that it leads to abstinence from intercourse. The physical symptom is more tolerable than looking at the failure of the relationship, or having sex with someone whom she no longer loves (see Case 2).

CONCLUSION

These cases have illustrated various factors involved in a psychosexual approach to the treatment of painful intercourse. Every patient comes with a different story, and it is only by working in ignorance with the patient that links may be made between physical and emotional factors in the causation of pain. Through this shared journey, the patient may be able to move on.

KEY POINTS

- Dyspareunia is pain that occurs during or after intercourse. It may have physical or psychosomatic origins, but there is a great deal of overlap between the two.
- It is important to remain a physical doctor and to exclude straightforward treatable physical conditions. This does not prevent the doctor adopting a concurrent psychosexual approach.
- The doctor needs to acknowledge the reality of the pain and to suggest that feelings might be involved.
- The doctor–patient relationship and a psychosexual examination can help the doctor to discover what *that* pain means to *that* patient and to establish links between physical and emotional pain.
- Dyspareunia may be a physical expression of unresolved feelings about the past, or a way of avoiding uncomfortable feelings in the present. It may be a way of avoiding sex in an intolerable situation.
- Dyspareunia does not necessarily need long term or lengthy intervention. It is often amenable to treatment in the context of a GP consultation or an out-patient appointment.
- This approach may prevent years of fruitless investigations and ineffective treatments.

REFERENCES

Cracciolo, R.N. 1998: Vulvodynia and vulvar vestibulitis syndrome. http://www.primenet.com/-camlla/vulvodynia.htm

James, M., Draycott, T., Fox, R and Read, M. 1999: *Obstetrics and gynaecology – a problem solving approach*. W.B. Saunders.

Skrine, R. 1997: *Blocks and freedoms in sexual life*. Oxford: Radcliffe Medical Press.

Tunnadine, P. 1970: *Contraception and sexual life*. Institute of Psychosexual Medicine.

15 Disorders of sexual preference and gender identity

Lynne Webster

Disorders of sexual preference
Fetishism; paedophilia; voyeurism, exhibitionism and frotteurism; sexual violence; sex addiction

Disorders of gender identity
Transvestism; gender dysphoria; intersex states; homosexuality

---

The typical clinician in primary care or outside specific psychiatric sub-specialties is unlikely to see many patients complaining about paraphilias or gender problems, compared with the numbers consulting with sexual dysfunctions. However, it is important to have some knowledge of these conditions and what can be offered to such patients, as the general practitioner's surgery, the genito-urinary clinic or the family planning clinic may be the first point of contact for people who are seeking more specialist help.

The request for help may come from either the patient or, more often, from their distressed partner. Some understanding of the condition is therefore necessary for the doctor to be able to offer appropriate support. A dismissive attitude or ignorance of referral options at this point might delay the patient's access to appropriate services for many years, as they can gain the wrong impression that nothing can be done for them and that no one is prepared to listen to their concerns.

However unusual, sometimes bizarre and sometimes distasteful the patient's complaint may be, or however difficult the clinician may find it to understand the world-view of someone with a gender identity disorder, each individual patient needs an objective assessment. Sometimes the patient is worrying needlessly about a common and harmless sexual preference that they have been too embarrassed to discuss with anyone else. In these cases, simple discussion, education and reassurance in the primary care or clinic setting can relieve much unnecessary suffering.

Those clinicians who have acquired the non-judgmental listening skills necessary for the practice of psychosexual medicine may find themselves sought out by patients with these less common sexual disorders as well as those with the more common sexual dysfunctions. It is for these reasons that it is advisable to have some familiarity with the classification, prevalence, presenting features and treatment of disorders of sexual preference and gender identity.

CLASSIFICATION

The International Classification of Diseases (ICD-10; World Health Organization, 1993) defines disorders of sexual preference, or paraphilias, according to three general criteria:

- The individual experiences recurrent intense sexual urges and fantasies involving unusual objects or activities.
- The individual either acts on the urges or is markedly distressed by them.
- The preference has been present for at least six months.

The Diagnostic and Statistical Manual (DSM-IV) of the American Psychiatric Association (1994) describes gender identity disorder as:

- A strong and persistent cross-gender identification (not merely a desire for any perceived cultural advantages of being the other sex).

TABLE 15.1

ICD-10 Disorders of sexual preference
• F65.0 Fetishism
• F65.1 Fetishistic transvestism
• F65.2 Exhibitionism
• F65.3 Voyeurism
• F65.4 Paedophilia
• F65.5 Sadomasochism
• F65.6–8 Multiple/other/unspecified disorders

DSM-IV Paraphilias
• 302.4 Exhibitionism
• 302.81 Fetishism
• 302.89 Frotteurism
• 302.2 Paedophilia
• 302.83 Sexual masochism
• 302.84 Sexual sadism
• 302.3 Transvestic fetishism
• 302.82 Voyeurism
• 302.9 Paraphilia not otherwise specified

- Persistent discomfort with his or her sex, or a sense of inappropriateness in the gender role of that sex.
- The disturbance is not concurrent with a physical intersex condition.
- The disturbance causes clinically significant distress or impairment in social, occupational or other important areas of functioning.

The ICD-10 and DSM-IV classifications give very similar lists and definitions of these disorders and can be used almost interchangeably (Table 15.1).

DISORDERS OF SEXUAL PREFERENCE

Fetishism

Fetishism is sexual arousal associated with objects, and takes its name from the anthropological term describing the worship of a sacred object. It is defined as:

- A period of at least 6 months of recurrent, intense sexually arousing fantasies, sexual urges or behaviours involving the use of non-living objects.
- Causing clinically significant distress or impairment in social, occupational or other important areas of functioning.
- The fetish objects are not limited to articles of female clothing used in cross-dressing or devices designed for genital stimulation, e.g. vibrators.

Another related diagnosis is 'partialism', where there is intense sexual fixation on a part of the human body or a particular feature, such as the foot or long red hair.

It is evident from the definition that there must be a spectrum of severity and a wide variety of fetishes. At one extreme there are mild, culturally acceptable and clinically insignificant fetishes. An example of this would be a man's enhanced sexual arousal at seeing his partner in particular items of clothing, such as stockings and suspenders. At the mid-point are the common fetishes such as rubberwear and leatherwear, which are catered for commercially by clubs, societies and internet sites, but which might restrict the fetishist's choice and range of sexual activities and partners.

At the far extreme there are bizarre fetishes, arousal associated with generally repulsive objects such as faeces and the compulsion to touch or steal fetish objects which can get the fetishist into trouble socially and legally (Case 1).

Case 1

Richard was a 23-year-old man of below average intelligence. His siblings were all independent and successful, but he still lived at home with his parents and was employed as a driver in his father's floristry business. He was shy and socially awkward, and though he had a circle of male friends who shared his sporting interests, he had never had a girlfriend. From an early age he had shown an interest in women's shoes, and at puberty this became associated with sexual arousal. He would steal his mother's shoes, especially those with high heels, to enhance masturbation. He came into conflict with the law when he started to visit shoe shops, asking to see high-heeled shoes and pretending he was buying them for a friend. This implausible story and his obvious agitation when handling the shoes aroused the suspicions of the shoe shop staff, who called the police after his third visit. He was cautioned, his parents were mortified and consulted his GP asking for help.

It is not fully understood how fetishes develop. Some are clearly fixations from infancy, such as the desire to wear nappies. Others seem to develop around puberty, with the almost accidental association of an object or material with sexual arousal, then reinforced by fantasy and masturbatory conditioning. This may partly explain why there are many more male fetishists than female, as the penile erection and orgasmic reward for the male is a more direct reinforcement than is possible for the female. Sociobiologists draw analogies with the imprinting seen in animals, whereas psychoanalysts would draw attention to the symbolism of the fetish object.

Clearly, people who are worried about a culturally acceptable and essentially harmless fetish need mainly understanding, reassurance, education and to be given permission to enhance their sexual lives with their particular preference in a way that can be creatively integrated into their sexual relationships. More troublesome fetishes that are blighting relationships or precluding the enjoyment of any other sexual activity may need treatment from a specialist, preferably a clinical psychologist with a special interest in this field. Early attempts to extinguish fetishes included unpleasant aversion therapies, such as presenting the stimulus along with electric shocks or emetic drugs. This has now evolved into more humane approaches, including masturbatory reconditioning and response prevention.

Key Points

- Most fetishes are mild and harmless.
- Some are serious enough to disrupt relationships and normal sexual functioning.
- Clinical psychologists can offer a range of cognitive and behavioural treatments that are often successful in modifying the fetishistic behaviour.

Paedophilia

This is defined in DSM-4 as 'a period of a least 6 months of recurrent, intense sexually arousing fantasies, sexual urges or behaviours involving sexual behaviour with a prepubescent child or children (generally aged 13 or younger)'. The definition also specifies that this must cause clinically significant distress or impairment in social, occupational or other important areas of functioning. This specification is a bit puzzling, as it implies that if someone is untroubled by their sexual urges towards children, then they do not meet the criteria for the diagnosis. Most clinicians take the common sense view that anyone with such urges can be termed a paedophile. A further diagnostic specification is that 'the person is at least age 16 years and at least 5 years older than the child or children'. This is clearly meant to exclude the type of innocent, mutually exploratory sexual behaviour that is commonly seen between prepubescent children. However, it does not take account of recent research, which has shown that sexual abusers of young children can often begin their activities quite early in adolescence, and certainly younger than 16 years of age.

It is extremely difficult to estimate the incidence and prevalence of paedophilia, as the activity is so clandestine and attracts severe legal penalties. Community surveys designed to find the proportion of the population who have been sexually abused as children consistently show a figure of around 10 per cent, which is likely to be an underestimate because of a bias towards under-reporting. Clinical and legal sources show that paedophiles are very much more likely to be male, though it is recognized that there are a small number of female offenders who sexually abuse children. Attempts have been made to categorize paedophilic behaviours, e.g. incest/non-incest, or heterosexual/homosexual, but in practice this is not very helpful. Interestingly, the majority of paedophilic men, whether their preference is for girl or boy children, tend to form heterosexual relationships with adult women.

What leads someone into sexual attraction towards children? The aetiology of paedophilia is unclear, but several predisposing and trigger factors are consistently seen in research on these offenders. If someone has themselves been a victim of sexual abuse in childhood, this makes them more likely to develop paedophilia than someone who has not had such an experience. Looking at the early life of offenders, a pattern of dysfunctional family attachments is often apparent, with neglect, emotional and physical abuse alongside the sexual abuse as part of the picture. Trigger factors very commonly seen at the time of the offence are the use of alcohol leading to disinhibition, and stress in other areas of the offender's life.

Therapists who work with paedophiles are very familiar with the 'cognitive distortions' that they use to deny aspects of their behaviour and justify themselves. Common examples are the belief that their activity has not harmed the child, that it was mutually enjoyable, that the child invited sexual contact by seductive behaviour and that the child was capable of giving consent. They may insist that the offence was an isolated impulsive incident when there is a clear pattern of premeditated seeking of opportunities to be close to children socially and occupationally, with a patient campaign of 'grooming' the child to win its confidence and trust.

Because of these factors, and the legal issues, assessment of paedophiles is not easy. It is best done by specialist teams within the forensic psychiatry and probation services, who can supplement history-taking from the patient with psychometric testing and thorough social assessment. Some centres use phallometry, where a strain gauge applied to the penis records arousal to a variety of test stimuli.

Similarly, treatment is usually undertaken in the same specialist settings either in prison or as outpatients. This may include hormonal manipulation with drugs such as cyproterone acetate to reduce libido (though no drug can change sexual preference), along with psychological programmes of behaviour therapy and relapse prevention, often using group therapy. Individual exploratory psychotherapy has a very limited role and seems to be less effective in changing behaviour. Despite the therapeutic pessimism that surrounds paedophilia, with some lifelong recidivist offenders being regarded as untreatable, treatment programmes are now being developed which seem to reduce the rate of re-offending. Research is now focusing on treatment possibilities for adolescent child-abusers caught early in their offending careers.

Paedophilia is a subject that arouses powerful emotions in the general public, as evidenced by the furore when a well-known paedophile is released from prison into the community. Healthcare professionals, despite their training, are not immune to these feelings of anger and revulsion. It is hard to apply the principles of psychosexual medicine, such as empathy and a non-judgmental attitude in these cases, and indeed they may not be appropriate as this can so easily draw the doctor into collusion with the paedophile's denial and self-justification. This is a good reason why referral to a specialist team is advisable. In primary care and in the general psychosexual clinic, problems of confidentiality can sometimes arise with these patients. As a general principle, the duty of patient confidentiality can be over-ridden if the doctor suspects that a child is at risk, and a statutory duty to inform the relevant authorities takes over.

Key Points

- Sexual abuse of children is common.
- Abusers themselves commonly have deprived childhoods.
- Risk factors include stress and alcohol consumption.
- Assessment and treatment is best done by specialist teams.
- Risk to children over-rides patient confidentiality.

Voyeurism, exhibitionism and frotteurism – the 'courtship disorders'

Voyeurism is defined as 'recurrent, intense sexually arousing fantasies, sexual urges or behaviours involving the act of observing an unsuspecting person who is naked, in the process of disrobing, or engaging in sexual activity'. In colloquial terms, the voyeur is the 'peeping Tom' who may find himself in court and in the local newspapers if discovered. Exhibitionism is similarly defined, but involves the exposure of one's genitals to an unsuspecting stranger. Frotteurism involves touching and rubbing against a non-consenting person.

These behaviours have been termed 'courtship disorders' because in developmental terms they seem to represent distortions of the socially acceptable sequence of attracting a partner, which normally progresses from seeing someone attractive, to trying to gain their attention and eventually initiating physical contact.

Little research has been done on these groups of offenders, because their behaviour often does not come to the attention of the law or the medical services. When it does, their offence is often treated as causing a minor nuisance to the public. However, this does not take into account the sense of intrusion, violation, fear and trauma that can sometimes be experienced by their victims. Offenders are usually male and commonly start before the age of 15 years. The urges are often lifelong and may be associated with other paraphilias, such as fetishes. Poor social skills are a common finding in this group (see Case 2), as is a history of sexual victimization in childhood. As with paedophilia, these offenders tend to use cognitive distortions to minimize the impact of their behaviour (e.g. 'What harm could I possibly be doing? I was only looking').

Treatment may involve a range of approaches, including cognitive and behavioural techniques, masturbatory reconditioning, response prevention and anti-androgens. Any element of obsessive-compulsive disorder may also require appropriate psychiatric treatment.

Case 2

Martin was born with a hare lip and cleft palate. Although this had been corrected surgically, throughout his childhood he had been teased about his speech and appearance. He had underachieved academically and by the age of 20 he was still painfully shy. His social life entailed going out drinking with a small circle of male friends from work. Though heterosexual in orientation, he was too self-conscious even to strike up a conversation with women at work or socially. He was somewhat over-protected by a very close and loving family. He began to drink more and more heavily, then on his way home from the pub he would hang around outside the neighbours' living rooms exposing himself and masturbating. Luckily for him, the neighbours complained to his parents rather than the police, and he was able to tackle the exhibitionistic urges by limiting his intake of alcohol, which had provided a powerful disinhibitory effect.

Sexual violence

Violence in the context of sexual behaviour can take place because of sexual sadism (with or without associated sexual masochism), or as part of an act of rape or sexual assault. Sadism is defined as 'recurrent, intense sexually arousing fantasies, sexual urges, or behaviours involving acts (real, not simulated) in which the psychological or physical suffering of the victim is sexually exciting to the person'. Masochism is similarly defined but involves the act of being humiliated, beaten, bound or otherwise made to suffer. Sexual sadism is particularly dangerous when associated with antisocial personality disorder, and this combination of factors is involved in many of the high-profile sexually motivated murders, as seen in the Fred West and other cases. Anyone presenting with significant levels of sadistic fantasy merits referral for specialist forensic psychiatry assessment. This is because the sadist often progresses to attempts to act the fantasies out with a victim.

Masochism seems to be more common than sadism, and fantasies of being submissive and dominated always figure prominently in any survey of sexual fantasies in the general population. At one end of the spectrum this is clearly a harmless adjunct to sexual activity, and patients who are worried about these fantasies can be reassured. Those with more insistent masochistic urges may seek out the rather clandestine but legal clubs, societies, magazines and internet sites that cater for those with the minority sexual preference for being spanked, whipped, bound and humiliated. This is generally only a problem if the activity causes distress by precluding other forms of sexual and relationship intimacy. At the more severe end of the spectrum, masochists may engage in behaviours that entail physical injury. As the law is currently interpreted, this may lead to prosecution 'in the public interest', even if the behaviour is in private and between consenting adults.

The sexual aggression involved in rape and other sexual assaults is difficult to categorize, as offenders are a very heterogeneous group and rape is a fairly common occurrence, with community surveys estimating that up to 25 per cent of women may have experienced rape or attempted rape. The area is further complicated by the current debate on 'date rape' and sexual harassment. Explanations of the rapist's behaviour may draw on psychodynamic, sociocultural, sociobiological and feminist theories, but it is clearly a difficult area to research when it is not even possible to reach agreed definitions of what constitutes non-consensual sexual activity.

'Sex addiction'

This term does not appear in any diagnostic classifications, but has gained currency amongst lay people and the psychological professions. It is generally used to describe any form of sexual behaviour which the patient feels to be compulsive in nature. This may take the form of an urge to visit prostitutes, to have extramarital sexual contacts, to masturbate frequently, to use pornographic materials and much other possible behaviour. The patient typically describes an increasing urge to indulge in the desired behaviour, which is resisted to some extent because of guilt feelings and the belief that the behaviour is damaging. The temptation grows until the behaviour occurs, followed by a relief from psychological tension, a surge of guilt, self-reproach and promises to change. The cycle of events is then repeated (see Case 3).

This cycle of behaviour, which has similarities to alcohol addiction or food binges, usually has fairly clear emotional and psychological gratifications for the patient. It may contain elements of excitement, danger and rebellion. It may help the patient to avoid intimacy and facing up to underlying depressive illness. It may be a true obsessive-compulsive disorder in some cases.

Assessment of each individual and their circumstances is clearly necessary, to provide an appropriate treatment programme. Much success is claimed for group approaches in the voluntary sector, with methods borrowed from the tried and tested Alcoholics Anonymous programme. These include Sex Addicts Anonymous, Sexaholics Anonymous and Sexual Compulsives Anonymous. Members are encouraged to face up to their powerlessness against their 'addiction' and place their trust in a higher power and the support of the group, to change their behaviour one day at a time.

Case 3

Rupert seemed outwardly confident and successful. At the age of 32 he was married with two small children. His job as an advisor on international corporate law was very well paid and entailed much foreign travel. He appeared attractive, physically fit and well groomed. Despite all this, he requested referral because of an intense feeling of self-loathing. Whenever he travelled away from home, he would stay in 5-star hotels and tune in to the pornographic videos available on the TV in his room for masturbation. Soon, this was not enough, and he would go out in foreign cities to tour the red light districts frequenting lap-dancing clubs. This had escalated to seeking out prostitutes and paying them for sex. He felt disgusted by his secretive behaviour and between trips he would promise himself that next time would be different, but he felt powerless to resist the attractions of the sex industry each time, and defined himself as a 'sex addict'. In individual therapy it emerged that he had had an emotionally deprived childhood, as both his parents had been blatantly engaged in extramarital affairs and took little interest in him beyond praise for his educational achievements. Inside, he felt profoundly unlovable and his sexual behaviour seemed to confirm this. In a paradoxically comforting way, it made him as bad as he felt himself to be. When he was able to address these painful issues, he found he was no longer troubled by the sexual compulsions.

DISORDERS OF GENDER IDENTITY

Transvestism

The International Classification of Diseases recognizes two types of transvestism: fetishistic transvestism and dual-role transvestism.

A diagnosis of fetishistic transvestism involves wearing 'articles of clothing of the opposite sex in order to create the appearance and feeling of being a member of the opposite sex', and this must be 'closely associated with sexual arousal. Once orgasm occurs and sexual arousal declines, there is a strong desire to remove the clothing.'

It can be seen from the diagnostic definition that this type of transvestism is much closer to being a disorder of sexual preference, with the fetish object being the wearing of cross-gender clothing, rather than being any sort of gender identity disorder. The assessment and treatment would therefore be similar to that of the fetishes already described, often with strong reassurance that this is a generally harmless sexual preference with no sinister implications about the gender identity of the patient.

In dual-role transvestism, the following defining elements occur:

- The individual wears clothes of the opposite sex in order to experience temporary membership of the opposite sex.
- There is no sexual motivation for the cross-dressing.
- The individual has no desire for a permanent change to the opposite sex.

From the definition of this disorder, it can be distinguished from transvestic fetishism quite easily by the absence of a sexual arousal motive for the cross-dressing. However, in clinical practice, the difference may not be so clear-cut. Some adolescent boys develop a transvestic fetish, masturbating while wearing female clothing, but seem to lose interest in this activity in their twenties or thirties, moving on to a typical pattern of dual-role transvestism. Similarly, although the definition states that the transvestite is not seeking gender reassignment, some individuals show a drift towards transsexuality as time progresses.

For the dual-role transvestite there is now a fairly extensive support network of voluntary groups and social organizations. These began with the Beaumont Society, which organizes group meetings and social events where men can attend cross-dressed in female role, in a safe and accepting environment. As most transvestite men are heterosexual, the Beaumont Society has also set up support groups for their wives and female partners, to promote tolerance and understanding of the condition. There is now a small industry servicing the needs of the cross-dressing community, with chains of shops and mail order catalogues providing wigs, clothing, corsetry, make-up and advice on everything needed for a man to produce a feminine appearance.

Clinically, this type of transvestism is perhaps best viewed as an absorbing hobby rather than a pathology. This case is argued strongly by the general practitioner and medical writer Vernon Coleman, himself a dual-role transvestite, who eloquently describes the pleasure and relaxation he obtains from dressing as a female, which gives temporary relief from the onerous role-expectations placed on the male in society. Attempts at eradicating the cross-dressing by any sort of treatment programme are usually futile. A more helpful approach is to de-pathologize the situation and encourage the patient to integrate the cross-dressing safely, comfortably and creatively into his life. Of course, this depends very much on his home circumstances and the views of any partner or family. Some female partners are almost incredibly understanding and supportive, helping their spouse choose suitable clothing and accompanying him to social events as 'sisters'. Others react with alarm and disgust, but can be persuaded to take a more tolerant view if the man promises to confine his cross-dressing to discreet venues, such as support groups. The most difficult negotiations occur when a female partner finds that her spouse has been cross-dressing in secret, sometimes for years, possibly concealing a hoard of female clothing in the house or even using hers. In these cases there can be an understandable breakdown of trust, which is very difficult to repair.

Cross-dressers may get into trouble with the law in some circumstances. If a man is detected wearing female clothing in public, and this causes any kind of scene, he may be charged with behaviour likely to cause a breach of the peace. Some clandestine transvestites resort to stealing items of female clothing rather than obtaining them openly by legitimate means, which can also end in arrest and conviction.

Key Points

- Cross-dressing may be fetishistic in nature, or may be unrelated to sexual arousal.
- Most transvestites are heterosexual males.

- Transvestites do not generally wish to have gender reassignment.
- An extensive commercial and social support network is available for cross-dressers.

Gender dysphoria

This term implies unhappiness with one's birth gender, and can cover a wide spectrum of human experience. In mild forms, there are the girls who are described as 'tomboys' and the boys with effeminate traits, who do not fit in very well with their gender peer groups, but nevertheless grow up without actually pursuing gender change, even if they retain some of their cross-gender interests and behaviour life-long. Societies differ in their degrees of tolerance of cross-gender behaviour, with some being quite rigidly prescriptive about gender roles and others showing a much more flexible attitude. Clearly, someone who feels that they are not entirely in tune with the gender role that society expects of them will suffer more or less depending on the culture that they live in.

At the other extreme, there are people who are so unhappy with their gender that they actively pursue reassignment. This is termed transsexualism and is defined as 'a desire to live and be accepted as a member of the opposite sex, usually accompanied by a sense of discomfort with, or inappropriateness of, one's anatomic sex, and a wish to have surgery and hormonal treatment to make one's body as congruent as possible with one's preferred sex'. Additional criteria specify that the wish must have been present persistently for at least two years, and that it is not a symptom of another mental disorder (such as a delusion occurring in schizophrenia).

Transsexualism is relatively rare, with an estimated prevalence in England of one in 34,000 men and one in 108,000 women, with male-to-female transsexuals outnumbering females-to-males by about three to one. There is no clear consensus about the causes of this disorder, as no biological abnormalities have ever been found consistently in this group, so various psychological theories, ranging from the psychodynamic to the sociocultural, have been mooted.

Some transsexuals present relatively early, with a history of severe gender dysphoria since infancy. They are often homosexual in orientation, and have rarely been married. Others have a later presentation, sometimes waiting until middle age before they ask for help. These patients usually have a history of many years of trying to conform to their anatomical gender role, including marrying and having children, and working in highly gender-specific jobs (e.g. the male-to-female transsexual who tried to conform by joining the Army and driving tanks). They may have tried dual-role cross-dressing and found this was not enough and often have a history of depressive episodes or alcohol abuse related to their unhappiness with their gender role.

As the treatment for transsexualism may ultimately result in irreversible surgery, careful assessment is clearly vital to exclude people with other mental illnesses such as psychoses or personality disorders, and those with unrealistic expectations of what gender reassignment can offer. Patients must be encouraged to think very carefully and deeply about the full implications of their planned course of action, and all possibilities of workable compromises and therapies that do not entail irreversible procedures must be explored. Most clinicians in primary care, unless they work in certain inner-city practices with a large transvestite and transsexual population, will rarely see more than a couple of transsexual patients in a working lifetime. Even the average consultant general psychiatrist is likely to have relatively sparse experience of this patient group. Assessment is therefore best done by specialist teams in recognized centres that have the necessary expertise, and can offer the multidisciplinary input needed for a full gender reassignment programme.

Such clinics are not common, and many patients will need referrals outside their area and may need to undertake a lot of travelling to and from appointments. If assessed as suitable, patients can expect to be prescribed hormones to achieve feminization or masculinization. This is not without risk, as relatively high doses of oestrogens or testosterone are required to initiate breast growth in men or cause the voice to break in women. Patients who smoke are at considerably higher risk of thrombosis when taking oestrogens in high doses, and all patients on hormone regimens will need regular monitoring of blood pressure, cholesterol levels and liver function tests. Once under way, some of these hormonally induced changes are irreversible. After surgery to remove the gonads, a long-term hormone maintenance regime is necessary to prevent osteoporosis and maintain the changes in the sexual characteristics.

Before referral for surgery, most clinics require patients to have successfully completed the 'Real Life Test', where they must live and work and be accepted in their chosen gender for at least two years. This entails an enormous social transition. Patients need great determination, strength of purpose and social support to achieve this, and some are helped by the various voluntary support groups now available, such as the Gender Trust and the F-to-M Network. Quite a number of them give up at this stage, finding the process too stressful and fraught with practical difficulties.

Those who are referred for surgery are therefore a very select group, and follow-up studies have shown that for these very determined patients the outcome of full gender reassignment is often good, with patients achieving contentment in their new gender role. For men, surgery entails removal of the external genitalia and the creation of a functional vaginal space. In experienced hands, the cosmetic and functional outcome of these procedures can be excellent. Some men also seek additional cosmetic procedures such as electrolysis to remove facial hair, surgical shaving of the cricoid cartilage to reduce the 'Adam's apple' appearance and remodelling of a masculine-shaped nose or chin.

Women usually seek bilateral mastectomy, hysterectomy and oophorectomy. Phalloplasty, the creation of a cosmetically and functionally acceptable penis, is more problematic. Some urological surgeons have expertise in this and offer a several-stage procedure that can be relatively successful. Recent advances in plastic surgery techniques developed in Holland using skin flaps from the thigh look more promising, but are not widely available.

As regards the legal status of transsexuals, they can fairly easily obtain documentation such as passports in their new gender, and change their name by a simple statutory declaration. However, in Britain, they are still unable to change their birth certificate, which means, amongst other disadvantages, that they cannot marry in their new gender. This has been unsuccessfully challenged several times in the European Court of Human Rights. Further challenges to this ruling are inevitable and it is likely that this will eventually lead to a change in the law. There have been legal cases brought concerning the right to treatment of transsexuals denied this by health authorities, and their claims have generally been upheld. There have also been a number of successful cases brought by transsexuals under anti-discrimination law in the workplace and in social settings.

Key Points

- Transsexuals require very thorough specialist assessment.
- Very few centres offer the full gender reassignment programme.
- Hormonal treatment has risks and leads to irreversible bodily changes.
- Patients must generally live in their chosen gender role successfully for two years before surgery.
- If patients are selected appropriately, the outcome of gender reassignment can be very good.

Intersex states

These are relatively rare conditions in which a child is born with indeterminate secondary sexual characteristics, or anatomical features of both sexes. Some are caused by chromosomal abnormalities such as Klinefelter's syndrome

(XXY), which affects about one in 700 newborn males. Most of these males are of normal masculine appearance, but some present at puberty with underdeveloped genitalia and a feminine distribution of fat on the breasts and hips. In Turner's syndrome (XO), which occurs in less than one in 5000 girls, there is a marked deficiency of oestrogens, with an absence of breast development and amenorrhoea.

Various inborn errors of metabolism can also cause intersex states. Testicular feminization syndrome (also called androgen insensitivity syndrome) occurs in karyotypic males. Insensitivity of target cells to testosterone in the developing foetus results in a child with an external appearance of female genitalia, but no upper vagina, uterus or fallopian tubes. Testes are found in the abdominal cavity, groin or labia. In congenital adrenal hyperplasia (the androgenital syndrome), a defect in cortisol synthesis leads to precocious puberty in males, but in females it causes masculinization of the external genitalia. This varies in degree, but the labial fusion and clitoral hypertrophy can be so marked that the child is sometimes assigned to the male gender at birth.

All these syndromes present very challenging problems for patients and their families. It is sometimes far from clear what is the most sensible decision about the gender to rear the child in, and mistakes about this can lead to much suffering and confusion about gender identity, particularly at puberty. Patients often need hormonal manipulation to induce and maintain the development of secondary sexual characteristics, and may need a series of painful plastic surgical procedures to achieve genitalia of an acceptable appearance and function. In addition to this, they usually need to come to terms with infertility. It is not surprising that they sometimes feel confused about their gender identity and can have difficulty forming successful sexual functioning in adult relationships. Careful planning and counselling of the patient and their family by a specialist paediatric team is essential in these cases, with a smooth transition to appropriate adult services after puberty.

Homosexuality

This is no longer seen either as a disorder of sexual preference or a gender identity problem. As far back as 1974, the American Psychiatric Association removed homosexuality from its list of diagnoses, but in other guises the category was retained until the most recent versions of psychiatric classification. Terms such as 'sexual orientation disorder' or 'egodystonic sexual orientation' have survived, to describe the patients who present with homosexual orientation but are very unhappy and distressed because of possible adverse social and other consequences that they perceive to be an inevitable part of this.

In the past, psychoanalytic, psychotherapeutic and behavioural methods have been tried to little avail in the attempt to change homosexual orientation. These have fallen into disrepute, particularly those behavioural techniques that used aversion by such things as electric shocks or emetic drugs in association with homosexual imagery.

Despite this, patients and their relatives still present with requests for treatment to cure homosexuality as though it were a disease, and are disappointed that such treatment is not available. Controversially, some isolated psychotherapists and some religious groups claim to be able to change homosexual orientation, but their results do not bear scientific scrutiny.

There is still much debate and dispute about the factors which contribute to the development of homosexual orientation. Twin studies have indicated a possible genetic component, so the search is on for a gene that determines sexual orientation, and neuroanatomists are busy dissecting homosexuals' brains to look for anatomical markers. Other theories place more emphasis on the social and cultural influences on the individual, but the current research effort is definitely biased towards a more biological view. This has mixed implications for the tolerance of homosexual orientation in society, as some may take evidence that sexual orientation is at least partly biologically determined as indicating that homosexuality is 'natural'. Others may see the opportunity for the future development of such techniques as antenatal testing for homosexuality, with the option to abort a homosexual foetus.

REFERENCES

American Psychiatric Association 1994: *Diagnostic and statistical manual of mental disorders*, 4th edn. Washington, DC: American Psychiatric Association.

World Health Organisation 1993: *The ICD-10 classification of mental and behavioural disorders: diagnostic criteria for research*. Geneva: World Health Organisation.

FURTHER READING

Ames, M.A. and Houston, D.A. 1990: Legal, social and biological definitions of pedophilia. *Archives of Sexual Behaviour* 19, 333–42.

Bancroft, J. 1989: *Human sexuality and its problems*. Edinburgh: Churchill Livingstone.

Coleman, V. 1996: *Men in dresses*. Barnstaple: European Medical Journal.

Di Ceglie, D. 1998: *A stranger in my own body. Atypical gender identity development and mental health*. London: Karnac.

Freund, K., Scher, H. and Hucker, S. 1983: The courtship disorders. *Archives of Sexual Behaviour* 12, 369–79.

Grubin, D. 1994: Sexual murder. *British Journal of Psychiatry* 165, 624–9.

Laws, D.R. and O'Donohue, W. (eds) 1997: *Sexual deviance. Theory, assessment and treatment*. New York: Guilford.

Levin, S.M. and Stava, L. 1987: Personality characteristics of sex offenders: a review. *Archives of Sexual Behaviour* 16, 57–79.

Tully, B. 1992: *Accounting for transsexualism and trans-homosexuality*. London: Whiting & Birch.

Part Three

Psychosexual Medicine in Clinical Practice

16 General practice

Roseanna Pollen

Psychosexual skills

Psychosexual work in practice

Politics and ethics

Other cultures

Practicalities of psychosexual work in general practice

General practitioners, in theory, should be adept at dealing with every possible kind of illness and patient. Jacks of all trades, it does not follow that we are masters of none, for the specialist skill of the GP is to use accurate diagnostic judgement throughout the entire range of illnesses as well as the ability to advise on effective management when our patients are under the care of hospital specialists. Consultants never entirely take over our cases and we retain the responsibility for appraising the appropriateness and proper conduct of any secondary care.

Herein lies the uniquely satisfying nature of our medical practice: we can participate as intelligent physicians and 'remote' surgeons in whole cases from all the sub-disciplines of medicine. Unlimited in its scope, general practice also allows for a degree of intimacy, a smallness of scale that could be seen as trivial and irrelevant in more specialized settings. We are often domestic in style as reflected in our buildings, furnishings and lack of white coats, in contrast to hospital clinics. Patients confide in us about all sorts of matters, medical or otherwise, and we can feel privileged or exasperated in turn by the limitless variety of problems that we take on. Psychosexual problems, like parenting problems, marriage and relationship problems suit the domestic scale of general practice. Our

unease in these areas arises from a primary sense of inadequate training or knowledge, apart from our own often unreliable personal experiences and a secondary awareness that we may be overstepping the boundaries of professional medical practice when we advise patients about such matters. Psychosexual therapy as a specialist skill need not be part of the armamentarium of every GP, but the ability to recognize psychosexual difficulty among our patients, and to differentiate the psychological, psychiatric and physical disease components of these presentations, is part of everyday practice (Hawton and Harrison, 1998).

Other authors in this book illustrate the work of specialists and the theoretical background to the scientific discipline of psychosexual medicine. The technique of psychosexual medicine as taught by the Institute of Psychosexual Medicine, although suitable for its extended role in the specialist referral clinic is, in fact, most at home in primary care. This chapter is about general practice and how an enhanced awareness of the doctor–patient relationship, particularly with regard to psychosomatic events in consultations, can enable the non-specialist to become more effective in the management of psychosexual difficulty. I will also discuss how specialist training can be incorporated into primary care.

PSYCHOSEXUAL SKILLS

To summarize what is discussed at greater length elsewhere in this book, the focus of psychosexual medicine is on how doctors may interpret what patients say or do in the context of a particular doctor–patient relationship and how this may throw light on their sexual difficulty. What sort of material is appropriate for such interpretations? The benchmark or standard for 'normal' patient behaviour during history-taking or examination is not closely defined. In general terms, however, we have expectations for any particular encounter with a patient and should be on the alert if we feel our expectations are not fulfilled, if we have a vague or sharp feeling that something is amiss. The vaginal examination, for example, may be almost a technical exercise when a patient undergoes 'routine' screening as part of her contraceptive care, and her behaviour during the examination may then be inattentive, whereas the woman with post-menopausal bleeding, who herself suspects cancer, may be apprehensive, awkward and otherwise difficult to examine, yet neither would be judged inappropriate.

The doctor may be alert to behaviour that suggests psychosexual difficulty, but it may not always be appropriate to make a comment about its sexual significance during a genital examination. Patients may learn to avoid an overly intrusive doctor and where your job demands that you are ready to diagnose and manage every kind of illness in primary care then a persistent bias towards the hidden psychological theme can be uncomfortable. It is through training and reflexive self-monitoring that the doctor learns more about her own style of working and the sort of doctor–patient relationships that she engenders.

The level of training and the amount of time and effort put in to acquiring such skills will vary according to the interest of any particular GP, but few can ignore it altogether. The rewards for acquiring these skills are great, for successful management of a sensitive problem in-house is extremely satisfying and, unlike the specialist, we may see our successes build upon themselves. Patients may return for other more humdrum problems and the rapport and trust between doctor and patient has obviously been strengthened. We live with our failures too, as in all areas of our work, and may face the discomfort of unknown outcomes when patients leave the list before their difficulties are resolved.

PSYCHOSEXUAL WORK IN PRACTICE

The specialist can see only those whom referring doctors choose to send, but the GP will find patients presenting psychosexual problems who would never ask for referral onwards and this in itself is a point of interest. The case-mix overlaps with that of family planning doctors, but the latter are less likely to see the elderly, for example, whereas in my experience this age group makes up a significant proportion of patients that I see with psychosexual problems. Patients do not need to fight for our attention, they do not have to go through the hurdle of asking for a referral and then waiting for the appointment; they do not have the anticipation and preparedness of the booked appointment. All this brings with it a certain amount of baggage that the specialist must deal with so that in contrast there is a freshness and immediacy about general practice that can be rewarding.

Specialist cases

It can in fact be most straightforward when a patient does request referral at the outset. If the doctor feels that she lacks the skills needed to deal with a problem, then acquiescence in the process of referral resolves the difficulty. If patients are seen in a clinic within the practice, then the boundaries are set; the doctor is undoubtedly an authority in contrast to usual shifts in power apparent in ordinary surgery consultations. These patients are relatively few among the population of those with psychosexual distress. Moreover, counselling and therapy has taken a knock in its status as a 'generally good thing' even among the middle classes that have traditionally been its keenest advocates. Men are now just as likely to ask directly for a prescription for Viagra as a referral for counselling.

General practice hardly ever allows you to switch entirely into specialist mode, even when you set up clinic sessions. Stray bits of routine practice, repeat scripts, advice about travel jabs or a relative's medical problems creep in to special sessions that would be more likely suppressed in a hospital out-patient consultation. The very paradigm of general practice is that of an integrated use of skills and attempts to split patients up into labelled cases managed by protocol rarely succeed in the way that the doctor intended.

Presentations

Problems with sex may be clearly announced as 'impotence', 'my sex drive has disappeared', 'I come too quickly', or they may be covert, presenting as difficulty with contraception, penile rashes, a vaginal discharge that is not apparently organic, fears of impending childbirth, fears of genital cancer and so on. What is unique about general practice is that the same patients may also appear in your surgery as the parents of sick children, patients needing prescriptions or certificates for minor illness, potential high risk screening targets for public health programmes and so on. In other words, any one patient is not contained within the limits of a psychosexual 'case'. Using psychosexual skills may then be discontinuous with any one patient precisely because the GP offers continuity of care, cradle to grave. 'Can I see you without talking about sex?' one patient asked timidly after we had spent several sessions exploring the reasons for her loss of libido and she was now worried about the more immediate problem of a cough. Moreover, the sexual partners of our 'cases' are usually known to the doctor and may come alone for their own illnesses and problems, during which consultations they may or may not make reference to their partners and their sex life.

We already advertise what sort of doctor we are and what kind of presentation is acceptable ahead of actual consultations (Norton and Smith, 1994). The timetable of short surgery appointments and the experience of sitting in a waiting room, overhearing those who negotiate with the reception staff for appointments, delivers a clear message that the GP is a busy doctor. If this does not make the patient think that a referral to someone who has more time is what is needed, it may push them to frame their problems within a very brief agenda. It then requires an effort of will on the part of the doctor to indicate that more could be said, and that time can be made available. The shortage of time can, however, be used to advantage by a patient who would feel uncomfortable in a longer setting, to engineer a very short and direct response from the doctor. 'My sex life isn't what it used to be but at my age its to be expected isn't it? I just want you to say if anything can be done, and if you say nothing will work then that's all right, I can tell the wife that.' Pursuing such patients with promises of more time may be counter-productive, but suggestive, open-door hints may plant the idea that more time could be made available, and that their assumptions are not necessarily correct.

We should not always castigate ourselves for economizing on time with patients if that is all they can manage at one visit. 'Can you see anything wrong doctor?' 'No everything seems fine and normal and healthy' sounds brief and unenlightening, but it is precise and appropriate, and significantly lacks the closing phrase, 'So you haven't got anything to worry about'. The patient is then free to think and to respond if they choose to do so, and the doctor can take note and comment on any continuing anxiety. Significant disease has been ruled out at this point, but the symptom has not been dismissed. Similarly, the GP can be an important witness to the trouble that a patient is suffering without necessarily intervening directly as an active therapist who always tries to put things right.

Urogenital disease and psychosexual distress

The typical work of psychosexual medicine is found in medical gynaecology or andrology. The patient presents with urogenital disease and at some point their psychosexual difficulty is revealed.

Case 1

Simone, a young graphic designer from Belgium, started off as the quick case that we can all feel comfortable with. She had typical cystitis, symptoms of frequency and dysuria. When she asked if she should see a gynaecologist as this was what she would expect at home, I felt rather pleased to be able to offer her 'expert' treatment in primary care. After the antibiotics, it was not a surprise that she had vaginal discomfort, doubtless thrush, not even needing a swab. Thereafter, nothing seemed to go right. By now the cystitis/vaginitis symptomatology was blurred and equivocal swabs and MSUs did not help. A late period raised a pregnancy scare that was happily unfounded. During her necessarily frequent appointments, where I felt that we had hardly got to grips with one problem before a new one arose, she looked increasingly harassed. She was uncomfortable during the vaginal examination for yet more swabs for bacterial vaginosis and there was some vaginismus. 'Does it hurt like this during intercourse as well?' I asked and she said resignedly, 'Yes, it's all been so difficult', without expanding on the subject. I thought that her answer was understandable given the painful pathology that she had suffered. Her composure remained cool and made me hold back from probing further. Our relationship was cast in a very clinical mode. Her chic 'continental' appearance and glossy styling visibly dulled as she became worn down by this catalogue of problems. Gradually, the series of minor infections came under control, but during one last episode of mild but proven thrush I took a swab test and found that she was no longer tense, although still visibly unhappy during the vaginal examination. I commented on how much she had had to put up with and, feeling relieved that she was more or less better, I could ask about feelings without her losing confidence in me as a medical expert. She responded in a low, slightly depressed voice, 'I just want all this to be right, I have so much responsibility really, you see I am working, I have a career but he is still an art student and can't earn much money. Its all down to me all the time'. I acknowledged her burden of responsibility and how the vaginitis had been really the last straw for someone who always had to be strong and healthy in this relationship.

Simone was not a psychosexual case hidden behind a spurious physical symptom, nor was she hysterical or neurotic. What this case illustrates is that individual patients with common diseases can be difficult or disturbing. Problems in their relationship or psychosexual make-up may not be made explicit until exacerbated by disease, and may be manifest through the genital examination.

Knowing too much

The GP can sometimes know too much and as much as primary care is the setting *par excellence* for fresh material, it can be confusing in its plethora of information. This may be given by patients' relatives or other members of the practice team who have heard different versions, and made different assessments of any one patient's current problems. I felt mystified when the girlfriend of a man that I had seen several times for impotence came to see me for termination counselling, mentioning him as her partner. She was as matter of fact and straightforward about it as anyone can be in these circumstances, with no mention of sexual difficulty or surprise or infidelity.

The wife who said off-handedly while taking her prescription for HRT that the sex side of things 'Doesn't bother us now' was puzzling, as her husband had been telling me how frequently they made love, 'But could I have Viagra to really do things properly?' There would have been nothing in his story that would make me doubt his version had I not had 'casual' access to his wife's side of the story. Did she know of our discussions and wished to warn me off? Whose story should I believe if both think that they are seeing me confidentially? More importantly, is one partner affecting my attitude towards the other against my better judgement? If I am sympathetic to a woman's account of her failing sex life, does this bias my attitude towards her husband when I see him for an unrelated matter? I would certainly look for an opening in the conversation if she had told me that he had a drink problem or was suicidal, but sexual problems are not clearly a doctor's territory. There are no easy answers to these quandaries.

POLITICS AND ETHICS

The holistic role of the British GP who may manage, in theory at least, any one patient's physical, emotional and social needs, is taxing at times. This all-inclusive remit can even allow ethics and politics to intrude uncomfortably into consultations. Women subjected to domestic violence who seek help with psychosexual distress are a case in point. Should the doctor interpret the material as presented, or should she make a stand and not only make explicit the exploitation in the relationship, but refuse to embark on any sort of therapy unless the violence is also addressed? More delicate still is the question of offering or refusing treatment to the man who is known to be the perpetrator of such violence where medical confidentiality precludes the doctor from saying, 'Your partner has told me that you have been abusing her'.

If children are involved, the priorities are usually obvious or rather the doctor will feel on safer ground protecting a child's welfare, compared with the ethical dilemma of deciding what sort of feminist viewpoint could be defended as part of good medical care of her patients. The usual answer is to say that a therapist should only deal with material that the patient presents in consultation, and this is generally good technical advice for therapeutic success. The continuity of family care of general practice does not always allow us to be so purist.

Case 2

Jayne is 28 and is married with two children. She is a slight woman and often late for appointments, apologetic and almost amusingly vague. She brought her youngest child late to evening surgery with a cough. After I had dealt with this, she said 'It's for me too, I don't know what is wrong with me. I don't feel like having sex any more with my husband, not since Kelsey was born. I wonder if something is wrong with me, is there some medicine to make me feel alright again? I never feel like having sex and if we do it hurts'. The nurse had taken her post-natal smear. I asked her if anything untoward had been found then and she thought back carefully, taking her time. 'Mmm, no-o', she said thoughtfully. 'There was nothing wrong'. Her face brightened and she sat up a little. 'It must be how I feel'. She went on to say that her husband had been shouting at her because he was out of work, and she thought he took it out on her because he was so fed up. She was quite certain that he would never come to any sort of counselling. 'He wouldn't ever think it had anything to do with him!' In our subsequent discussion, I elicited her fear that the marriage could end, and her irritation and anger with him. She agreed that she did love him with all his faults, but she felt he was unreasonably stubborn. 'If he won't do anything about this, do you think that I should give you medicine so that you can try and solve all these problems on your own, without him being involved?' I asked. She looked yearningly at her baby crawling happily on the floor. 'I couldn't leave him ever, for the kids' sake', she said with feeling. 'Of course', I said and maintained a supportive stance with very mixed feelings.

Whatever the doctor feels about family values and feminism, her first duty is to address the problem that the patient has brought, rather than to engage on a consciousness-raising programme. But if we badger our patients about changing their smoking habits because such behaviour is harmful, it may also be defensible to pay attention to the harmful effects of women's subordination in the causation of depression.

OTHER CULTURES

People do not belong wholly to cultures as if they were closed systems of fixed beliefs, particularly when they are living in Britain, often in multicultural areas that offer a diverse and changing experience of family life and socio-cultural traditions. There is a liberal bias commonly found among sympathetic doctors in post-colonial Britain that almost over-compensates at times for past wrongs. Doctors can accord an excess of value to minority ethnic traditions and cultural values as static institutions that should never be called into question. Such views can sometimes lead to the neglect of the personal issues that beset our patients, and are usually more immediate and pressing than the group ethics of their own particular culture (Gatrad and Sheikh, 2000; Gilroy, 2000).

My own practice is in an area with a large population of patients of Bangladeshi origin. Although it is possible after working for many years in the same area to generalize, the diversity of that experience means that I cease to be surprised by those that deviate from the strict rules of Muslim-Bengali culture. A married Bengali woman with two children who asks for a coil in order to delay her next pregnancy may be the next patient after the woman from an apparently similar background who cannot contemplate using condoms, let alone anything more certain, and already has seven or eight young children, 'Because of my religion'. It should not be forgotten that it may be easier for a patient to cut short a lengthy and difficult 'counselling' session with a doctor about, say, abortion, by pulling out the culture card and stating that such practices are simply not allowed for such as themselves. It does help to know that world Islamic institutions are not as strict as some of our patients may imply with regard to the ethics of fertility control, but it is not necessary to have a compendium of world cultures and religions in your head to be able to detect something about the doctor–patient relationship that does not ring true, or hints at ambivalence when discussing such choices.

The availability of translation and advocacy services does not do away entirely with the sense of difference that can be awkward or painful in consultations with patients from different cultures. Many doctors work with patients who, though British in their ethnicity, are in fact from a very different cultural background from themselves and on reflection you may find that you already have developed skills that allow you to sift the so-called 'normal' for any group from the unusual and abnormal.

It is important to remember that any individual patient may occupy a different position in relation to cultural beliefs compared to others from the same population and it is not unusual or impossible to feel or believe in two things at once that are apparently contradictory. It is easy to be empathetic to the woman who is vehement in her anger about the painful mutilation of female circumcision that is hindering her fertility or impending labour. It is harder to feel comfortable dealing with her sadness over the loss of sexual excitement and pleasure that ensues when the circumcision is reversed, and even more difficult when her husband complains that his sexual pleasure is diminished by her newly created wetness and openness. His feelings may be due to his adherence to religious correctness, which implies that he is overlooking her distress or he may be overwhelmed by her altered behaviour and excitement about babies (rather than just sexual pleasure), now that her vagina and womb are literally open to insemination and all that that entails.

Case 3

A young man from a politically troubled African state told me that he must have Viagra because he could not give his girlfriend more than four or five orgasms a night. I felt unwillingly drawn into the public stereotyping of powerful oversexed large African men. In fact, despite his commanding physical presence, it was obvious that he was timid and depressed, lonely and sad about lost relatives and children that he was unable to bring to the UK. He was in effect impotent or lacking in sexual pleasure and unable to feel strong enough to sustain a new relationship in exile. An exact knowledge of average orgasm-rates in his home country were irrelevant here. I saw him several times and talked about his depression. His relationship ended, but not long afterwards he was proud to bring his new girlfriend to register with my practice, and they seemed very much the happy couple. I found it difficult to find out their true feelings when she underwent several terminations in the next two years. Several more years later she herself came to see me and said that she had lost all her sexual feelings in the past three months. As she had mentioned her worry over her job in the same consultation, I related her loss of libido to her recent anxiety state. This did not seem to get us anywhere. 'It's not that doctor, I am not worrying any more over that'. Her manner was very winning and charming as she spoke softly, smiling in an engaging manner with her lilting accent and gorgeous African print robe that was all quite beguiling. I asked about her boyfriend and their relationship. It seemed she was avoiding a discussion about him because she hated to criticize, being such a tolerant and pleasant person. She talked about how he was always ready to make love to her and again I felt distracted by my thoughts as to what might be accepted as enough or too much or too little for this exotic couple. Her manner was a bit less animated during this description, so I ventured that it sounded as if he or their love-making was always the same, no matter what mood she might be in. Her perfect charm broke down and she agreed that he tended to overlook her wishes and feelings. I interpreted that she was cross with him and holding out because his demands undervalued her and what she had to offer. She spoke eloquently, drawing a carefully observed picture of an introspective and anxious man. He had bought herbal medicine and had made her take it, she said. It had had no effect and he had avoided any discussion about her feelings, 'I was really upset with him for that'. I praised her for her sensitivity and said that her sympathetic personality could nevertheless include some righteous anger without endangering the relationship. It was obvious that she was going to persist with making things work, but she would no longer blame herself alone for their mutual loss of sexual pleasure.

The continuity of care in general practice makes it much harder for a doctor to set boundaries for the kinds of medicine that they practise. Whereas it is obvious that we cannot perform major surgery, gaps in the secondary care system mean that it is often the GP who has to limp along, managing problems that are strictly speaking outside our range of skills or with less than adequate resources for the work in hand. Heart-sink cases are a complete chapter in the textbooks of general practice and for the most part we work comfortably enough within the limits of our skills (Gill and Sharpe, 1999). Our case books of psychosexual medicine are, however, more likely to include those patients that do not fit the guidelines of brief interpretive psychotherapy, but are vaguely defined both in the goals that we seek to achieve with the patient and the methods that we might use.

PRACTICALITIES OF PSYCHOSEXUAL WORK IN GENERAL PRACTICE

The independent contractor status of GPs may have altered for better or worse through several reorganizing phases of the NHS, but it still allows individual doctors to shape their own style of medical work with a degree of flexibility that can be envied by salaried practitioners. The specialist clinic can therefore be realized within general practice for those doctors who are trained and enthusiastic about any particular special interest, such as psychosexual medicine. With the advent of vocational training and the parallel decline of local authority clinic work, well-baby and antenatal clinics are now accepted without question by most practices as well as other medical clinics. They are, of course, dependent on teamwork with health visitors and midwives who are not usually employed by the practice and can only come at certain dedicated clinic times to the surgery. Contraceptive work and well-woman screening are often absorbed into everyday surgeries rather than the specialized clinic, either by patient choice or because the practice organization prefers opportunistic work to clinic sessions. Much of this work is delegated nowadays almost wholly to the practice nurse.

Another factor that affects the provisions of psychosexual services in general practice is whether any particular surgery uses personal lists or mixed lists of patients. Large practices with mixed lists might be the most suitable setting for specialized clinic work and the smaller practices or those that have personalized lists are not likely to be comfortable with partners setting up specialized sessions.

Specialists in general practice

The important point is that any doctor who feels the urge to extend the use of their specialized training within general practice must think carefully about the effects that running a clinic-style session will have on the rest of the practice. She must first ask herself why it is that specialized clinic work appears attractive to herself in the context of general practice. Is it the dissatisfaction with trivial complaints, the disappointment with low status general practice *vis-à-vis* hospital specialists? How will patients view you if you advertise your special psychosexual clinic within the practice? Doctors can make a name for themselves even within the small scope of a GP surgery as 'the children's doctor', 'rheumatologist', or 'minor-ops doctor'. The major advantage of setting aside time for a clinic is just that – the time is protected, circumscribed and dedicated. Psychological work is time consuming and demanding of the doctor's attention and it is frustrating, often, to find that time just does not allow you to give of your best to distressed patients in the middle of morning surgery, at least not without immense cost to other patients, partners or yourself. In favour of clinics is the fact that you are providing a service to your partners and patients in a very difficult area where specialist clinics are often thin on the ground and waiting lists are long. A large practice with its full complement of nurses is likely to generate enough referrals for a regular clinic session. In a smaller practice the same effect can be obtained by setting aside, say, a 30-minute session on an ad hoc basis when referrals arise (Stuart, 1993).

The fully trained doctor will feel an alignment with colleagues who work in special sessions. On the other hand, being used to working within 'normal' consultations, she may feel uncomfortable in the sudden liberty and insecurity of a longer session, where the specialist expectation must be realized without the usual props, such as a special suite of rooms that clearly announce to the patient that they have embarked on a different type of medical care.

How do patients know what you are doing if there is not a clearly advertised clinic session, nor any of the visual clues that communicate to patients that they are being referred from the basic primary care relationship to one that is partially removed from general practice? Referring nurses and doctors can tell patients that one of the partners is interested in this sort of problem and they can therefore build up the picture of the specialist. Self-referrals can be a bit more awkward. The overt presentation, 'Could I be referred? I've got this problem with sex' may elicit the response 'Well I have a special interest in this and I sometimes set aside a longer appointment to see how I could help'. While this apparently is very convenient, it gives the patient very little choice (Carter, 1997). It is difficult for the patient to say 'Well the reason I said can I be referred is because I never imagined you as the sort of doctor that I could talk to about this'. What I am suggesting is that the usual preliminary inquiry that you would use when referring any type of patient, in order to find out their hopes, fears, expectations and needs, is appropriate even when you have yourself in mind as the specialist (Coulter, 1998). The doctor can still be left in the dark, and this is just as true for referrals to other doctors as to yourself. Is the patient asking for themselves or to please someone else, or to spite someone else, to prove someone right or wrong? The point to be made is that GPs are GPs and the adoption of a specialist's mantle can be hazardous, or may destabilize or critically change the doctor–patient relationship in a very powerful way.

Supervisory role

With or without special sessions or referrals, the GP who has completed further training in

psychosexual work can work as a supervisor or facilitator to the primary care team in a more or less explicit way. This relationship will be affected by whether or not you are ever likely to be able to accept a referral. Offering supervision may be read by colleagues as a way of deflecting unwanted referrals, whereas if you never see other partners' patients it cannot be read in that way. The dilemma is, 'Am I pleasing my colleague by feeding her interesting cases for her 'hobby' specialty, or am I burdening her when she is already extending herself?' Clear communication and set parameters to this sort of work in-house allows you to avoid many such pitfalls. Within my four-handed practice, working full time with a personal list, I feel that I can manage one long case-session a week, two at a push, but more than that will crucially reduce my availability to general primary care appointments.

Confidentiality

Whatever style or level of work you choose, any exploration of patients' psychosexual difficulty is likely to yield disclosures of intimate material that is of a different order to run of the mill medical details or even general psychological problems. Patients' expectations about confidentiality are likely to be much higher; they will have a lower threshold for anxiety about confidentiality when describing their sex lives to you. Patients embarking on a disclosure about their sexual difficulties will more often say something about not wanting their partner to know about this discussion than for other problems. In fact, for some areas of general practice there is almost a reverse expectation of confidentiality. The reception staff may be friends or local acquaintances, and it is obviously important to be sensitive to this. GPs will be used to issues of confidentiality to a degree that is often quite sophisticated because of their more frequent contact and closer social relationships with patients.

The ethical limits are even less clear when the doctor has an urge to share interesting case material with clinical colleagues. This can be a very necessary and useful debriefing exercise after emotionally traumatic encounters, or it may be a simple request for help with a difficult case, supervision or reassurance. On the other hand, it can reveal a tendency to wish to distance oneself from patients, or even to indulge in salacious gossip. There is something amiss if you need to advertise the fact to your colleagues that patients often make astonishing or intimate disclosures to you, but it can require effort of will to contain a fascinating or exotic account. However, keeping secrets and a proprietorial attitude towards one's patients may be just as pathological.

Practice nurses' work

Most practices these days employ practice nurses and it is likely that the bulk of routine smear tests and contraceptive work will be directed to them. This means that the opportunity to use a 'routine' vaginal examination as part of a psychosexual assessment may be lost or at least altered by the shared knowledge (for patient and doctor) that such examinations are usually re-routed to the nurse. It is sometimes a special dispensation to ask the receptionist to set aside surgery time for the doctor to do a smear and this gives added weight and meaning to the moment of examination. Many women are slack about their routine smears without their being any hidden psychopathology, but those that avoid them persistently, even when reminded, are betraying some difficulty. Those who refuse to see the nurse in favour of the doctor may also be letting you know in advance something of a psychological nature. Where the suggestion that the patient should book their routine smear test with the nurse is countered with, 'Oh I'd rather you did it doctor', then the doctor must ask herself if the patient is overly dependent, or if she might be racist for she knows the nurse is black or Indian, or if she is worried about genital disease or infection. The patient may add that the last time she had a smear with the nurse it was painful. The doctor must consider whether or not the nurse is adequately trained or if the patient has vaginismus during clinical examinations. A delicate path must be trod so as not to undermine the professional status of the nurse or to become a doctor who collects overly dependent patients.

Sometimes the doctor must work at second hand, without the benefit of a vaginal examination, even though it would be anticipated as being revealing but where repeating the examination might appear to be odd. However, it may be appropriate to offer a second examination without implying that the practice nurse's assessment was inadequate. The doctor can suggest that, 'As you still have a problem would you like me to have a look as well?' since anyone can miss something or fail to reassure, despite their best efforts.

There is an argument to be put that if nurses are doing the bulk of this routine work, then training in psychosexual medicine would most efficiently be awarded to the nurse. How far the technical role of the nurse extends to a practitioner role that includes the diagnosis of genital disease and psychosexual therapy depends on the individual nurse's interest and expertise and must be accompanied by careful monitoring of the boundaries of professional and diagnostic territories. For the most part this is unproblematic, but such shared cases can highlight interprofessional difficulties that already exist in the practice where, for instance, the nurse feels aggrieved by traditionally hierarchical professional relationships. Doctors may deflect, consciously or otherwise, difficult and heart-sink patients to the nurse rather than embarking on a vaginal examination in surgery time with someone whom they feel may expose emotional and psychosexual difficulties that the doctor would rather not deal with. Each may undermine or competitively encroach on the other's clinical role. It is obvious that openness, dialogue, discussion and sharing of particular experiences with difficult or interesting cases, can do much to increase a mutually supportive working relationship between nurses and doctors in this area (Applebee, 1997). The same sorts of issues arise where a female partner gets the bulk of the gynaecological work of the practice and the desirability of making a female doctor available to patients should not be abused by inappropriate referrals of difficult patients to that partner by male colleagues.

Supervision and continuing seminars

The nearer you are to the hospital consultant model of specialist, especially where psychological work is involved, the more there is a need for regular supervision and meetings with other specialists. It could be argued that supervisory seminars or sessions with a supervisor overweights the notion of 'specialist', whereas the training of the Institute of Psychosexual Medicine could be said to enhance the non-specialist skill of being a doctor who can pay attention in a medical setting to psychosexual distress. However, the ability to keep up a freshness of attitude and to maintain a method that is in many respects counter-intuitive to the standard medical model of disease and cases needs some input. Occasional meetings may be of greater benefit than mandatory audit. Peer review through seminars, perhaps even if only on an annual basis with doctors who do the same sort of work, may be the best primary method of clinical governance. The benefit of a well-led supervisory seminar is that it is possible both to examine and to enhance the appropriate clinical skills of the attending doctors.

KEY POINTS

- The skills of psychosexual medicine help the GP to deal with psychosomatic problems.
- The level of training and the amount of time and effort put in to such skills will vary according to the interest and needs of any particular GP.
- Psychosexual therapy as a specialist skill is not required of every GP, but the ability to recognize psychosexual difficulty is an essential part of everyday practice.

- Psychosexual problems may present as physical symptoms and become manifest at the time of genital examination.
- The GP can be an important witness to the trouble that a patient is suffering without necessarily intervening directly as an active therapist who always tries to put things right.
- People do not belong wholly to cultures as if they were closed systems of fixed beliefs. The personal issues of our individual patients are usually more immediate and pressing than the group ethics of their own particular culture.
- Psychosexual skills can be used in general practice at a variety of levels from very short unplanned consultations to long special sessions for referred patients.
- The provision of care for patients with psychosexual problems can be adapted to the different arrangements in group practice, and may involve other members of the primary care team.

REFERENCES

Applebee, K. 1997: *Troubleshooting in general practice.* London: Royal Society of Medicine Press.

Carter, N. 1997: Keeping focused in General Practice. *Institute of Psychosexual Medicine Journal* 16, 11–12.

Coulter, A. 1998: Referrals to specialist clinics. In McPherson and Waller (eds), *Women's health.* Oxford: Oxford University Press.

Gatrad, A.R. and Sheikh, A. 2000: Birth customs: meaning and significance. In Gatrad, A.R. and Sheikh, A. (eds), *Caring for Muslim patients.* Oxford: Radcliffe Medical Press.

Gill, D. and Sharpe, M. 1999: Frequent consulters in general practice: a systematic review of studies of prevalence, associations and outcome. *Journal of Psychosomatic Research* 47(2), 115–30.

Gilroy, P. 2000: *Between camps: nations cultures and the allure of race.* London: Allen Lane, The Penguin Press.

Hawton, K. and Harrison 1998: Sexual problems. In McPherson and Waller (eds), *Women's Health.* Oxford: Oxford University Press.

Norton, K. and Smith 1994: Implications for the clinical setting. In Smith (ed.), *Problems with patients: managing complicated transactions.* Cambridge: CUP.

Stuart, M.R. 1993: *The fifteen minute hour: applied psychotherapy for the primary care physician.* Westport CT: Praeger.

17 The contraceptive clinic

Merryl Roberts

CONTRACEPTION

'It is a truth universally acknowledged' (Austen) that a woman entering a contraceptive clinic must be in want of expert advice about contraception. Contraception is defined as the intentional prevention of pregnancy. Therefore, women coming to these clinics are seeking to control their fertility. It is commonly assumed that because of this such clinics are simple and rather boring.

THE ROLE OF THE CONTRACEPTIVE CLINIC

In practice, contraceptive clinics are much more complex, both in general practice and community sexual health settings. As the term 'Sexual Health' indicates, a wide-ranging variety of services is offered to the patients who attend.

Contraceptive clinics strive to be client friendly, and this is reflected in their atmosphere. Opening times and appointment systems are tailored to the client need. Young people like clinics that are informal, sympathetic and confidential. They need to be able to drop in with a morale-boosting group of friends at the end of the school day, and feel welcomed and respected. The staff of these clinics need to be experts in child protection issues, as well as contraception. Busy women who are struggling to balance work and home need clinics that open during the lunch break, and at the end of the working day. Women at home with young children like morning clinics they can combine with shopping, or evening ones, if they can find a baby sitter.

Members of staff in community clinics are traditionally part time and female, and many contraceptive clinics in general practice are run by practice nurses. Indeed, nurses have a traditionally strong role in the field of contraception across all of primary care. These nurses are highly specialized, able to run clinics on their own, working to protocols. Many patients feel that they can more easily confide in a sympathetic nurse than a busy doctor, and nurses hear many sexual problems as they take smears or discuss the pill. Some nurses are content to identify a sexual problem and refer the patient on, but more and more nurses are training in the field of psychosexual medicine in response to these needs. All fields of medicine depend on teamwork between the different healthcare disciplines, and in the contraceptive clinic there is an especially strong partnership between doctor, nurse and clerical staff. Clinics where this mutual respect falters are rarely successful.

Contraceptive clinics offer much more than expert advice on all forms of birth control, although doctors and nurses are prepared to spend a great deal of time discussing these. They also give advice about sexually transmitted diseases, infertility, pre-conception planning, as well as menopausal and pre-menstrual problems. Women bring worries about menstruation, pelvic pain, chronic vulval irritation or painful sex. More and more men are attending contraceptive clinics, either to obtain condoms, or to accompany their partners. This is often an opportunity for them to seek advice for themselves.

THE PATIENT–DOCTOR PARTNERSHIP IN CONTRACEPTIVE CLINICS

The atmosphere of a contraceptive clinic engenders a different relationship between patient and healthcare worker. The balance of power between patient and receptionist, doctor and nurse, appears to be more equal than in many other medical settings. A contraceptive patient is never a supplicant; she comes to discuss *her* needs, she will listen to your advice, but feels quite free to reject it. Mostly, she wants you to listen to her, give her accurate information so that she can make an informed choice, and respect her decisions. She feels comfortable enough, and powerful enough, to be pretty certain that you will. One major difference between mainstream medicine and contraceptive clinics is that the decision to attend is made purely by the patient. An ill patient has little choice, she or he needs medical care; a woman seeking contraceptive advice comes because she chooses to. If she doesn't like what she gets, she will go elsewhere: from general practice to a community family planning clinic, and vice versa. Often, she comes and goes just as she wants, moving between community clinic and the GP, like a lucky dip. No one lectures her if she suddenly reappears after a long break. She's the boss. Such choice, such power, is not readily available in today's NHS, and it makes it easier for women to feel confident enough to broach their own agenda.

Case 1: The golden goddess

A peaceful summer's evening, and I had my consulting room in the family planning clinic to myself – a rare treat. I wasn't training. All the nurses were busy somewhere else. Picking up the next set of notes from the box on the outside of the consulting room door, I called a name, and in strolled a tall, smiling, attractive, brisk and efficient young woman. As I introduced myself I looked at her notes, and observed that this was her first visit to our clinic. She smiled even more, revealing even, sparkling white teeth, and said that she usually got her pill from her GP, but, as she now worked near the clinic, it was easier to come here. It seemed a very ordinary, relaxed, routine consultation, 'How can I help you?' I said, looking at her. Her smile tightened, and suddenly, the relaxed feeling in the room changed and I became aware of a lot of anxiety. My antennae twitched. She fenced, nervously 'Lots of girls in the office come here...', she replied, glancing at me, '...they say you are all very nice.' Mmm, I thought, is this an appeal for me to be 'nice', whatever that means, a statement that she was 'nice', or a warning to me that she had a hidden agenda, which was not at all 'nice'. I sat back in my chair, put my pen down, and waited.

Her smile seemed to be stretched tautly across her face; above it, her eyes were wary. 'I am on pill X', she rattled, 'Like it very much...need some more...that's all...nothing really...', her voice tailed off. Once, in my greenhouse, I had found a small bird, trapped. By the time I had caught and released it my own heart was racing in panicky sympathy. I felt just like that now, obviously picking up on her feelings of panic – but why should she be afraid? 'You seem...worried about something...', I said, tentatively, and realized that I was indeed treating her gently, nicely; was I afraid of hurting her, like the bird? The smile wavered. Outside in the corridor, a baby wailed, a nurse laughed, and there was a loud clunk as yet another set of notes arrived in the pending box on my door.

The smile was now somewhat frozen, but still there. She took a deep breath.

'I would like to have a smear', she said. I waited. 'I got a letter from my GP's surgery, but the nurse couldn't do it...she said that I was too small. She sent me to the GP, but he couldn't do it either. He gave me something to calm me down, to take before I went back, but...I thought perhaps...I felt such a fool', she finished, savagely, furiously. Into my peaceful room had stalked the contagious angry terror of the non-consummator. I waited. 'I tried to tell my mother', she said, still hanging on to the vestiges of the smile, 'although heaven knows, she has got enough on her plate'. Now the words were pouring from her. 'My father has a bad back, and he is, well...always has been really, well...can't blame him I suppose, but you never know where you are with him, pretty short-tempered. My sister argues with him. But I...well, I'm like my mother – anything for a quiet life.'

In a few short sentences she had painted a vivid picture of a 'good' girl, a victim mother, angry father and, that stalwart of non-consummating women, the rebellious naughty sister. I was filled with admiration. It can take ages to get this far in a psychosexual clinic. This girl was as aware of the pressure on time as I was. She continued 'Anyway, I sort of told my mother, and she said that I was probably too small. I might need an operation'. My door clunked again, reminding me that time was short.

What should I do? The number of patients waiting was growing; I could hear a restless hum. I was tempted to refer her to the psychosexual clinic. Perhaps I should ask her to come back when I could make more time? However, I was acutely aware this girl had already failed twice in her own eyes. To send her away would surely only reinforce her failure. I decided to take the bull by the horns. 'Too small for intercourse', I said, in a matter of fact way. Her eyes filled with tears. 'He can't get in at all – I *must* be too small.'

'Why don't we have a look', I said.

She nodded, after all, this was what she had come for, but she looked very frightened. She undressed slowly, reluctantly and got up on the bed with her knickers still on. I didn't say anything – she said, 'how silly', and took them off. She sat, cradling her knees. I waited, leaning against the couch. I was certainly allowing her to take and keep control. We were about to perform a very physical examination, to look at a vagina, which is 'too small'. And yet I know that vaginismus is about fantasies of the internal world, albeit suppressed and unrecognized. It is also about power, loss of control, fear, pain, ownership, and the sexy self. These are powerful and threatening emotions, so much so that they are easier to express as a physical symptom. The difficulty for the doctor or nurse is to find a bridge, so that the patient can link the mind and body.

Hugging her knees, clearly terrified, she tried to recover her bright smile.

'You are good at hiding feelings', I said, 'You are obviously afraid, yet still you smile.'

'I'm an ostrich', she said, 'I'll go out rather than face a scene!' 'I expect that's how you deal with your anger at your father, suppress it, shut it in.'

'To be angry at Dad is to play his game', she said.

'Ah', I said, 'you shut him out then, that's another way of expressing anger. It's interesting that you are shutting yourself, your boyfriend and the doctor out of your vagina as well.'

She thought about that.

'Do you know, when I get upset I go into my room and close my door – it's the same thing, really? I would like to move away from home, my sister has. But, I know my mother would really miss me, she depends on me . . .'

'You seem torn', I said, 'whether to be a good daughter, a victim, belonging to your mother, or your own person, doing what you please, owning your own flat, owning your own vagina. I think that you are fed up with doing what other people expect and want – even perhaps your boyfriend.'

She looked at me, 'I feel such a fool', she said again, ruefully. She had said it before, and I hadn't really picked it up.

'An angry fool', I said. 'Looked at dispassionately, sex is a pretty foolish thing.'

'Can you do a smear?' she asked, urgently.

'If you like', I said. Physically, of course, the smear was completely unnecessary; this girl was still a virgin. Emotionally, it was clearly very important. A rite of passage, perhaps claiming ownership of her vagina. Just what normal, grown-up women do. I had a vision of her workplace, her colleagues moaning on about having a smear taken and her desperate wish to be like them.

Still, we had begun to look at emotions, and she had turned me back to the physical. I raised the back of the couch until she was propped up, quite high. I showed her the speculum and the cervical spatula. She gazed at them with horror.

'Have you put your own finger inside?' I said.

'NO', she said, 'never'.

'Why not try now', I said. She was very tense, and I thought she was going to weep, but she gradually inserted her own finger, and then two, tightening and relaxing the muscles as she gained confidence. I gave her the speculum, and explained what to do. By now we were both in a hurry. Bit by bit, she herself inserted it, crouched over herself, she opened it, and allowed me to peer inside. To my relief, I could see the cervix. I took a smear. We were both beaming. Still with the speculum inside she said, 'I'm not small at all'.

She still comes to the family planning clinic for her pills; we discuss whatever she wants briefly at each visit. Should women be good or bad? Is anger dangerous? She has consummated. And recently moved out into her own flat.

By coming to a family planning clinic and booking herself in for a short routine appointment, she had exercised her own choice. We had not 'sent' for her. Perhaps, if I had been her GP I would have acted differently, but I was a clinic doctor, aware that she came with a heavy baggage of failure, and I didn't feel that I could add to that. She was not 'my' patient in the sense of general practice; she was using me and this setting of a purely contraceptive clinic. If she failed again, she would never need to face us again. This gave her a position of more power, which I felt had helped her to confide her problem and deal with it. The very nature of the clinic was important in helping her. This was a short appointment, and I actually didn't spend much over the normal time with her. A short appointment time is generally perceived to be a disadvantage when dealing with sexual problems, but it can be just the opposite, concentrating everyone's mind.

MIND AND BODY IN THE CONTRACEPTIVE CLINIC

The goddess presented with a clear physical request, a smear test, and a physical symptom, a vagina that was too small. She also presented with a lot of anger, hidden behind a smile, and the need to control the consultation. All these presenting complaints are interrelated, and important. They can't be separated; they have to be addressed at the same time. Both the physical symptom and the emotional terrors are real; they exist together, and must be treated together, although the vital process of building a bridge between them can be difficult. For the goddess, the opportunity of talking about emotions whilst preparing for a physical, vaginal examination began to build the bridge. As it does for many.

Sex is the ultimate mind–body experience. For sex to be pleasurable and successful, both mind and body need to work well together, a problem with one will affect the other. A contraceptive clinic exemplifies this; there it is understood, and discussed, that feelings about a type of contraceptive will affect a woman's sex life – choosing a method of contraception is far more than a purely intellectual choice. It is but a short step to talking about feelings about sex in general. The purely physical, the fitting of a cap for example, merges with the purely emotional, a dislike of touching herself internally, to produce a discussion about perceptions of the vagina, and its sexual role.

WHAT IS A CONTRACEPTIVE CONSULTATION ABOUT

In theory, every patient attending a family planning clinic has a cast iron calling card. She is coming to obtain contraception, that is, she already accepts that her body is her own responsibility, hers to control. In theory, *she* owns her vagina, can put a cap in it or not, *she* owns her uterus, can grow a baby in it or not, *she* controls her hormones, can alter her whole cycle or not. Doctors and nurses may naively think that the consultation is all about contraceptive advice. Our patients are very well aware that the real reason they attend is to have a good sex life, without getting pregnant. Sexual intercourse is the not-so-hidden agenda; any discussion of contraception must involve sex and this makes sexual difficulties easier to talk about, if the doctor or nurse is able to listen and pick up the patient's clues. This hidden agenda of sexuality brings women into the clinic who are not as confident about their own body, do not feel they own their vagina, and feel uncertain about their sexual selves. For these women, presenting with a 'physical' contraceptive problem is a way of seeking help for a hidden sexual one.

The very fact that the contraceptive clinic is separate, that this doctor or nurse is not 'my' GP or practice nurse, helps some patients. In general practice, sexual problems are often revealed to a locum GP, the newest GP Registrar, or a GP not normally seen. It is clearly easier to talk about such embarrassing issues to a relative stranger, someone you don't have to see again. There are times when the feelings revealed are difficult for both patient and GP to cope with afterwards.

Case 2: The furious vaginal discharge

> The evening clinic was busy, and running late. Everyone was tired. The cleaner was clanking her buckets hopefully. I was training a GP Registrar to insert IUDs, and thinking of my supper. A nurse strode into the consulting room. 'There's a really unpleasant woman out there', she said, clearly angry. 'She has no appointment, and is demanding to see you, says her GP told her to come. She's been really rude to everyone. She shouted at Y, who is upset.' My heart sank. 'Bring her in', I said, with resignation.

In stormed a small, determined lady with short, spiky hair and a furious expression. She glared at the nurse, who pursed her lips. Next to me, my trainee quietly moved his chair backwards, and pretended he wasn't there. The room glittered with anger. I thought that I didn't blame her GP for sending her over, and wished I had a computer screen to look at. She sat on the edge of her chair, hands on her knees, leaning forwards aggressively. I wanted to go home, and stayed silent.

She went on to the attack. 'My GP told me to come. He said you might be able to help. I've got this terrible vaginal discharge, nothing helps it, I'm waiting for an appointment with the gynaecologist, but it's not for ages.'

I wondered why such a chronic condition had presented with such urgency in a family planning clinic, so late at night. I knew the GP, and was sure he had done everything necessary. I felt fed up, and puzzled.

I said: 'I'm just wondering why you needed to be seen tonight, couldn't wait?'

She spat back: 'Because I am completely fed up with it, that's why!'

Behind her, my nurse's face was a picture of disgust, next to me my trainee looked at his watch.

She went into great detail about her discharge, how it smelt horrible, she had to wear pads, all the smears and swabs, the creams, pessaries and tablets which hadn't worked, how it was ruining her life. It sounded repulsive, and I really didn't want to know, but I had a feeling that she wouldn't be fobbed off. Besides, I knew that all this inappropriate anger, the strange urgency, must mean something. The women was intimidating, she had frightened the staff – was she afraid herself?

'Better have a look', I said, and we moved to the couch. I shook my head at the nurse and trainee. I didn't need them, and pulled the curtain around us. She got up reluctantly. 'It's horrible', she said. I pulled the curtain, laid out a selection of swabs, snapped on some strong gloves and, with some trepidation, opened her vulva. Normal. I inserted a speculum. An immaculate, clean, vagina. I felt stunned. I realized that I had bought into the fantasy of the 'horrible' vaginal discharge. She was looking at me with apprehension.

'What do you think?' she said, anxiously.

What to do? The repulsive discharge was a fantasy, but just saying it didn't exist wouldn't help. I took the speculum out, and examined her internally. No tenderness, normal uterus. There was a very tense atmosphere, as she waited for my verdict.

However, the intimate nature of the genital examination, the intimate space created by pulling the curtain around the couch, had created a more intimate atmosphere between us. Closing her legs, I leant against the couch and gazed at her seriously. How could I create that bridge, to help her make the connection between what she was feeling emotionally and how she perceived her physical vagina to be? All I really had was her inappropriate anger, and what I considered to be her fear. In my favour was the extreme urgency of her presentation, which made her more vulnerable, I felt. There is something to be said for an open door policy. I decided to risk even more anger, and put these feelings to her. 'I think that you *feel* that your vagina is dirty and horrible. I think that you are very, very angry, *at* something, and probably afraid, *of* something', I said. 'I feel puzzled, myself. But, I have to say, that your vagina is as clean as a whistle. However, I feel something is going on inside you, to make you so sure that your vagina is so dirty.' That said, I stayed still and waited. To my surprise she did not get even angrier. Instead, she sat up, wrapped her arms around her legs and, still on the couch, began to talk about her husband, who had recently been diagnosed with diabetes, and wouldn't accept it. He had been abroad on a business trip, and she was sure that he had picked up something nasty sexually, because his penis was sore and red, but he wouldn't see his doctor. He wouldn't talk about anything, and she was convinced he had 'given her' something. Her pain spilled out. What could she do? They weren't having sex any more because he was just avoiding it. That evening, they had had a row, he had gone out somewhere, she felt she couldn't bear it any more, so she had gone to the doctor, and her doctor had sent her across to the clinic. She couldn't tell her nice doctor about the filthy infection, no wonder he couldn't cure it. 'There is no infection', I repeated, 'if your husband had a sore penis it might be because of thrush, common with diabetes; if he was avoiding sex, that could be due to problems with getting an erection, could be also due to the diabetes. You are angry, and afraid, and so is your vagina.' She looked at me, suspiciously. 'No infection?' she repeated.

'No'. There was a long pause. 'It's late', I said. 'You can come back and see me again if you like.' But, she never did. Later, I met her GP in the corridor. 'Thanks for seeing Mrs B', he said. 'You sorted it out anyway. What did you give her?'

Mrs B couldn't tell her GP about her 'filthy' infection, she was ashamed of it, and knew him too well. She was able to tell me, a stranger, in a clinic which is all about sex, and whom she need never see again. Did she make that connection, between her anger at her husband and his supposed STD, and her dirty vagina?

IDENTIFYING SEXUAL PROBLEMS IN A CONTRACEPTIVE CLINIC

Since the contraceptive clinic is basically all about sex, and women can bring such a wide variety of problems to the clinic, it is hardly surprising that there are many ways in which sexual problems are presented.

Physical symptoms, for example, the chopping and changing of contraceptive methods, blaming of 'hormones', a vaginal discharge where none is present, dyspareunia when the scan and vaginal examination are normal, chronic vulval 'thrush' in the absence of the typical discharge or a positive swab, all of these should cause the clinician to think of a sexual problem. One enormous advantage of a contra-

ceptive clinic is that so many of these 'calling cards' involve a vaginal examination, that intimate examination when defences are weak, and sudden revelations can occur. The woman who always manages to avoid having a smear test. The one who, on the couch, says apologetically, 'I'm sorry, I haven't had time for a bath'. Or, 'What an awful job you have, doc'. The women for whom a smear test is a cause for great tension, or who turns her face to the wall to avoid looking at you. These are all clues as to what she feels about her body, and often to how she feels about her sexual self.

To a clinician, a sexual problem can be considered as part of a differential diagnosis, mind and body examined together. The base of the 'bridge' is already in place.

Case 3: Miss A

'It's Miss A again', said the nurse, plopping a thick pile of notes on my desk. I flipped through the notes with a sinking feeling. I had never seen her myself, but Miss A had seen most of the doctors and nurses in quite a few of our contraceptive clinics over the past few months. She was a 'clinic hopper', and probably a 'GP hopper' as well. She had never settled on a form of contraception; everything seemed to cause problems. Her notes were peppered with complaints about weight gain, bloating, lower abdominal ache, aching legs, a vaginal discharge and dyspareunia. She had been fully investigated and nothing abnormal had been found, but she had been given Canestan and Diflucan anyway. She had tried lots of different contraceptive pills. The cap put her off. Condoms irritated her. She had been given diet sheets ('I eat practically nothing'), and advised to add exercise ('I don't have the time/I'm too fat to wear a swimming costume'). We had referred her to her GP ('I'm sure he can sort out your tummy pain') and he bounced her back rapidly to us. ('They know all about that sort of thing in the contraceptive clinic'). A gynaecologist had been suggested.

Plump and hot, she plonked herself down in the chair, and gazed gloomily at me. 'Here I am again', she began 'like a bad penny'. She didn't smile, and I too felt gloomy and depressed. 'I'm sure it's my hormones. My stomach feels terrible, and I've got that discharge back. Perhaps it's that new pill Dr P gave me?' The sheer size of her notes intimidated me, but the pattern was familiar. The continuing dissatisfaction with contraception, non-existing vaginal discharges, it seemed like a typical way of presenting a sexual problem. I found a note that said: *Denies any sexual difficulty. Blames discharge.* 'You've certainly had a lot of problems', I said, as I began to try to sort through her notes, all her swabs, smears, ultrasound scan etc., trying to think what to do. 'I'm at a loss', I said, 'none of the tests seemed to show anything up.' She sat there, big and passive; I felt heavy and hopeless myself. 'Did you get to see the gynaecologist?' I could see a way out here. 'No', she replied, 'not yet.' Hope sprang within my heart. 'Perhaps we should wait until you have seen him?' She became agitated. 'What', she squawked, 'I can't wait, I *can't* wait.' I sat back, somewhat surprised by this sudden show of emotion. 'I am getting married next month', she said, 'You've *got* to sort it out by then!'

Forgetting her thick notes, which I had been using so successfully as a defence against her, I put my pen down and just looked at her. I felt her despair. 'It must be dreadful for you', I offered. She looked at me as though I was a simpleton. 'You can say that again. Time something was done!' 'It must be causing problems with sex', I said. 'Yes', she replied readily, 'it's so painful, we have more or less stopped. Mind you, he is very good, very understanding. Well, he's a long distance lorry driver, and we've been saving as much money as possible, so he's not here all that often. We're going to Barbados for our honeymoon. All inclusive.' At that, she sounded close to tears. I felt close to tears as well. 'It's the first time I have met you', I said, 'So, I don't know what you feel about all this. It seems to me that you are dreading this honeymoon, for starters. It must be upsetting your boyfriend as well.' 'He's lovely', she said, 'he couldn't be nicer, very different to . . .', and she fell silent, as I sat and waited.

The silence seemed to last a long time; we could hear all the normal noises of the clinic around us, making our silence even deeper. I found that I was holding my breath, taking care not even to move. I seemed to be afraid of putting her off: whatever was going through her mind must be important. More silence. The muscles in the back of my neck ached. Hesitantly, slowly, she told me of her first fiancé, who had been killed in a car crash two weeks before the wedding. She held onto my hand, and wept as she described her guilt at finding someone else, at enjoying sex with somebody else – a guilt which got worse and worse as the wedding approached. She had become afraid that she would call out her first love's name when she climaxed. Barry didn't understand her fear, just went off with his lorry; well, she could hardly discuss her first love with him, and they were so different. 'Do you know', I said, 'it seems to me that in a strange way you are angry with Barry, for driving his lorry about the country, full of cheer, and coming home, full of life, and love, and lust for you, when your first love is dead.' She cried, and then calmed down. Then she said, 'But I don't see what all this has to do with my discharge'. 'Yes', I replied, 'we mustn't forget your discharge', and we went to the examination couch and drew the curtain. I examined her in this intimate atmosphere; she watched me, anxiously. 'Do you know', I said, 'that this is absolutely normal, there is no discharge, and everything is healthy.' 'Are you saying that it is all in my mind?' she said. 'Well', I said, 'you said to me that your mind felt guilty at enjoying sex; perhaps all these problems are your body's way of expressing guilt.'

'Or even to protect me from being hurt again', she replied. She had begun to make the connections between physical and emotional pain; the bridge-building had begun.

THE VAGINAL EXAMINATION AND THE DOCTOR OR NURSE–PATIENT RELATIONSHIP

Physically touching a patient is always a powerful moment, and it is no accident that strong rules and taboos surround this, to protect both doctor and patient. Examining the genitals, whether in men or women, is especially powerful, and is thus regulated even more strongly. The Royal College of Obstetricians and Gynaecologists have issued a booklet of guidelines (RCOG, 1997), which recommends the use of chaperones. They also recommend that any problems identified be discussed after the examination, with both doctor and patient safely seated at the desk. However, in clinical practice, a vaginal examination will often lead to revelation of inner feelings, which will be lost if the clinician is so clinical as to ignore any feelings at all. It is vital to treat these expressions of feelings in a completely professional way, and chaperones are no bar to doing this. A doctor or nurse can observe what is happening in an objective, clinical and thoughtful way, and interpret this to the patient, either beside the couch, or at the desk. Where sexual problems are so often presented as physical genital symptoms, what effect the genital examination has on both doctor and patient is vitally important, both in diagnosing the problem and understanding it.

CONCLUSION

Contraception is about sex. Sex is a mind–body experience, and this is mirrored in the clinics, where physical problems affecting sex and emotional sexual difficulties intertwine. In such a setting, doctors and nurses who are aware of the possibility of sexual problems will quickly find that they are hearing them. Observing what is happening within the room, how the patient is behaving, what effect this has on the doctor or nurse, listening carefully and observing the genital examination for psychological pointers as well as physical signs, all help the clinician. Much can be done in a short time, but training in an IPM seminar helps to increase skills and make the best use of the time available.

KEY POINTS

- Sexual problems are commonly confided in contraceptive clinics.
- It is important that clinicians working in these clinics keep sexual problems in mind when thinking of a differential diagnosis.
- The combination of mind and body medicine already exists within a contraceptive clinic.
- Discussion of a contraceptive method often involves talking about sex, which allows a problem to be discussed.
- Short appointment times are not necessarily a drawback to helping sexual problems. Much can be achieved in a short time.
- A vaginal examination, even if routine, can lead to disclosure of a sexual problem.
- The way a woman acts during a vaginal examination gives strong clues to the way she feels about her body.

REFERENCES

Austen, J. *Pride and prejudice*, ch. 1.
Royal College of Obstetricians and Gynaecologists 1997: *Intimate examinations. Report of a working party.* London: RCOG Press.

18 The genito-urinary clinic

Tessa Crowley

> Psychological aspects of genital infections
>
> Homosexual patients
>
> The patient and HIV

Genito-urinary medicine (GUM) clinics have developed from the network of clinics set up after the First World War to deal with sexually transmitted infections (STI). The venereal disease regulations of 1916 stated that treatment was to be confidential and free of charge. These principles still apply today. Over the years the type of problems presented at GUM clinics have changed and now cover a broad range of sexual health disorders. The prevalence of syphilis and gonorrhoea in the United Kingdom has decreased dramatically over the last century. However, other sexually transmitted infections, such as genital warts, *C. trachomatis* and herpes have increased. HIV has taken centre stage. Where once we could predict bacterial incubation periods and prescribe antibiotics that resolved infection, today we are faced with viral latent infections and possible long-term carriage. Other names often used for these infections are 'the pox', 'the clap', 'VD'. Names that are associated with feelings of stigmatization, guilt and shame. Therefore it is not suprising that there is a psychosexual morbidity associated with acquisition of STIs.

- GUM clinics offer complete confidentiality.
- The number of people attending GUM clinics continues to rise.

PSYCHOLOGICAL ASPECTS OF GENITAL INFECTIONS

People who come to GUM clinics do so for a number of different reasons, but the single common thread is sex. Tom Main, the analyst and founder of the Institute of Psychosexual Medicine, wrote that: 'sex is something more than a body matter, more than bodily acrobatics: it is also a matter of high passionate feeling and the giving and getting of intense bodily and mental pleasure, the most intimate relationship of all. The sex act is therefore above all *psychosomatic* and that is why doctors meet the problems they do, for they have easy access to the body as well as to the mind.'

Sex is about physical and mental pleasure when things are going right, but when things go wrong where do people go? Departments of genito-urinary medicine are easily accessible and they deal with a range of sexual health issues. Many people with sexual problems may present for the first time to a GUM clinic. It has been reported that up to 20 per cent of women and 37 per cent of men attending these clinics have a sexual problem (Goldmeier *et al.*, 2000).

GUM clinics offer self-referral and easy access to a free, utterly confidential consultation with a medical professional who is used to talking about sex. This is the reason people choose to come to us. They bring with them the emotional baggage of sex gone wrong. From minor anxieties, which can be readily addressed such as 'Have I caught something?' to the more complex issues associated with, 'It hurts when he puts it in', 'I can't come' and 'I can't do it anymore'.

The presentation of a sexual problem in a GUM clinic can be overt or covert. Patients attending these clinics have a spectrum of presenting problems but only a small proportion will disclose sexual dysfunction as their primary complaint. In one study only 11.6 per cent of 163 GUM patients presented sexual dysfunction as their primary complaint, although this entire group wished to discuss their sexual problems (Crowley, 1998). The fact that some people had attended on many previous occasions and had undergone frequent and repeated examinations and investigations without disclosing bears witness to the difficulty patients experience in discussing these problems. Sexual problems may only be disclosed if the doctor is perceived as sympathetic. When the problem is clearly stated by the patient, the appropriate therapeutic interventions may be offered. These may be pharmacological, surgical, behavioural or psychodynamic. However, it can be difficult for the patient to acknowledge sexual difficulties even to themselves. It may also be difficult for a busy physician to hear the underlying problem. Doctors often perform innumerable examinations and screening tests, when a different approach might have allowed the patient to share their anxiety. As Balint said 'he who asks questions will get answers – but hardly anything else'. 'Listen to the patient; he is telling you the diagnosis' (Balint and Norell, 1989). Winnicott suggested that in infants ill health is identical with doubt about oneself and that this is true of the psychosomatic sufferer at any age. It is a matter of the balance of the forces of 'good' and 'evil' within (Winnicott, 1988). The health of the body, in so far as it is noticed, is translated into fantasy, which is felt in terms of body. He gives the example of guilt being expressed as vomiting or conversely that vomiting (secondary to a physical cause) may be felt to have betrayed the secret inner self. Is it possible to think more simplistically that people might express their feelings through their bodies? We do this all the time by physical stance, expressions, pitch and tone of voice. Anxiety is defined as 'a state of uneasiness or tension caused by apprehension of possible future misfortune or danger. A state of intense worry often accompanied by physical symptoms such as shaking or intense feelings in the gut.'

We are familiar with the sensations before an exam; the frequent need to use the lavatory. There is a perfectly sound physiological explanation. Anger, rage or irritation can cause the heart rate to increase and the clenching of fists. When someone is overcome with fury they are described as 'white lipped' and 'red with rage'. There is gut-wrenching pain that accompanies loss, particularly death. Grief can be seen as weight loss and failure to thrive. When these powerful emotions cannot be acknowledged because they threaten the status quo (whether it is the relationship or that person's belief system) can they not be expressed in other ways? This might be as 'the pain in the neck' or the headache that absolves one from sexual performance. It might be far easier to have a penis that refuses to become aroused, a vagina that won't let him in or a vulva that is too sore to bear being touched than to think about the conflict. Understanding this can be difficult for the patient. Once one begins to understand it is possible to move on. Movement from the somatic to the psyche is a change that can be illuminating, but it can also be painful. To facilitate this change, the doctor can produce the space in which the unconscious thought could move into consciousness.

The doctor–patient relationship is the therapeutic tool that we can use in these cases. We observe, evaluate and interpret it. This relationship is the dynamic interaction between two people. In the consultation we are part of the dynamic process, interacting with the patient, monitoring his or her feelings and responses together with our own and pulling back to try to understand what is happening. We try to think constructively about the issue at hand and use it as a therapeutic tool (Neighbour, 1993). In the ideal world, we would be able to do this within a pleasant room set up for this purpose, with enough time to allow a gentle pace and reorganization of our thoughts before the next patient. However, most problems turn up in the day-to-day work in a busy clinic where time is an issue. Whilst the majority of GUM clinics support the idea of the provision of psychosexual services, only 42 per cent currently provide one (Keane *et al.*, 1997).

Focusing on the doctor–patient relationship allows us to help the man or woman who comes into the clinic with their soreness, their recurrent discharge, their penile or testicular pain, their herpes, their thrush, their genital discomfort, their 'despair' with the whole business of 'down below'. Using this training we can facilitate their understanding of the problem and allow the focus to be relocated. Whether this is the woman acknowledging her 'soreness' with her partner or a man sharing his grief at his partner's miscarriage or simply allowing the expression of hurt and shame at

having caught something they thought only 'dirty' people got. It is easier to be potent and powerful and prescribe as is expected of us by the patient and ourselves. People with painful genitals (for whatever reason) will experience negative feelings about their sexual function. Patients sometimes need to be enabled to share their fantasies of being dirty or damaged with us. We can diagnose the illness and treat the body and often this is enough, but sometimes it is not. We can suppress the recurrent herpes, but not the feelings about having it. We can give a man an erection with pharmacology, but cannot guarantee that he will be able to achieve the intimacy with another person that allows him to have sexual intercourse. There are many pressures on a doctor in a busy clinic. Acknowledging our own ignorance and tolerating the not knowing is much harder, but often it is so much more rewarding for both the patient and the doctor.

Case 1 illustrates some of the difficulties encountered on the conveyer belt of a routine clinic. It also demonstrates the fact that the psychosexual work can be done in this setting. The presenting complaint in this case was 'soreness', one of the commonest symptoms we deal with.

Case 1

There was another doctor sitting in with me. I asked Miss X how I could help.

'I just dropped in because my boyfriend said it was the doctor's job to sort me out.'

I felt a frisson of irritation. 'I've been going to my doctor for months now and he hasn't helped at all. It's thrush. I get it all the time. He gets blotches all over every time we have "it". It is really sore. It clears up when he uses the cream but it comes back every time. I've used all the pessaries and all the creams. I've even tried three different types of tablets. The last one the doctor said was my last chance. He said if this didn't fix it nothing would. He said I was stuck with it. We're getting married in a few months time and it's gone on too long so I thought that I'd come down here and get it sorted out. It happens every month. It spoils everything, he gets so sore every time.' My feelings waxed from a sense of 'Oh recurrent thrush no problem', and waned to 'who am I kidding, this is a no hoper'. There was desperation in the way she spoke. Doctors were no good, what on earth was I expected to do? I felt overwhelmed. Was this a clue to what she felt? 'It sounds as though you've been having a bad time. I'm surprised that you're still having sex.' 'We don't really, not any more, it's really getting him down. We're getting married in a few months', she repeated. A sense of urgency entered the room. 'Tell me what happens to you when you have the thrush.' 'Nothing happens to me, only to him.' So we talked about how sore he got and both agreed that it was awful. What a bad time he had of it. He was an invisible presence and we worried about him. It took me a few moments to realize I was being distracted from her. I was irritated with this man. 'Has he come with you?' 'No he wanted to wait and see what you found on me.'

My irritation mounted. 'That sounds as though you feel as though it's all your fault.'

'Well it is isn't it? It's him that gets sore not me.' 'You mean you are so infectious inside?' 'Well it all started with me. Everything was fine for two years and then suddenly I got thrush and its never been right since.' The sense of frustration was huge. I wondered how was I going to manage this girl who had been sent to make her man better. What was it that we were not looking at? Doctors had been doling out medicines without looking. Her GP had not examined her. The practice nurse had taken a swab on two occasions. I decided to be totally honest. I was conscious of the early timing of this disclosure. 'Let's look at what I can do for you today. I can screen you for infections. But as this problem has been going on for so long I doubt if I can come up with a cure today. But we can look at the problem together and go from there. I'll start by examining you if that's OK with you.' She relaxed some more. There was a sense of her being more in the room and there was less of her boyfriend's presence. She climbed on to the couch easily as my colleague managed the light. We looked together at her healthy normal vulva and vagina. She seemed cut off, yet there was a sense of expectation. I passed the speculum easily as she stared at the ceiling.

'I felt as though you expected me to find something nasty inside? I expect it must have been a shock for you suddenly having something go wrong down here?' She looked at me. 'Yes I couldn't understand how it got there. I mean after all we had been together for two years.' I said tentatively, 'I suppose you must have worried where it came from?' There was a painful silence. 'Yes, I thought he had been with someone else. He thought the same.' 'In fact it broke your trust in each other?' She nodded. I was still standing at the foot of the couch. She lay exposed and vulnerable, but she felt really present. Their lack of mutual trust lay between them. How was I to go from here?

She got dressed, telling me about what had happened two years ago. How the doctor had dismissed her fears and given her pessaries. How damaged she had felt inside. How horrified that something had infected her. Since then she had worried about her vagina in some way being damaging to him. How afraid she had been that he could not love her any more. I listened but had to finish the consultation as our time was up; I had of course overrun. I suggested that she could come back to see me for a longer appointment. I had to rush off, as I was late for a teaching session with the students. Another doctor had to give her the microscopy results. I was very aware that this was unsatisfactory and I thought she would not return.

I was aware of being under pressure to perform. My sense of frustration at not being there quite long enough perhaps mirrored her experience both with the doctor and this man who sent her down to be fixed. There was the unacknowledged irritation with him that I felt. There was hopelessness at the recurring nature of the soreness. Yet I felt that we began to work. It was mostly rushed, she was not sure that she wanted to play. I let her down by rushing off. I had serious other commitments to students who I felt I also let down. I had an obligation also to the doctor sitting in. Despite all this I felt that we had connected and begun to do some work. My aim then was just to start, but was it fair to do so when so limited by time? In fact she did come back for a long appointment that she had arranged and we were able to work together.

- It can be easier to 'feel' the words than to say them.
- Recurrent thrush means more than just a recurrent yeast infection.

HOMOSEXUAL PATIENTS

Patients who attend GUM clinics have a detailed sexual history taken. The purpose of this is to ascertain risk of acquisition of infection so that they can be managed appropriately. When I teach the medical students I tell them to ask all patients whether the sexual partners are male or female. This is usually greeted with various degrees of resistance and I find that role-play is helpful in illustrating the problems that can arise in the consultation when the doctor assumes that all people should be considered to be heterosexual. The group work is to think about the range of emotional responses that will be evoked by this attitude in those people who have same sex partners. There are always some students who worry about offending the 'normal' person, but who have not considered that their attitude is judgemental and offensive to particular groups of patients. If the doctor cannot acknowledge difference, how can the patient discuss their sexual problem?

Until fairly recently, homosexuality was treated as a sickness or a sin. Male homosexuality was a criminal offence in Britain until 1967 and was classified as a psychiatric disorder until 1974. There is still a discrepancy in the legal age of consent between heterosexual and male homosexual sex. Towards the latter part of the twentieth century there was a movement towards accepting that homosexuality is part of a broad range of sexual expression. As early as 1905, Freud described the concept of infantile bisexuality. In his three essays on the theory of sexuality, he explored the development of the choice of sexual object. He wrote 'a persons final sexual attitude is not decided until after puberty and is the result of a number of factors, not all of which are yet known' (Freud, 1977). Whilst there has been a growing acceptance of same sex relationships, a great deal of ambivalence and resistance still exists within the general population. Heterosexual behaviour is still presented as the more acceptable. The attitudes of our culture are internalized and are brought into the doctor–patient relationship. There is a commonly held belief that men who have sex with men have many more partners than those who have sex with women. Some work points to a tendency of lesbian women to have relatively stable long-term relationships. Together with the advent of HIV, this might explain why homosexual men have been a more visible presence in the GUM clinic than lesbian women. However, there is also substantial evidence that lesbians have, in general, satisfying sexual lives. Some clinics now offer sessions exclusively for these people.

Sexual dysfunction can occur irrespective of sexual orientation. The problem occurring in a same sex relationship may be of the same type as occurs in a heterosexual relationship, such as anorgasmia, erectile dysfunction, dyspaerunia, loss of desire or problems with arousal. However, there is a difference in prevalence. Lesbian women tend to present loss of desire and aversion to oral sex more than vaginismus and dyspareunia. One of the commonest problems in gay female relationships is loss of sexual desire. If women are socially conditioned to initiate sex less often, two women in a relationship may be expected to place less emphasis on frequency of sex (McNally and Adams, 2000). Problems associated with STIs provoke similar emotional responses, but may have a different impact in a same sex relationship. One woman who saw me for recurrent herpes found it very difficult to maintain her sexual relationship, despite having an understanding and supportive partner. It was her own difficulty around oral sex more than the fear of infecting her partner that was the main problem. Gay men may have problems dealing with the fear of acquiring HIV. Penetrative intercourse is often not the main focus of activity for gay couples and they may have a more varied repertoire than their heterosexual counterparts. Thus there might be problems unique to particular sexual practices that need to be considered in a different way. The doctor might need to recognize and challenge his or her own assumptions about homosexual behaviour. Anal intercourse is not exclusive to gay men, nor do all gay men practise it. Some men need to explore their negative feelings about this practice and understand the earlier prohibitions that are still operating. Some of this may be difficult for the doctor to listen to and it is important to recognize this (Crowley, 1995). Internalized homophobia in the patient can underlie the presenting problem, such as loss of sexual interest. The incorporation of anti-homosexual messages from parents, peers and the background culture can impede sexual functioning in gay clients. Some of these issues are illustrated in the following case.

Case 2

I saw B whilst I was still attending training seminars. I had seen him before when I treated his anal warts. This time he asked me to check inside for warts. As he got on the couch, he said 'Don't you find your job disgusting?' I said perhaps he was saying something about how he was feeling. He looked surprised and said 'perhaps'. I noticed that during the examination I said his anus looked 'pretty'. Perhaps there was a need to reassure him that this was an OK area and that this doctor was OK with it? I noticed that inserting the proctoscope was difficult and said 'You seem to be finding this uncomfortable. I wonder if it hurts when you have anal sex?' He told me he did not have penetrative sex any more because it hurt since the warts were diagnosed. He talked about anal sex and how he had previously enjoyed it. He told me of his initial disgust when he had done self-enemas. I found myself thinking that nothing he said surprised me, but I was aware that the atmosphere in the room was uncomfortable. I wondered why I seemed unable to discuss this problem. The atmosphere was becoming more uncomfortable. I was ignoring a problem that was being presented through the genital examination. What would I have said if this was a woman with dyspareunia?

'Tell me, where is the pain?' He talked about pain just inside the anal canal that made it tight, almost as though there was a blockage there. We discussed the examination and the fact that I had found everything to be normal, but that it did not feel normal to him. I wondered what he expected me to find. He said, 'Surely some scars after all that wart treatment'. I became aware that this all felt rather exciting, but also slightly dangerous. I said, 'Lots of scar tissue sounds rather fragile'. 'Yes', he said, 'it must be quite damaged and look horrid.' I reassured him, but said, 'It sounds so delicate it must be frightening to put a penis near it'. He said he thought that it might rip through his rectum, causing bleeding and pain. I said, 'It sounds almost life threatening; anal sex sounds terribly dangerous for you'. He looked relieved as he agreed. We were then able to explore how this meant he could avoid intercourse. He was able to talk about his fear of HIV and his inability to insist on condoms and how he was not quite sure of his new partner. Subsequently, he did manage to negotiate the practice of safer sex with his boyfriend.

I was excited about this male dyspareunia and took this case to my seminar training group to examine it more closely. After presenting it, I was surprised at the silence, disbelief and even hostility I encountered. There was something stopping us working as a group and focusing on the problem. The leader stepped in and highlighted this difficulty and allowed us to acknowledge that we all had different experiences of different patient populations. She pointed out that there were some strong negative feelings about this man's sexual acts. It was only after the group recognized and acknowledged this that we could look at the doctor–patient relationship properly.

I had assumed that my group worked as often with male homosexuals as I do. I had denied my own initial resistance to working with this man and this resistance was re-enacted in the group. The resistance I believe was society's attitudes to homosexuality; the denial of it and the discomfort were both mine and my patient's. He had not been able to tell his parents, as he knew they would be revolted; his father spoke openly of his disgust for buggery and his mother would be unable to cope. I nearly didn't listen hard enough to his pain and fear, partly because in genito-urinary medicine the message is very much about the risks of anal sex and partly because both his and my internalized parent were in agreement that anal sex is wrong.

- Prejudice can prevent the doctor working.
- Differences need to be acknowledged.

THE PATIENT AND HIV

Testing for HIV is an every day event in GUM clinics and the vast majority of people have negative results. It is a serological infection, which can be transmitted via the exchange of bodily fluids. The commonest route of infection is by sexual contact. Vertical transmission also occurs. The health advisor counsels those who describe significant risk behaviour and issues covered include informed consent, confidentiality, prognosis, available treatments, transmission dynamics and safer sex practices. If a diagnosis of HIV is made, there are now well-described guidelines to be followed for the management of the disease, with much practical and psychological support available. The course of this infection has changed dramatically with the introduction of antiretroviral drug therapy. There has been a huge decrease in opportunistic infections and a shift from in-patient to out-patient management. HIV-infected people are living longer and the quality of their life has improved. These people live with HIV infection, and the impact of this on their day-to-day lives and relationships has been demonstrated by the personal disclosures of a number of people in the public eye. It is not surprising that sexual dysfunction is commonly reported in this group and it can be due both to direct and indirect physical manifestations of the disease process, to the emotional impact or a mixture of both (Newsham *et al.*, 1998). Knowing that one can potentially infect the person with whom you are having sex can make it impossible to enjoy the moment.

A patient who had been HIV positive for a number of years had a new male partner. He had no problems with his erection until the moment he tried to penetrate his male partner. His fear of passing on the virus became overwhelming at that moment. For other men, this might present as anorgasmia.

The first woman whom I tested for HIV and found to be positive was a warm, caring individual who had acquired the infection abroad from a long-term partner. I saw her occasionally over the years and she managed her illness with great courage. Once she talked about contraception and we explored various methods. None suited and finally in exasperation she broke down in tears. She explained how plastic and rubber barriers made her feel contaminated. That she felt unable to allow herself to merge with her lover and how much she missed that closeness. Safe sexual practices can be experienced as intrusive in the intimacy of sex.

To make love one needs to feel loveable, and the disease process or the treatment side-effects can cause dramatic changes in physical appearance. Poor body image and psychological symptoms, such as anxiety and depression, are incompatible with feelings of sexual desire.

The anxiety around the fear of acquiring this infection is enormous. The term 'worried well' is applied to the many people who present to GUM clinics requesting screening, despite being in a very low risk group. Some will return repeatedly for tests following almost any episode of unprotected sex. It is as though they must be punished for having misbehaved.

People in this category require careful counselling, usually by a health advisor or psychologist, in order to clarify what their underlying problem is.

The fact that HIV infection can be asymptomatic for years means that some people carry the unvoiced belief that they are infected from an event in their past. Often it is a sexual encounter that they regret. This may be because it was a casual affair that was an aberration from their normal monogamy. The secret rankles and their guilt is translated into a potential fatal illness. Education, information and a tolerant non-judgemental approach are usually enough to resolve the anxiety. Sometimes it is because the sexual encounter was experienced as abusive. People who have been sexually assaulted a number of years ago often present requesting HIV screening in GUM clinics. In these cases it has been important to deny the assault and push it out of full consciousness. Presenting themselves for screening is an opportunity to access counselling and discuss the other issues involved and hopefully to move on. If the request can be thought about and spoken, then work can be done. It is more difficult when the anxiety is presented through bodily symptoms. The patient who is unable to articulate his or her fears, such as is seen in the next case, poses particular problems. It is then that the psychosexual work needs to be done.

Case 3

P had been to the clinic on five separate occasions over a period of a few months. He complained of an itchy sore penis. Nothing was ever found on his investigations. He was in a long-term happy relationship. He had been given numerous creams by his GP and ourselves, all to no avail. He was fed up. He described the soreness. 'It is there all the time and it gets worse after I have sex. All the creams are useless.' I thought he wanted to say that the doctors were useless too. He sat as though to say, 'Go on then make me better'. He denied any other sexual activity. I went through the routine of examining and testing him, knowing I would find nothing. I gave him his negative results and he sat there. He said with annoyance, 'Well what is it doctor, I am not imagining this'. I reassured him that of course the discomfort was real and that it must be spoiling things for him and his wife. He dismissed me with, 'No, sex is fine, it is just this soreness'. I tried to tease out of him some hidden anxiety, but failed. I gave up and found a cream that he had not tried before. For a moment, we were both hopeful, but I had to be honest. I said that I did not think it would work any more than the others, but he could try. If it did not help, he could come back and we could look at it from a different angle. He looked suspiciously at me and asked what I meant. I struggled as I tried to describe a possible link with the body and the mind. I talked about how we can perceive discomfort in different ways depending on how we feel inside ourselves. He left and I felt dismissed. I thought, 'I've failed'.

He returned with his soreness one month later. This time I didn't try so hard and we established that when he left the cream off things seemed a bit better. We agreed to stop the cream. There was a long silence. I wondered what he had been doing about the time the soreness started. 'Nothing' and then he paused. I remained silent. He had been in Romania, delivering a lorry load of aid to the children. He looked at me and said he had not slept with anyone else. The atmosphere in the room changed as he told me about the children and how ill they were. They were so unused to people, some had never been out of their cots. How awful their lives were. Not like his baby daughter's, she was 6 months old and he adored her; she had every thing they did not have. He had helped build a school out there. Each day the children had come out to watch, but had been scared and shy.

Finally, they had begun to sit with him. He was close to tears as he described this. There seemed to be so much pain in the room between us. I sat still listening. Most of them were HIV positive; he felt helpless, and he had to do something because they had so little, not like his daughter. I said that some people might be worried about catching HIV. He responded quickly with the fact he knew there was no risk to him. Then he paused and said that they were often covered with sores or cuts and, if they hurt themselves in the playground, he and others often washed and dressed their cuts. 'But I'm not worried for me.' Very carefully, I suggested that perhaps he was worried for his daughter. He had conceived her after the visits and he knew about vertical transmission. He sat looking at his hands and then up at me. He said that yes, he was scared that he might have HIV. That would mean that his baby might end up like those others after all. He looked frightened and relieved. I tested him. He came back a week later for his result, which was negative. His penis was better.

P knew all about the transmission dynamics of HIV. He worried his fear would be dismissed as he himself dismissed it. He therefore found it impossible to articulate. The grief that he had experienced for the dying children had been difficult to acknowledge. He had no risk factors for STDs, but had chosen to come to our clinic because his penis was sore. After all, our clinics are well known to deal with sex and HIV. The fear that he might not only have given his daughter life but also a terminal illness was too awful to bear.

- People with high-risk behaviour for acquisition of HIV should receive significant pre-test counselling.
- Anxieties about sexual issues may present as requests for HIV tests.

CONCLUSION

Sexual dysfunction occurs at all ages and in all varieties of patients. Doctors who can hear what they are saying will be told. Specialist sexual dysfunction clinics have a place, but they might lead to fragmented care. There is a need for training about sexual dysfunction across disciplines. Some patients who come to GUM clinics do so because they see it as a place where shameful secrets can be left, where there will be people who can bear the parts of themselves that society has labelled as problematic or unacceptable. The labelling and classification of people and their problems serves a purpose at times. In the practice of medicine, the diagnosis can be reached through the recognition of the patterns of symptomatology. In psychosexual medicine we cannot categorize our patients. Each case is unique unto itself. Labels can distract attention from the person to whom they are attached. We need to look beyond the shadow they cast.

A paper on 'Explorations in the uses of language in psychotherapy' reminds us of the sharp rise in anxiety as the medical attention falls on delicate matters (Havens, 1996). Drawing on Proust, the author states that the medical person looks into the flame: he does not stand aside to watch the shadows. The psychosexual doctor has to do more than just look into the flame; she or he has to risk putting a hand in to touch the patient. The pattern in this work is not elucidated by medical examination and history-taking. Neither does the doctor or patient alone reach understanding. No change in this field can occur without each doctor and patient working together. By this I mean the creation of the therapeutic space. This is the field of play into which the doctor and patient can enter safely and be creative.

The use of language in our work is of importance, as Ruth Skrine suggested in her book *Blocks and Freedoms in Sexual Life*. The words our patients and ourselves use are important in the process between us (Skrine, 1997). Words are powerful; attached to them are huge feelings that resonate in the tuning forks of our bodies. Sometimes it is easier to 'feel' the word than to speak it. The soreness and irritation, the pain, the endless tears become a continuous discharge. Our job is to translate feelings into words and words into feelings. Assisting at the delivery of the unspoken idea, just as Socrates was a midwife for the birth of latent knowledge. We can do this in the day to day work on the conveyer belt, but only as long as we do not use the existence of specialist clinics to excuse us from the work.

T.S. Eliot wrote

Birth and copulation and death,
that's all the facts when you come down to
    brass tacks ...

As doctors we deal with birth and death, the beginning, the middle and the end. Birth is a beginning and death is an ending, but the middle is about being alive. Sex or sexuality is an important part of most people's lives. As doctors, I hope we will remember this and, when needed, pay it tribute.

KEY POINTS

- Psychosexual problems are frequently presented in GUM clinics.
- Acquisition of a sexually transmitted infection may cause a psychosexual problem.
- Screening tests might be used to avoid discussing sex.
- Don't assume that your patient is heterosexual.
- Anxiety about HIV can present as a psychosexual problem.

REFERENCES

Balint, E. and Norell, J.S. (eds) 1989: *Six minutes for the patient: interactions in general practice consultation.* London and New York: Tavistock/Routledge.

Crowley, T. 1995: The doctor, the patient and the intrusive other. *Institute of Psychosexual Medicine Journal* 10, 6–8.

Crowley, T. 1998: Sexual dysfunction as presented in a routine genitourinary medicine clinic compared with that within a specialist psychosexual clinic. *Sexual Dysfunction* 1, 25–9.

Freud, S. 1977: Volume 7, *On Sexuality.* In Richards, A. and Dickson, A. (eds). Penguin Books.

Goldmeier, D., Judd, A. and Schroeder, K. 2000: Prevalence of sexual dysfunction in new heterosexual attenders at a central London genitourinary medicine clinic in 1998. *Sexually Transmitted Infections* 76, 208–9.

Havens, L. 1996: Explorations in the uses of language in psychotherapy. In Groves, J.E. (ed.), *Essential papers on short-term dynamic therapy.* New York: New York University Press, Ch. 13.

Keane, F.E.A., Carter, P., Goldmeier, D. and Harris, J.R.W. 1997: The provision of psychosexual services by genitourinary medicine physicians in the United Kingdom. *International Journal of STD & AIDS* 8, 402–4.

McNally, I. and Adams, N. 2000: Psychosexual problems. In Neal, C. and Davies, D. (eds), *Issues in therapy with lesbian, gay, bisexual & transgendered clients.* Milton Keynes: Open University Press.

Neighbour, R. 1993: *An awareness-centred approach to vocational training for general practice.* Dordrecht: Kluwer Academic.

Newsham, G., Taylor, B. and Gold, R. 1998: Sexual functioning in ambulatory men with HIV/AIDS. *International Journal of STD & AIDS* 9, 672–6.

Skrine, R. 1997: *Blocks and freedoms in sexual life. A handbook of psychosexual medicine.* Oxford: Radcliffe Medical Press, 126–31.

Winnicott, D.W. 1988: *Human nature.* London: Free Association Books.

19 The gynaecology clinic

Sue Field

Women with sexual difficulties present to the gynaecologist in several ways:

- If the presenting complaint is difficulty with sexual intercourse, this is usually thought by the patient and her GP to be due to a physical cause, often because of pain.
- The sexual problem seems to date from a gynaecological or obstetric event and is felt to have a physical basis.
- The gynaecological complaint is a 'calling card', easier to present than the underlying distress due to her own or her partner's sexual difficulties.
- The sexual problem emerges during routine history-taking or by awareness of verbal or non-verbal clues during the consultation or vaginal examination.

PHYSIOLOGY, PSYCHOLOGY OR PATHOLOGY?

The patient presents a physical symptom and expects a physical explanation and treatment, and often meets a doctor with a similar physical agenda. However, it is artificial, unhelpful and ultimately impossible to separate mind and body. Psychology, pathology and physiology interact in a way unique to each patient to produce sexual symptoms, for example:

- Pathology can directly cause sexual difficulty, which resolves when the physical problem is treated.
- Abnormal physical findings may be coincidental and unrelated to the sexual problem but are easier (for the doctor and the patient) to deal with.

- Failure of arousal and tension in the pelvic floor muscles can give rise to pain during intercourse, both superficial and deep, and cause or perpetuate physical symptoms and signs.
- Because the symptom is related to her genitalia and sexual function, the woman has feelings about it and these feelings dictate the meaning she gives to the symptom and how she seeks help.
- The physical problem may serve a purpose (perhaps not consciously), e.g. an excuse to avoid sexual contact that was unrewarding or a way to express 'unacceptable' feelings of anger against the partner. This will influence how the patient responds to treatment.
- Women who have little knowledge of or confidence in their female and reproductive function – have never explored their bodies or used tampons – are more likely to develop fantasies and fears affecting both their sexual enjoyment and the way they react to symptoms, and to expect their partner – and the doctor – to be responsible for solving the problem.
- Those who have learned to express feelings as physical discomfort will also be more likely to end up in the gynaecological clinic.
- There is increasing evidence of the interaction between ovarian hormones and neurotransmitters, and feelings may be caused by physical as well as psychological means.
- The treatment of gynaecological problems, particularly operative treatment, may have physical and psychological effects on sexual function.

THE CONSULTATION

The setting and the patient's expectations influence the doctor–patient relationship. The gynaecologist's primary obligation is to detect and treat pathology, and physical symptoms and findings must be valued. It is more difficult for the 'expert' doctor, used to clear-cut diagnoses and confident in their surgical skills, to accept that, in psychosexual understanding, with each new patient they are ignorant. With the pressure on to come up with all the answers, it is hard to avoid generalizing and putting people into neat diagnostic pigeonholes, and instead to struggle with each patient to piece together her individual 'truth'.

Previous chapters will have described how useful the psychosomatic genital examination can be in trained hands. In the gynaecology clinic, patients may misinterpret attempts to discuss or interpret their reactions during vaginal examination in terms of their sexual problems, particularly if the doctor is male. Guidelines from the RCOG state that the only time that it is appropriate to discuss sexual function during vaginal examination is when attempting to reproduce the discomfort of a woman complaining of dyspareunia (Royal College of Obstetricians and Gynaecologists, 1997). Comments made after the examination is over, as the doctor is washing his/her hands and the chaperone has left, can be useful – 'You seemed to find that unusually difficult – I wonder why . . . ?' but leaving it until the patient is fully dressed and back in the consultation room may miss the moment.

Patients are often resistant to suggestions that their emotions might have something to do with their symptoms ('Are you saying it's all in my head?'). Referral (however appropriate) to a psychosexual clinic often results in non-attendance. A pragmatic approach, combining investigation and treatment of the physical agenda, while doing psychosexual work without labeling it as such, is usually helpful. It may only be when exhaustive physical investigation and treatment have failed to cure the complaint that the patient is willing to delve more deeply into the psychosexual aspects of her problem.

Case 1

A young woman in her early twenties was referred because of profuse vaginal discharge and loss of feeling during intercourse. This seemed to date from cryotherapy for a cervical ectropion – but my clever interpretation that she might feel frozen inside fell on deaf ears. The vaginal examination, during which she was calm and relaxed, showed a mucous discharge, recurrence of the ectropion and a tender mass to the left of the uterus. She agreed that sex had sometimes been uncomfortable and not as enjoyable as previously – perhaps an ovarian cyst causing pain? Everything seemed very physical. She was referred for a scan and a review appointment in the gynaecology clinic arranged for repeat cryotherapy. The scan showed no mass (?constipation), and her ectropion was duly treated. When she came back no better, despite her cervix being nicely healed and swabs negative, review in the psychosexual clinic was arranged.

This time, she attended with her husband. She revealed further details of their sexual problem – she felt too wet and this led to reduced sensation and pleasure for both partners. The breakthrough came when I sat back and admitted there was nothing else I could think of to do physically – lack of arousal could cause loss of feeling – perhaps the way she felt about sex could have something to do with it. Was anything else going on about the time this started? 'Well, that was when he had the affair...'. Tears, anger – she had been so desperate to keep him that she had bottled up all these feelings and gone ahead with the wedding plans rather than lose face in front of the family.

Subsequently, they split up, and with a new partner sex was enjoyable. She still had a discharge, but accepted this was normal for her.

A case of her body expressing the tears she had bottled up? Or was I closer to the mark with the frozen feelings, but she wasn't ready to hear? Or perhaps her body was betraying her by showing the changes of arousal towards this man who had hurt her and who was being effectively punished by loss of sexual enjoyment.

In this chapter, the most common sexual complaints that present in the gynaecology clinic will be discussed, with consideration of the ways in which mind and body interact to produce sexual problems.

ANATOMY, CONGENITAL ANOMALIES

Fantasy or fact?

Worries about normality of the vulva and vagina may present at the gynaecology clinic. Patients with non-consummation and vaginismus often report fantasies of a barrier in the vagina or of being too small. Occasionally, they *do* have a congenital abnormality such as a vaginal septum or a hymenal band, illustrating the importance of the physical examination. If they present early, as teenagers with difficulty

using tampons or first attempts at intercourse, removal of the physical barrier usually results in resolution of the problem. However, those who present many years down the line often have superimposed psychological and psychosexual problems that have led them to avoid seeking help and deterred doctors and nurses from examining them – and these are not so easily dealt with.

Complaints that one or both labia minora are 'too large' are becoming more frequent with greater exposure to multiple sexual partners and comparison with photographs and diagrams. This anxiety may surface at puberty and may resolve as the labia majora develop fully or it may be more noticeable after childbirth or weight loss. Often there are physical effects with discomfort wearing tight clothing or horse-riding, and examination confirms the labia to be uneven, or larger than average. Most gynaecologists are understandably reluctant to operate on 'normal' anatomy, but the author's experience is that this is more akin to a request for plastic surgery. Body dysmorphic disorder must be excluded: this psychiatric condition is characterized by preoccupation with an imagined defect or grossly excessive concern about a minor abnormality. Surgery to reduce the labial size is quick and easy and the patient is usually delighted with the results.

It is more difficult to deal with complaints that the vagina is too large, especially when this is unrelated to childbirth and no abnormality is found on examination. The real symptom is of reduced sensation during penetrative vaginal intercourse and this complaint may come from either or both partners. During arousal, venous engorgement and the formation of the 'orgasmic platform' means that the vagina moulds snugly around the penis with increased pleasurable sensation for both partners, so lack of arousal may underlie this complaint. Unreal-istic expectations and ignorance may contribute to the disappointment. The underlying problem may be a true mismatch in size. We are all different – as there is a normal variation in penile and vaginal size, occasionally a man at the smaller end of the scale may encounter a woman at the larger end. A confident and loving couple will find ways to accommodate this difference and gain mutual pleasure, but it is the meaning each individual attaches to the symptom that determines whether a psychosexual problem develops – 'Am I too small/not man enough for her?' 'Am I too demanding/a loose woman/made wrong?'

Case 2

A nulliparous girl in her early twenties had requested gynaecological referral because she felt her vagina was too big and she had no sensation during intercourse. She was a plump lass, wearing a tight trouser suit and seemed to fill the room. The consultation was difficult with little eye contact and her discomfort at being there was obvious. She told me that she had had two boyfriends who had commented that she felt 'too loose' during sex and she had felt deeply humiliated by this. She felt no pleasure during penetration although foreplay and arousal were apparently not a problem. She wanted to know if anything could be done – an operation to tighten things up. All attempts to look at her feelings were fruitless. I did comment that she seemed to be taking all the blame and responsibility and maybe they were lousy lovers, 'Not man enough for you?' This fell on deaf ears; all she wanted to know was could anything be done?

So I examined her. Once again she was very tense and looked at the wall, her legs rigid and knees just parted. My comments on how difficult this seemed for her were met with silence. As I touched the entrance to her vagina, she flinched. Far from having a large vagina, she had quite marked vaginismus. 'It doesn't seem as though you have no feelings', I said, 'You seem to have some very negative feelings about yourself . . . Is this what it is like when you have sex?' But she denied this, asking again if it was too big and could I do anything. I didn't feel I could suggest she examine herself.

I retreated into reassurance, as there genuinely wasn't anything that I could do surgically and rather lamely sent her off with a leaflet on pelvic floor exercises and no follow-up. After she had left, I realized how tense I had been and felt rather shell-shocked. I also felt guilty that here was an obvious psychosexual problem that I hadn't been able to fully understand and wrote offering her a further appointment but she did not reply. I realized just how powerful she had been, keeping the consultation to her agenda, making me feel responsible and active but being left disappointed and unfulfilled herself – like her sex-life perhaps? Whatever was behind these defences was too big for her to admit to and me to get to – her need for love perhaps, or her sexuality – and had to be kept controlled and hidden.

SUPERFICIAL DYSPAREUNIA

Pain on penetration may be due to vaginismus, which in itself may be primarily a psychosexual problem or may be secondary to or perpetuate a physical problem. It is important to exclude dryness due to lack of arousal or post-menopausal atrophy – using lubricants produces wetness, but not the other manifestations of arousal such as the cushioning and sensitizing effect of vasocongestion.

Skin bridges and fissures

Patients sometimes complain of a tender skin bridge at the fourchette, possibly a variant of normal anatomy. The primary problem may be psychosexual, causing vaginismus or dryness and subsequent friction on this area, leading to superficial grazes which are acutely tender and perpetuate the problem. If intercourse was initially pain-free, it is easier to assume a psychosexual cause – the anatomy was always like that, but it didn't always hurt. There are conditions labelled as 'fragile fissuring vulva' or 'fossa navicularis syndrome', where the skin does appear to be abnormally fragile and prone to fissuring, possibly linked to friction from tight clothing, especially sportswear. There may or may not be scarring, but tenderness or splitting is found on stretching the skin. This usually responds to advice about clothing and application of 1 per cent hydrocortisone ointment, but occasionally excision of the area involved is suggested – this may leave a scar that can be equally tender.

Skin bridges can also be the cause of superficial dyspareunia after perineal suturing after childbirth or prolapse repair, and surgical restoration of normal anatomy may be necessary (Paniel, 1999). However, many women fear they have been 'stitched up wrong', when the real problem is dryness and vaginismus. Examination and particularly self-examination to demonstrate how well things have healed can be combined with exploration of their feelings about the delivery and motherhood.

Recurrent candidiasis

Vulvovaginitis due to infection with Candida is common. The itch and discharge may cause anxieties about dirtiness, smell and sexually transmitted disease and embarrassment leads to inability to discuss the problem with the partner and delay in seeking help, thus worsening the problem. The symptoms are ignored or inadequately treated by the patient for many months allowing chronic irritation and inflammation to develop, which may only be symptomatic when intercourse is attempted. Repeated attacks seem to reduce the resistance to further attacks, and the inflammation may persist long after the swabs become negative. Attempts at intercourse in a tense and unaroused state because of fear of pain perpetuate the inflammatory response and increase the risk of recurrent symptoms. Management with repeated doses of anti-fungal agents weekly for six months, with a mild steroid cream to soothe the inflammation, may be necessary. It may take some time for sexual confidence to return, and psychosexual support and encouragement to try self-examination and maximize arousal helps.

Vulvar vestibulitis

This is a syndrome characterized by entry dyspareunia, vestibular erythema (most noticeable around the openings of the vestibular and paraurethral glands) and extreme tenderness to light pressure, classically with a cotton bud.

The aetiology is uncertain. Sensitization of the pain fibres seems to occur, secondary to chronic inflammation due to trauma (intercourse) or infection (chronic candidiasis). Not surprisingly, there is severe sexual dysfunction, and attempts at intercourse in a tense, unaroused state only perpetuate the problem. Treatment with topical steroids and/or local anaesthetic cream may be combined with amitryptilene to down-regulate central neurotransmission, but works best when combined with psychosexual help to break the pain–tension vicious cycle (Schover et al., 1992).

Lichen sclerosus causes itching and sexual problems due to dryness of the vulva, narrowing of the introitus, skin bridges, loss of anatomy and burying of the clitoris in adhesions. It can occur at any age, and the classical white plaques are usually easily spotted if the patient is examined. Unfortunately, younger women may self-medicate for 'recurrent thrush' for many years before the true diagnosis is made. Treatment with potent topical steroids relieves symptoms and may restore anatomy in early cases, and is best managed in a specialist clinic.

Lichen planus is another itchy skin condition that can cause chronic vulval inflammation and dyspareunia. There is an erosive form that affects the vaginal mucosa and can cause painful adhesions. Again this is often mislabeled as 'thrush'. These conditions underline the importance of a good clinical history and examination in any woman complaining of physical symptoms and referral to a specialist Vulval Clinic if anything looks abnormal or symptoms fail to respond to treatment. Case examples that demonstrate the wide range of emotion that can cause pain are given in chapter 14.

DEEP DYSPAREUNIA

During female sexual arousal, the vagina expands and the uterus moves up out of the pelvis, causing 'ballooning' of the upper vagina. If intercourse takes place without these changes, the woman may experience pain, often described as 'feeling as if something is being knocked'. This sensation can be reproduced by moving the cervix during pelvic examination.

A careful history and examination will usually reveal clues to the underlying psychosexual problem: suppressed fear 'My mother died of cancer of the womb'; repressed grief about loss of the baby through termination expressed as tears on touching the cervix during internal palpation; anger at the partner who is pushed off and frustrated because he 'hurt her again'. In this context it is useful to consider domestic violence ('Does he hurt you in other ways?')

and previous child or adult sexual abuse which can present in the gynaecology clinic as recurrent urinary or vaginal infections, dyspareunia or unexplained pelvic pain.

Any gynaecological pathology that reduces the mobility of the uterus or means inflamed tissue is touched during penetration will cause pain, but will usually cause symptoms at other times and positive physical findings on examination. Laparoscopy is invaluable in excluding conditions such as endometriosis. This condition can be difficult to diagnose on the basis of history alone, and the extent of the disease does not correlate with the severity of symptoms. The pain of endometriosis classically occurs in a cyclical pattern, worse before and during menstruation, often associated with bowel irritation. However, deep dyspareunia may be the only symptom of an isolated lesion in the Pouch of Douglas, and in a woman with no problems with interest, arousal or orgasm and no obvious psychosexual triggers, laparoscopy is justified. A negative laparoscopy may aid resolution of the problem if specific fears about pathology are put to rest, and makes it easier to engage the patient in consideration of the psychosexual aspects of her problem. A diagnosis of endometriosis with implications for fertility and side effects of treatment may bring it's own psychosexual consequences to explore.

Pelvic venous congestion is a cause of chronic pelvic pain that causes post-coital aching (as distinct from true dyspareunia) which lasts for hours to days, but also pelvic discomfort worse premenstrually and on standing. This condition is linked to the effect of ovarian hormones on the blood vessels and cured by abolishing ovulation. Links have been proposed with 'stress' and depression and a history of sexual abuse, or possibly failure of resolution of vasocongestion during sexual arousal without orgasm – cause and effect are difficult to prove. A combined hormonal and counselling approach seems to be most effective.

Irritable bowel syndrome is linked with deep dyspareunia, possibly due to increased visceral sensitivity to stretch, or somatization. The presence of typical bowel symptoms and absence of gynaecological symptoms and signs gives the clue.

BLADDER PROBLEMS AND SEX

Post-coital cystitis

Recurrent bladder infections can be triggered by the mechanical effect of penile thrusting, which encourages bacteria from the introitus to spread up the short female urethra. Some women are particularly susceptible to recurrent urinary infection, either because they harbour more pathogenic bacteria or have reduced resistance. Anatomical variation in the site of the urethral opening may be a predisposing factor. Vaginismus will direct the angle of penetration more anteriorly, causing increased friction on the urethra and bladder base, and this will be exacerbated by lack of arousal. This may be the primary problem or may develop as a result of the repeated infections even when intercourse was initially enjoyable – the infections are seen as a 'punishment' for sexual enjoyment, there is anger at the partner who has all the fun while she suffers the after effects. General advice on hygiene for both partners to minimize any spread of bowel flora to the vulva and on voiding after intercourse can be combined with prophylactic antibiotics either nightly or after intercourse. This will be most effective when combined with consideration of the psychosexual elements.

Leaking during intercourse

It is not unusual for women with bladder neck weakness to describe involuntary loss of urine during penetration, and those with detrusor instability may experience urgency during arousal and leakage at orgasm. This loss of control, with it's connotations of babyishness and dirtiness, is very distressing to some and often not volunteered unless directly asked about. Damage to the anal sphincter at childbirth can produce incontinence of flatus or faeces during intercourse, which is even more difficult to admit to and cope with. Fortunately, treatment directed at the underlying bladder or sphincter dysfunction is usually effective (Cardozo, 1988).

Loss of fluid similar to prostatic secretion has been described at orgasm in some women (so-called female ejaculation) without other bladder symptoms and is thought to be due to stimulation of glands embryologically similar to the prostate in the G-spot. Once again, it is the meaning attached to the symptom and the feelings about it that dictate the effect on the couple's sex life – this varies from extreme anxiety at the prospect of leakage, causing avoidance of all sexual contact, to a philosophical towel on the bed – the male partner, used to the mess and wetness of ejaculation, is typically much less concerned.

THE FERTILITY CLINIC

Couples having difficulty conceiving experience many powerful emotions – shame, guilt, blame and anger, grief. The desperate desire for a child may be an avoidance of underlying relationship or personal problems.

A complaint of infertility may be the first time the couple have felt able to present nonconsummation, either due to her vaginismus or to his erectile problems or severe premature ejaculation. In around 5 per cent of couples the infertility is due to coital factors alone, and they may be relevant in many of the 25–30 per cent with 'unexplained' infertility. A detailed and sensitive psychosexual history and examination is essential, with the emphasis on what actually happens during sex. Perhaps surprisingly, some women with vaginismus may be able to undergo digital and speculum vaginal examination, but still be unable to let their partner's penis in.

The chances of conception increase the more frequently intercourse occurs – but couples 'trying for a baby' tend to reduce the frequency in the hope of maximizing their chances of conception. The emphasis on reproduction rather than fun can lead to psychosexual problems in either or both partners. It has been estimated that up to 35 per cent of couples attending for infertility investigations and treatment have sexual difficulties, with 10 per cent of men unable to perform mid-cycle and 20–25 per cent of post-coital tests negative for semen (Balen and Jacobs, 1997).

THE COLPOSCOPY CLINIC

Despite increased information and publicity, the finding of an abnormal smear and referral for colposcopy causes anxiety in many women. They may be unable to take in or fully understand explanations of 'pre-cancer' or 'wart virus', assuming that they have cancer and that their life and fertility are under threat. Because they have had no symptoms and the cervix is hidden and unfamiliar, the diagnosis comes as a shock: there is no way for them to monitor or recognize the presence or seriousness of disease, giving feelings of loss of control and confidence, and fantasies about how horrible and frightening their abnormal cervix must be (Kavanagh and Broom, 1997).

The colposcopy clinic itself can trigger the revelation of psychosexual problems. It used to be routine to ask about number of sexual partners and age at first intercourse, thereby confirming the woman's fears that this was a punishment for promiscuity and sometimes provoking tearful revelations of childhood sexual abuse. All the feelings triggered by a normal vaginal examination can be magnified by the experience of colposcopy with the loss of control and passivity of using stirrups and exposure, often to several members of staff, combined with fear of cancer and treatment.

Seeing her cervix on the monitor can replace the woman's fantasies of horrible growths with the reality of small areas of white skin. Worries about being 'burned' by the laser or anxieties about healing after a biopsy or loop excision can be dispelled by the same means when she returns for follow-up, but may contribute to

sexual difficulties until the 'all-clear' is given. Long-term sexual difficulties are uncommon nowadays, perhaps reflecting improved awareness of the implications of an abnormal smear. However, some women will be particularly vulnerable, including those with limited understanding or to whom the diagnosis has some specific meaning, often those whose anxieties and fantasies prevent them attending for screening, treatment or follow-up.

EFFECTS OF GYNAECOLOGICAL PROCEDURES

Sterilization

Female sterilization is an increasingly popular method of contraception. Prospective studies have shown no increase in psychological or psychosexual distress after sterilization in the majority of women, and freedom from worries about pregnancy may lead to more frequent and enjoyable intercourse (Oates and Gath, 1989).

It is now well recognized that regrets are more likely if the sterilization is done at a time of stress, e.g. immediately after delivery or at the time of termination of pregnancy, and such situations are now rare. A sterilization may be requested in the hope of improving pre-existing relationship or sexual problems or because of failure to find a suitable alternative contraception, rather than from a true desire to have a permanent procedure. In her desperation to get what she sees as the answer to her problems, the patient may hide or belittle relationship problems – the doctor may feel the pressure and be alerted to the possibility of a hidden agenda. She may reveal underlying resentment or scorn in the way she responds to routine questioning about the possibility of her partner having a vasectomy instead. The woman who requests an operative procedure may be someone to whom control and certainty are important, or who passively wants someone else to take responsibility for her fertility – any subsequent sexual problems may be due to her underlying personality traits.

The loss of fertility can cause difficulties when sexual activity was endured because of the hope of pregnancy or there is underlying guilt at sexual enjoyment 'just for fun'. A decision to opt for sterilization may be made rationally and women may be surprised at the strength of subsequent feelings of bereavement at the loss of the possibility of further babies, particularly if they felt pressurized by their partner or medical staff into having the procedure.

Hysterectomy

From an anatomical viewpoint, removal of the uterus and cervix changes the relationship between bladder, bowel, ovaries (if conserved) and the vaginal vault. Extensive dissection can disrupt the autonomic nerves of the pelvic plexus, causing changes in sensation and theoretically compromising sexual response. It has been suggested that subtotal hysterectomy, where the cervix is not removed, is less likely to result in dysfunction both sexually and of bladder and bowel. It has also been suggested that removal of the cervical mucous glands may reduce vaginal lubrication (Thakar et al., 1997). These theories have not been borne out by studies comparing hysterectomy with endometrial ablation and subtotal with total hysterectomy, which show rather that women find their sexual enjoyment is unchanged or improved after simple hysterectomy for benign disease. In fact, several areas in the anterior vaginal wall including the 'G-spot' have been shown to be sensitive to sexual stimulation with the cervix less so, and 'internal' orgasm is still possible after removal of the uterus and cervix. Simple hysterectomy will not affect the sensitivity of the clitoris, vulva and introitus, so important to most women's sexual enjoyment, and cervical secretions make little or no contribution to vaginal lubrication during sexual arousal. There is no doubt, however, that some women (and their partners), whose internal sensations involved pressure on a retroverted, fibroid or prolapsed womb, will notice a difference after hysterectomy which may be distressing if they are unprepared for this.

Removal of their womb has emotional significance for most women, involving as it does loss of fertility, the monthly rhythm of periods, and feelings about femininity and sexuality. There may be relief at freedom from the nuisance of bleeding and pain, worries about contraception or unwanted childbearing. Other women will go through a bereavement reaction, sometimes surprising their rational selves by the strength of their emotions over the loss of an organ that was causing problems, diseased or superfluous. These 'illogical' feelings may be repressed, but surface uncomfortably during sexual contact. The sense of loss may be expressed as a fantasy of a 'black hole', an emptiness or 'something missing' inside, worries about where the sperm go and that the top of the vagina remains open, so that intercourse might somehow involve poking around the bowel or bladder. These images may lead to avoidance of sexual contact or lack of arousal, which then means they really do 'feel nothing inside' thus setting up a vicious cycle of disappointment and further avoidance. Discussion during vaginal examination, including self-examination, will help to replace fantasies with reality. It is important to remember that the partner may have his own fantasies and fears which may result in him being less forceful or even losing his erection during penetration, all contributing to loss of sensation in the woman (Tunnadine, 1996).

Some women without pathology seem determined to have a hysterectomy and reject alternative treatments. Underlying this may be a deep unhappiness with their femininity, possibly due to sexual disappointment or a desperate need to control the messy emotional business of hormones, bleeding, weakness – all easier to express as physical complaints focused on the womb. In their determination to get rid of the offending organ, they may escalate their subjective complaints and the gynaecologist feels great pressure to operate. Confrontation is unhelpful and one tactic is to agree in principle, then talk about it. A comment such as 'It's not much fun for you being a woman . . . ' may open up a discussion of feelings and expectations, and attention to the clues during vaginal examination can also be helpful. Ultimately all that may be possible is to ensure that she appreciates what hysterectomy can and cannot achieve. Relationship problems, low self-esteem, a stressful life and pelvic pain and dyspareunia without organic cause are unlikely to be cured by hysterectomy, but no more periods and no more pregnancies can be guaranteed. Unrealistic expectations will contribute to later regrets and ongoing symptoms.

Oophorectomy, hormones and libido

Hysterectomy may be combined with removal of the ovaries, and even if the ovaries are conserved, they tend to fail some 4–5 years earlier after hysterectomy than they would have done naturally. Women who have had a hysterectomy may be less likely to be aware of or ask for help with menopausal symptoms, including loss of interest in sex or vaginal dryness. For the woman still menstruating, the sudden dramatic drop in oestrogen levels of a surgical menopause means that symptoms are often more severe than those of the natural climacteric, and because they are used to higher levels of circulating oestrogen, they may need higher than usual doses of hormone replacement therapy. Adequate levels of oestrogen are important in sexual behaviour, affecting brain function, and the senses of smell and touch so important in finding the sexual partner attractive, as well as peripheral response to sexual stimulation. It is always worthwhile checking the serum FSH level in any woman who has had a hysterectomy and presents with sexual problems to be sure that she is on adequate hormone replacement (Khastgir and Studd, 1999).

The ovaries also produce around half the total circulating androgens in women, and oophorectomy reduces androgen levels below those experienced after natural menopause. While there is no evidence linking levels of androgens to sexual behaviour in menstruating women, some women on oestrogen-only HRT do report loss of libido that dates from loss of their ovaries, with no other obvious psychosexual problems. Possibly some women are used to relatively higher levels within the normal range, or are more sensitive to the effects of testosterone on sexual desire. Androgen replacement may be useful in these women and can be achieved using testosterone implants or tablets in combination with oestrogen. An alternative is to use tibolone, which closely mimics ovarian function, having oestrogenic, androgenic and progestagenic actions. There is no reason why tibolone cannot be used in hysterectomized women, but younger women whose ovaries have been removed may need additional oestrogen supplementation to prevent hot flushes.

Of course, hormones have only a small part to play in the complex interaction between mind, body and partner that translates into a satisfactory sexual experience. A woman on adequate doses of oestrogen and testosterone may find her increase in dreams and fantasies does not translate into increased frequency of intercourse – and may then be more open to a psychosexual approach to consider why she doesn't want to have sex with her partner.

Effects of gynaecological cancer

A diagnosis of gynaecological cancer strikes to the heart of a woman's sexual and female identity. Often, the impact on sexuality is not fully appreciated until the initial pre-occupation with the shock of diagnosis and issues of survival and coping with treatment have passed, and the patient is pronounced cured or in remission. It has been shown that sexual dysfunction develops early and is unlikely to resolve over time without specific treatment (Crowther et al., 1994).

Studies looking at sexual function after gynaecological cancer have tended to concentrate on the ability to have penetrative intercourse rather than the overall quality of physical intimacy and pleasure which is more important to many couples after a life-threatening illness (Bos, 1986). Women may press for reconstructive surgery or continue to have unrewarding coitus because of a desire to please or keep their partner or to pretend they are 'back to normal', or may use the cancer as an excuse to avoid intercourse which had never been enjoyed.

Treatment may involve radical surgery (removal of uterus, ovaries and upper vagina, vulval skin and clitoris or total exenteration), radiotherapy or chemotherapy with accompanying changes in physical function and body image. Physical effects of treatment on sexuality may be general, such as fatigue, nausea or diarrhoea, or specific, including changes in sensory perception, loss of uterine and cervical sensations, reduction in vaginal capacity and lubrication, loss of orgasmic capacity, hormonal effects on libido, limitation of movement due to scarring or lymphoedema, urinary incontinence. Women undergoing radiotherapy are encouraged to persist with intercourse or use dilators, but without understanding the feelings around this, it is not surprising that the advice may be ignored. It may be difficult to disentangle in each individual woman how much her symptoms are due to physical changes and how much to her feelings interfering with desire and arousal.

These feelings may include change in her and her partner's perception of herself as a woman, as a sexual, attractive and desirable being. Anxieties that sex may have caused the cancer (not unfounded in the case of cervical malignancy) and may therefore transmit it to the partner or cause recurrence are not uncommon, as are worries that radioactivity may harm him. Associated feelings of guilt about punishment for past sexual misdeeds (particularly if enjoyable) may combine with anger and blame towards the partner who 'gave it to me'. However, couples who have previously been confident and secure within the relationship and with their sexuality will be more motivated, able to communicate and experiment to work out for themselves a satisfactory way of achieving mutual sexual pleasure.

The bodily changes involve loss not just of organs but of fertility, menstruation, hormones and the sadness and anger of this bereavement can be difficult to express, particularly to the doctors who 'saved her life' or family who feel she should be grateful and get back to her old self. She and her relationship and sex-life will never be the same again – for a while, the relationship of adult–child or carer–patient that prevails during acute ill health makes intercourse seem inappropriate. This may persist in one partner's mind longer than the other's. Many couples report a shift from quantity to quality, the emphasis transferring from intercourse to other ways of expressing affection, with improvement in the relationship and real intimacy.

Because of feelings of shame surrounding the genital area and sexuality, some women will find it very difficult to discuss these areas with an existing partner or to expose her scars and feelings to a new partner, and young single women are particularly likely to develop problems.

There is a need for detailed factual information both before and after surgery or radiotherapy, with frank discussion of possible effects on sexual function available for both partners. They may not be able to take this in immediately and written information, including how to ask for help, can be taken away for future use. The doctors reviewing the patient at follow-up visits may feel reticent to ask about sexual matters, perhaps feeling guilt at being the 'cause' of any problems and not confident in their abilities to manage them. A psychosexual approach could involve uncovering the feelings interfering with arousal and enjoyment, questioning assumptions and giving permission to the couple to 'work it out for themselves' and the therapeutic use of the psychosomatic genital examination to help them come to terms with the physical changes and appreciate what is reality and what is fantasy.

CONCLUSION

Training in psychosexual medicine is invaluable for the gynaecologist. We may feel that there is not enough time in a busy clinic to deal with the hidden agenda. But useful psychosexual work can be done in a brief consultation ('It only takes a moment to switch on a light...') or during a routine vaginal examination and much time saved by avoiding unnecessary repeat visits, investigations or surgery.

KEY POINTS

- Gynaecological pathology and treatments can directly cause sexual difficulty, and discussion of sexual matters should be considered in every gynaecological consultation.
- Psychosexual problems may cause or perpetuate physical symptoms.
- Patients' feelings about their reproductive organs influence their presentation and attitudes to treatment.
- Separation of mind and body is unhelpful and often impossible – treat individuals, not bodies.
- Attempting to understand the 'hidden agenda' saves time by avoiding unnecessary intervention and follow-up.

REFERENCES

Balen, A. and Jacobs, H. 1997: *Infertility in practice.* London: Churchill Livingstone.

Bos, G. 1986: Sexuality of gynaecologic cancer patients: quality and quantity. *Journal of Psychosomatic Obstetrics and Gynaecology* 5, 217–24.

Cardozo, L. 1988: Sex and the bladder. *British Medical Journal* 296, 587–8.

Crowther, M.E., Corney, R.H. and Shepherd, J.H. 1994: Psychosexual implications of gynaecological cancer. *British Medical Journal* 308, 869–70.

Kavanagh, A.M. and Broom, D.H. 1997: Women's understanding of abnormal cervical smear test results: a qualitative interview study. *British Medical Journal* 314, 1388–91.

Khastgir, G. and Studd, J. 1999: Hormonal replacement therapy after hysterectomy. *Contemporary Reviews in Obstetrics and Gynaecology* 11(2), 119–27.

Oates, M. and Gath, D.E. 1989: Psychological aspects of gynaecological surgery. *Clinical Obstetrics and Gynaecology* 3(4). London: Balliere Tindall.

Paniel, B.J. 1999: Surgical procedures in benign vulval disease. In Ridley, C.M. and Neill, S.M. (eds), *The vulva.* London: Blackwell Science.

Royal College of Obstetricians and Gynaecologists 1997: *Intimate examinations. Report of a working party.* London: RCOG Press.

Schover, L.R., Youngs, D.D. and Cannata, R. 1992: Psychosexual aspects of the evaluation and management of vulvar vestibulitis. *American Journal of Obstetrics and Gynaecology* 167, 630–6.

Thakar, R., Manyonda, I., Stanton, S.L. *et al.* 1997: Bladder, bowel and sexual function after hysterectomy for benign conditions. *British Journal of Obstetrics and Gynaecology* 104, 983–7.

Tunnadine, P. 1996: Psychosexual aspects of hysterectomy. *Journal of Obstetrics and Gynaecology* 16, S6–9.

20 The psychosexual medicine clinic

Helen Hutchinson

Case 1

Mrs A has been attending the family planning clinic since her marriage three years ago. She has met Dr B several times, and has found her easy to talk to. On this occasion Mrs A has come for a cervical smear, and has specifically requested that Dr B should take it. In the consultation the doctor notices that Mrs A appears much more tense than usual. Discovering that this is her first smear, she asks if Mrs A has any questions before they proceed. Mrs A shakes her head. Once on the couch Mrs A seems very anxious, but when Dr B comments on this the only response is a half-smile. However, when the doctor asks Mrs A to separate her legs, she actually moves them tightly together. Dr B observes, 'It seems difficult for you to tell me how scared you are about this test – but your body is showing me how frightened you are. I wonder if there are also difficulties in your sexual relationship which you find it hard to talk about?' And so, then and there, with Mrs A sitting huddled on the examination couch, the story of her unconsummated marriage is revealed. The doctor and the patient have already started to work together on the problem.

Mrs A had chosen the doctor in whom she wished to confide her problem, and also the timing of her confidence. She chose to use a request for a smear as a way to reveal her difficulties, although this choice may have been less than conscious. There can be little doubt that, from the patient's point of view, these constitute the ideal conditions in which to work on her problem. Indeed, it was for just such situations – the presentation of sexual difficulties within the context of the doctor's ordinary work, be it general practice, family planning, GU medicine or gynaecology – that the training provided by the Institute of Psychosexual Medicine was developed.

However, not all doctors have an interest in this area of human interaction, and fewer still have been trained to deal effectively with such problems within the time constraints of normal medical practice. The psychosexual medicine clinic acts as a resource for referral: for those patients whose initial choice of confidant has been unable to take matters further, and for those with particularly complex problems which need more time than is likely to be available in the primary care setting, or the busy hospital outpatient clinic.

In this situation the relationship between the patient and the doctor is clearly different. The patient cannot choose the doctor in whom he wishes to confide; neither can he choose the timing of his revelations. Both doctor and patient know, from the outset of their first consultation, that they are there to focus on the sexual difficulty; there can be no escape, for the patient who gets cold feet, into a pretence that the real reason for his appointment was to discuss his sore throat, or bad back, or whatever.

THE EFFECTS OF REFERRAL ON THE PATIENT

So what sort of reactions do patients have when a referral to a psychosexual clinic is suggested? Some feel relief that their problem is being taken seriously, whilst others worry that perhaps their difficulty isn't really important enough to justify referral to a 'specialist'. Some may be anxious about having to talk about such private matters to a stranger; others welcome the opportunity to discuss, with just such a stranger, with whom they will not have an ongoing association, feelings which they would feel uncomfortable sharing with their 'cradle-to-grave' GP. Many, having plucked up the courage to reveal their problem, often after a considerable period of suffering, are most distressed at the idea of having to wait some time before they can be seen at the specialist clinic. Some believe that such clinics will insist on the involvement of their partner, and may worry that the partner will not cooperate, or that they will be forced to share, with that partner, feelings, fears and doubts which they wish to keep to themselves. Many are put off by the title 'psychosexual', believing that they are being sent to see a psychiatrist and that the implication is that they are mentally ill.

Some of these anxieties can be addressed if the referring doctor is willing to take time to explain the nature of the clinic to the patient, and an explanatory leaflet, sent from the clinic to the patient as soon as the referral is received, can be helpful. Such a leaflet may also acknowledge patients' fears about confidentiality. The idea that information about their private, sexual life will be written in hospital or clinic notes, and that detailed accounts will be sent back to the GP (to be read by others in the practice?) can be most alarming.

THE EFFECTS OF REFERRAL ON THE DOCTOR

The doctor, too, is changed by this role of 'specialist resource'. It is more difficult to be a co-seeker for truth, alongside the patient and equally unknowing at the outset, if one has been labelled 'an expert'. Medical specialists, in general, provide diagnoses and give treatments to relatively passive patients, whose only real choice may be over which, if any, treatment to accept. This is far removed from what we have come to understand as the basis of psychosexual medicine, which requires at least half the work to be done by the patient.

The doctor is likely to know more about the referrer than she does about the patient. She may trust this particular doctor to refer suitable patients, or be aware of a tendency to try to 'dump' impossible cases at her door. She may especially wish to impress a certain referrer with her cleverness, empathy or understanding. Any of this can affect the doctor–patient interaction before the two even meet.

When they do meet, it is the doctor's task to rapidly establish a working relationship with the patient, knowing that he has not been able to positively choose her as the doctor to whom to confide his difficulties. And there are unlikely to be any second chances. In primary care, if the doctor fails to pick up some of the patient's communications in a particular consultation, she can reasonably assume that the patient will return at some point in the future and she can try again. The patient who has not felt understood in the psychosexual clinic is unlikely to return for a further appointment.

Each doctor working in a referral clinic needs to decide whether to attempt to give the patients some idea of what to expect at the clinic before they attend. Should she send a letter or leaflet explaining the way she works, or is it better to allow this to emerge as the consultation progresses? Could too much prior information interfere with the work? On the other hand, perhaps too little will lead to a patient who is so anxious about what may happen at the clinic that no work can be done at all in the consultation.

The doctor must also decide on a policy for those who do not attend, or who cancel at short notice. For many patients their ambivalence about attendance is a mirror of their sexual difficulty. Ideally, this can be acknowledged, and eventually worked with, in the later consultations between doctor and patient. However, in the referral clinic, the doctor does not just have a responsibility to a particular ambivalent patient – there is an equal responsibility to

those other patients on the waiting list who miss out while the reluctant attender is given another chance. Some services try to tackle this issue by including in their patient information leaflet a recognition that it can be difficult to find the courage to attend, but that the first step is usually the hardest. Others will make direct statements about the needs of patients who are waiting to be seen, and have a policy of only accepting last minute cancellations in an emergency.

Clinic doctors also need to balance the interests of the patient and those of the referrer. How much should be included in the doctor's letter back to the referring clinician? Some write very full accounts, believing that in this way they educate the referrer about how they work and ensure suitable referrals in the future. Other doctors feel that great detail about very private and personal matters is inappropriate, believing that the patient is likely to have told, in their initial consultation, as much, or as little, as they wish that particular doctor to know.

SURVEY OF DOCTORS WORKING IN REFERRAL CLINICS

The Institute of Psychosexual Medicine (IPM) is a training organization, not a service provider. Doctors who have undertaken the training, and passed the assessment leading to Membership of the Institute, will be using their skills in their ordinary work setting and some will also be working in psychosexual medicine clinics. The IPM does not run these clinics, although it will provide enquirers with a list of clinics in which IPM members are known to work.

In order to be able to present the reader with reliable information about the organization of psychosexual medicine clinics, the author undertook a questionnaire survey of IPM-trained doctors working in such clinics at the end of 1999. Replies were received from 62 doctors, some of whom were working in more than one clinic, although not all questions were answered by all respondents. The IPM has a current membership of between 120 and 130 fully qualified (through membership assessment) doctors, about 75 of whom are registered as running referral clinics. The questionnaire survey should, therefore, provide a representative account of just what goes on in these clinics. Any numbers or percentages given in the rest of this chapter will refer to this survey, unless otherwise stated.

THE DOCTORS

This work is predominantly done by women. Only five of the surveyed doctors were male, a similar proportion to the current members list. Only 15 per cent of the doctors surveyed regarded psychosexual medicine as their main area of medical work, whereas 50 per cent regarded this as being family planning, 20 per cent worked mainly in genito-urinary medicine and 15 per cent in general practice. Thirty-eight doctors only saw psychosexual patients in NHS settings, six only saw private patients, and the remaining 18 worked in both the NHS and the private sector. The information that follows refers to the NHS clinics.

Half the doctors were working in referral clinics for only one session each week, with a further third undertaking two sessions. Only three doctors did this work at anything approaching half-time (four or five sessions). Reflecting this, 40 per cent saw less than 50 new patients a year, and less than 10 per cent saw more than 150.

The doctors were largely middle-aged, two thirds being in their forties or fifties. There may be some cause for concern with regard to the future of these clinics if younger doctors find it difficult to make the time for the training, or find that their working schedule does not allow space for some sessional work.

The IPM regards the appropriate qualification for referral work as the Membership (there is also a diploma qualification for those using their skills in their own clinical work). The further training that leads doctors towards the Membership involves greater examination of such processes as defences in both doctor and patient, and a greater awareness of unconscious factors operating in the patient. It can be difficult for doctors to meet such cases in their normal work setting and some are tempted into running referral clinics before their training is completed. This may happen not just as a result of the doctor's desire to gain more experience, but also because of pressure from the employer. When an IPM doctor retires from a special session, there is a real risk that the service may be lost forever if a new recruit is not found immediately. Fifty-five per cent of doctors responding to the survey had not begun to work in specialist clinics until after they had passed the Membership assessment. Twenty-five per cent had started one or two years ahead of this, suggesting that they were indeed looking for the greater experience necessary to prepare them for the Membership. The other 20 per cent had been seeing referrals for some considerable time before passing the Membership examination. The seminar training system developed by the IPM (see the Appendix) does not provide 'supervision' of the doctor's work. When doctors start to take referrals before they have qualified, it may be that they should establish an appropriate supervision system – this should be the responsibility of the employing authority. It may be difficult to organize in areas where doctors are working in isolation – less than half the doctors surveyed worked in services that employed other IPM doctors.

Although 70 per cent of the clinics are able to accept self-referrals, the vast majority of patients have, in fact, been referred by a doctor or other professional. The clinician who is considering such a referral needs to know about the provision of psychosexual medicine clinics in his area.

CLINIC AVAILABILITY AND ORGANIZATION

The IPM list of clinics in which its Members work includes clinics in all NHS regions. However, the reality is that the vast majority are in London and the Home Counties, and in many areas provision of services is very thin on the ground. This adds further to the difficulties of the patient, who may have to travel long distances to be seen, involving considerable time off work, and for a reason that he may not wish to reveal to his employer. Many use up their holiday allowance in order to be able to visit the clinic discreetly.

Once a referral is received, 30 per cent of clinics contact the patient and require them to make a positive move to obtain an appointment, either by returning a form or phoning the clinic. Those who employ this strategy believe it considerably reduces the number who fail to attend a first appointment. Thirty per cent simply send an appointment and accept the 'do not attends' (DNAs), whilst the other 40 per cent send an appointment and ask the patient to confirm that they will attend. DNAs are common in all areas of medicine that relate to emotional issues. They are, perhaps, even more common when the area involved is the essentially private one of sexual expression. Patients may lose their nerve after a referral that they had agreed to; others may only have agreed in the first place to please the referring doctor. Some psychosexual doctors have found higher DNA rates (or failures to make an appointment when this responsibility is given to the patient) when the referral has been made by a hospital doctor than when it has been made from primary care. It may be that the patient is particularly anxious to please the hospital doctor; it may be that, having already been referred to a specialist and not found an answer to their problem, they despair of ever finding a solution; it could be that hospital staff do not explain fully how they think the psychosexual clinic might help; and it could be that the hospital clinician actually sees the clinic as a dumping ground for awkward patients, and that this view is communicated to the patient.

It has already been suggested that, for the patient who has plucked up the courage to confide his sexual difficulty to a doctor, the waiting time to see another doctor can be a considerable trial. Unfortunately, few clinics are able to see patients very quickly after referral. Only 14 per cent of surveyed doctors were able to see a new patient within a month. A total of 70 per cent would normally be able to offer a first appointment within 3 months of a referral. Four doctors, however, had waiting lists of greater than 6 months, the longest being 18 months! Five services had received some recent increase in funding to attempt to reduce waiting lists; an equal number had experienced recent actual or proposed cuts to their service.

The location of the psychosexual medicine clinic is within a family planning centre in 65 per cent of cases. In a further 12 per cent, the clinics are held in gynaecology outpatients. These traditionally female settings may be presenting yet another hurdle to the approximately 50 per cent of referred patients who are men. Nine per cent of clinics are held in GU or sexual health services, 6 per cent in general practice; two are held in urology clinics (as part of an erectile dysfunction service), and one each in a psychiatric outpatient clinic, a private hospital and a rehabilitation unit.

Twenty-nine doctors work alongside others. Eighty per cent of these are other IPM doctors, either qualified or in training; five work with nurses who have had similar training, five with behavioural therapists and two with psychiatrists. (Some services had several different professionals involved.) With multidisciplinary teams it is more likely that the patient will have an initial assessment interview before being allocated to a particular professional for ongoing therapy.

APPOINTMENTS AND DURATION OF TREATMENT

The vast majority of doctors surveyed give the patient a first appointment and allocate subsequent appointments on an ad hoc basis at later visits. A few give an early initial appointment for assessment, with further consultations being arranged some weeks later according to the length of the waiting list. Three doctors allocate a series of appointments at the outset of treatment.

The time allocated for first appointments was 30 minutes in 12 per cent of cases, 30–45 minutes in 44 per cent, and up to an hour in a further 44 per cent. This may seem to be great luxury to those used to the short consultations of primary care, but clearly some time has to be spent at the outset on developing a working relationship. Subsequent appointments tend to be shorter.

The work done in psychosexual medicine clinics is short term and focused on the sexual difficulty. Sixty per cent of the doctors see the majority of their patients only three or four times; a further 30 per cent usually have five or six meetings. Most have a few patients who need a more prolonged relationship with the doctor, but in all cases this a small proportion of the total. The largest group seen for a prolonged period (25 per cent) were the patients of a doctor who is also a trained and practising psychotherapist, presumably seeing some very complex cases.

The focus of the work in psychosexual medicine clinics, as in other settings, is the study, by the doctor, of the doctor–patient interaction and particularly of that interaction at the time of the genital examination, with subsequent interpretation of the doctor's understanding of these events to the patient. The patient is then free to use these interpretations to gain insight into the origins of his particular difficulties. Many doctors do, however, sometimes make use of other skills in their work in referral clinics. Fifty-five per cent would either prescribe, or advise the prescription of, sildenafil (Viagra) in some cases; 55 per cent would prescribe or advise other 'physical' treatments for erectile dysfunction; 65 per cent would sometimes make use of simple behavioural techniques, for example, to overcome 'performance anxiety'; 65 per cent sometimes get involved in 'relationship counselling', with the emphasis temporarily removed from the sexual. Over a quarter of respondents will at times be involved in all four of these related activities, whilst only two said they never use any of them.

SUITABLE PATIENTS FOR REFERRAL

The most important factor when deciding whether a patient is suitable for referral to a psychosexual medicine clinic is the extent to which he accepts that sex is a psychosomatic event; that bodily sexual reactions occur in response to feelings, and that other feelings can block these reactions. If the patient is unable to accept that attendance at the clinic will involve the examination of his feelings, then referral is pointless. He must also understand that *he* will be doing the work both during and between the consultations – this is not a situation where the patient turns himself over to the doctor to be 'cured'.

It has already been made clear that the work in these clinics is short term and that the doctors have been trained to look very specifically at the sexual area of the patient's life. Most have no psychiatric training, or training in marital therapy. It follows that, to be helped by such doctors, the patients should be functioning reasonably 'normally' in most areas of their lives, but with a difficulty in the sexual arena. Most psychosexual doctors would not have anything to offer patients with personality disorders, patients who are currently psychiatrically ill, couples with relationship difficulties, or people with gender dysphoria. Since the work involves talking about feelings, the doctor and patient also need to be able to communicate in the same language; interpreters can rarely convey the nuances of emotional expression which can be so important in understanding the patient's problem.

The clinic doctor is clearly dependent on the referring doctor providing appropriate information about the patient – much time may be wasted by both patient (including the time he spends on a waiting list) and doctor if unsuitable referrals are accepted. It is sometimes possible for the psychosexual doctor to recognize an inappropriate referral from the letter. The clinic doctor rejected the following referral, for example, without seeing the patient: 'This 58-year-old lady often talks about her sexuality, and that she has no feeling 'down below' any more, and is desperate for help with this. She was apparently fine psychologically up until three years ago, when she lost her job. At that time she saw a psychotherapist whom she now talks about in very unfavourable terms, saying that she hypnotized her against her will, then sexually abused her and caused a large number of apparently unrelated bodily symptoms. She has been seen by the psychiatrists who think she probably has a severe personality disorder of the paranoid type, or possibly a paranoid psychosis.'

This patient was clearly unsuitable for treatment in a psychosexual medicine clinic because of her underlying psychological disorder. However, she also illustrates the need for the psychosexual doctor to protect herself from accusations of sexual 'abuse'. With this patient's history of allegations against the psychotherapist, the use of the genital examination, so much the focus of psychosexual work, would obviously be potentially dangerous for the doctor. Sometimes the doctor needs to protect herself not from allegations of abuse from a patient, but from personal abuse *by* a patient. The following referral was also turned down, by a doctor who worked in an entirely female environment and who recognized that she would be unwise to try to use the genital examination as a psychosomatic event with this patient: 'This man would like help with his premature ejaculation. He has a diagnosis of personality disorder, and is frequently depressed. Since the breakup of his marriage, finding a new relationship has been his major concern. Unfortunately he made advances towards one of our practice nurses which resulted in us deciding he should only see male doctors at the practice. This has aggravated him quite a lot. I would suggest that if you have access to a male counsellor, this might be more appropriate for him given his recent history.'

Sometimes the referring doctor, whilst having several pieces of information about a patient, appears not to have put them together. A consultant gynaecologist asked a psychosexual doctor to see one of his private patients to talk

over her request for a hysterectomy. The patient was 20 years old and the gynaecologist was concerned that she 'might in the longer term come to regret the procedure'.

The gynaecologist reported that the patient had always seen her menses as an 'unnecessary intrusion' in her life. She was clear that she never wished to have a sexual relationship with either a male or female partner, nor did she want to have children. She described a very negative attitude to periods from an early age, certainly from before puberty. Elsewhere in the letter the consultant stated that the patient also wanted breast reduction, but felt this might be more difficult to arrange than hysterectomy.

The psychosexual doctor replied that she did not feel she was suitably qualified to help this patient, and suggested she should be referred for assessment by a psychiatrist with an interest and expertise in gender dysphoria.

Even mental health professionals may sometimes have a strange view that sexual difficulties are in some way separate from the overall psychological difficulties of their patients. A senior psychologist referred a patient to whom he was planning to offer 'a course of interpersonal therapy' to tackle her obsessional jealousy of her husband and her obsessional tidying of their home. The psychologist felt the origins of her problems were in her relationship with her mother, from whom she had learned to feel inferior and unlovable. However, he also wished to refer her to the psychosexual clinic, as she was unable to experience orgasm with her husband, although she was orgasmic on her own.

The psychosexual doctor replied that it would seem clear that the patient's inability to enjoy orgasm with her husband was due to her great difficulty in trusting herself to anyone, and in feeling safe and secure with anyone. If it was possible to effect some changes in these areas during her psychological therapy, then the orgasmic difficulty was likely to resolve; if not, then the doctor would be pleased to see the patient at this stage, but not before.

It is not always possible to predict unsuitability for treatment from the referral, however.

Case 2

C was a 19-year-old student, referred by her GP with a problem of vaginismus. The doctor commented C was enjoying her life as a student, and her academic studies, but was very upset by her inability to have intercourse in a previous relationship, and keen to seek help. The psychosexual doctor felt this was a very suitable referral, with an apparently well-motiv-ated patient, and arranged to send an appointment.

Before C received the appointment, however, she turned up at one of the doctor's family planning clinics, saying she needed to meet the doctor before she went home for the long summer vacation. She told the doctor that she had never been able to use tampons and had been unable to allow penetration by her previous boyfriend. She thought her difficul-ties were due to her father's negative attitudes towards boyfriends, and to problems in her relationship with her stepmother (her real mother had died of breast cancer when C was 2 years old).

The doctor offered to examine her. This resulted in copious tears when the doctor's fin-ger touched the introitus. With the vacation about to start, the doctor decided to withdraw at this point, rather than risk starting to look at issues which would then not be able to be pursued in the following three months. She arranged to see C again at the beginning of the autumn term, but was later interested to see that in her notes from this first consultation she had described a sense of 'little girl frustration' about C's tears.

The following term the doctor saw C five more times at weekly intervals (much more fre-quently than she usually sees patients). It gradually became clear to the doctor that C was behaving like a small child in their consultations, constantly demanding more and more attention and forever repeating 'it isn't fair' in relation both to her sexual problem and to her relationships with both family and friends. The doctor felt increasingly that she was dealing with an emotional 2-year-old, lost in an adult body and with an adult intellect, and won-dered whether C's difficulties actually went back to her mother's death. Fortunately, she was able to arrange, with the help of the GP and financial assistance from the university, for C to have psychotherapy during her remaining two years as a student.

Sometimes, however, what may seem like an 'impossible' case from the history may turn out to benefit considerably from brief psychosexual therapy.

Case 3

Mr D was a 60-year-old former lorry driver who had been unable to work since he had had a coronary artery by-pass operation. He had asked for help with his erectile failure in a new relationship. He was not prepared to consider any physical treatments for his erectile fail-ure, and he was taking several drugs with the potential to cause impotence as a side effect. The psychosexual doctor receiving the referral letter thought that it was unlikely that she would be able to help much in restoring Mr D's erections, but that she might be able to help him to consider alternative ways of sexual expression, and so she duly sent him an appointment.

When he was seen at the clinic, Mr D reported that he had persuaded his GP to discon-tinue all but one of his impotence-inducing drugs. He was quite clear that he had had no problems with his erection prior to nine months before, when he had met his new partner. It emerged that when Mr D described his erections as failing, he meant that he would lose them after about 30 minutes of 'foreplay', and could then not regain the erection. Even so, there had been a recent occasion when he and his partner had been able to spend all day in bed, with intermittent, satisfactory lovemaking. Mr D's real problem was that his new girlfriend was black, and Mr D had lots of fantasies about the sexual prowess of black men, fearing he would compare unfavourably with his partner's previous lovers. He was able to look at these fantasies with the psychosexual doctor and after three appointments he was much less pre-occupied with his sense of relative inadequacy.

PROVIDING INFORMATION FOR REFERRERS

Considering that appropriate referral is considered so important by doctors working in this area, it is curious that only 30 per cent actually have a leaflet giving information for referrers. The rest presumably rely on word of mouth, and on previous 'successful' encounters with a particular doctor's patients, to ensure suitable referrals.

Eleven colleagues provided the author with copies of their leaflets for referrers. Ten of these gave details of what they regarded as unsuitable patients for referral. Eight specified a personality disorder and nine a current psychiatric illness. Five mentioned deep-seated problems leading to conflict with the law, and five suggested that there was more appropriate help available for those where the sexual problem appeared to be but a part of a much wider difficulty in the couple relationship. Four pointed out the impossibility of working when there wasn't a common language between doctor and patient. In four cases the leaflet specified what sorts of problems could be tackled, and provided a list.

Seven of the leaflets emphasized that what was on offer was brief therapy, and six made the point that it was not necessary to suggest that both partners attend the clinic. Eight explained that physical examination of the patient was likely. Most gave information on when and where the clinics were held and the names of the doctors involved, and also on how to make a referral, but only three gave information on how long the patient was likely to wait for an appointment. All made some suggestions on possible alternative sources of help for those patients who were considered unsuitable for the psychosexual medicine clinic. (The commonest suggestion was Relate for relationship difficulties, followed by urologists for erectile problems with a predominantly organic basis. The Portman Clinic, as a possible resource for those with deep-seated difficulties resulting in fetishes, exhibitionism, etc., was mentioned in four leaflets.) Five leaflets spelt out that the patient must accept that their difficulties probably had an emotional origin, and six made the point that they should be otherwise functioning well. Three doctors stated their willingness to discuss potential referrals over the phone.

PROVIDING INFORMATION FOR PATIENTS

Only slightly more of the surveyed doctors provided information for the patients about what to expect at a psychosexual medicine clinic (38 per cent). The advantage of providing such information is that a patient who knows what to expect is likely to be less apprehensive, and so more likely to work, from the beginning of the relationship with the doctor. A simple explanation can be given of how feelings can affect bodily reactions, and it can be emphasized that the patient can expect a body–mind approach to his problem. The short-term nature of the treatment can be spelt out, and information can be given about the length of appointments and expected intervals between appointments. Reassurance can be given about the confidentiality of the consultations, and it can be emphasized that it is not necessary to involve a partner unless this is wanted by the patient. It is also possible to suggest that other sources of help, for example Relate, may be more appropriate in some cases. The sort of doctor they will meet can be explained – a 'body' doctor with an interest in sexual problems rather than a psychiatrist.

Many psychosexual doctors fear that there may be real disadvantages in providing the patient with too much information about the clinic. The patient and doctor are unable to start out together with a 'blank sheet' and the patient may misinterpret some of what he has been told, so complicating the succeeding doctor–patient interactions.

Eleven doctors provided copies of the information given to patients; in eight cases this was in the form of a leaflet, and in three in the form of a letter providing additional information as well as the appointment time. In six cases the leaflet was sent to the potential patient on receiving the referral and the patient asked to make an appointment if, after reading the leaflet, he felt the clinic could help with his particular difficulty. In the other cases the information was sent with the appointment.

As with the information for referrers, no leaflets contained all the information a patient might want or need. Eight gave the names of the doctors; three mentioned that the doctors had received training with the IPM, with a further six describing the doctor as a specialist or consultant in psychosexual medicine, or as having had special training in this area. Eight included the prefix 'psycho' at some point, with only one spelling out that the doctor was not a psychiatrist. Six made it clear that this was *brief* therapy, and nine gave the duration of the appointments. Two included the likely interval between appointments.

Only three leaflets explained that a physical examination was a likely part of the consultation, with four more saying that the 'physical aspects' of the problem would be 'assessed'. Three specified the need to talk about feelings with the doctor; another five said that the 'emotional and psychological aspects' would be 'explored'.

Five leaflets were explicit about confidentiality; five stated that there was no need for the partner to attend, and two made a general comment about understanding how difficult it could be to take that first step of actually attending the clinic. Three gave the waiting time for an appointment, and most explained how to cancel an appointment, if necessary.

ARE THESE CLINICS AN EFFECTIVE USE OF NHS RESOURCES?

This question is not, at present, answerable. Obviously many people do benefit from this sort of therapy and the effect on their lives extends far beyond the purely sexual. This can be seen from some of the case studies in this volume and from others reported in the *Institute of Psychosexual Medicine Journal* and in other books on this subject (Lincoln, 1992; Tunnadine, 1992; Skrine, 1997). However, it is much more difficult to look at an unselected group of referred individuals and reach some idea of the benefit of therapy, although some attempts have been made (Bramley, 1983; Stainer-Smith, 1996).

There are many problems in trying to assess the value of the clinics. If we are trying to measure *cost*-effectiveness, then all patients who are seen at the clinic must be included in any analysis, including those who are clearly unsuitable for this sort of treatment (a further reason for doing our best to ensure appropriate referrals). Then we must consider how to assess 'success' in this area. Is it the end of a 'symptom', or is it a greater satisfaction and contentment for the patient in his sexual life? Mr D's symptom (Case 3) was unchanged at the end of his treatment, but he was much happier with his sexual relationship. It is also necessary to decide who should make the judgement about success – the doctor or the patient?

A group of IPM doctors have been working to produce a scheme that can be used to assess the usefulness, to the patients, of psychosexual medicine clinics. They have agreed that only the patient can decide whether they have benefited from their attendance (although preliminary studies suggest that there is in fact good correlation between patient and doctor views on this). Since directly asking the patient in the consultation is considered to have an unknown effect on the continuing doctor–patient relationship, the only way to ask patients is via a questionnaire. Designing a simple questionnaire that patients clearly understood took considerable time and effort.

It is not generally considered ethical to send questionnaires to patients without their prior agreement and, since the doctors hope to show change over the course of therapy, with a first questionnaire to be completed just before the first consultation, this consent has to be sought before the patient ever meets the doctor. It is hardly surprising that, in these circumstances, the proportion of patients agreeing to take part is low. It is also possible that those who do agree are atypical and particularly anxious to 'please' the doctor (which may be reflected in their questionnaire responses). In order not to bias the way the doctor interacts with the patient, it is also important to try to ensure that the doctor does not know which patients are participating. Considerable effort continues to attempt to resolve the many difficulties that have arisen and it is hoped that it will, eventually, be possible to give some sort of objective view of the usefulness of these clinics. For the time being, perhaps encouragement can be found in the fact that doctors continue to refer to the clinics, having seen the changes that have

been brought about in their patients who have attended in the past.

KEY POINTS

- The fact of referral affects both patient and doctor.
- Clinics offer *brief* therapy focused on the sexual aspects of the patient.
- Patients should be functioning normally in other areas of their lives and accept that their emotions may be playing a part in their problem.
- Referral is not appropriate for those with personality disorders or mental illness.
- It is *not* necessary to encourage the partner to attend.

REFERENCES

Bramley, M. 1983: Non-consummation of marriage treated by members of the Institute of Psychosexual Medicine: a prospective study. *British Journal of Obstetrics and Gynaecology* 90, 908–13.

Lincoln, R. 1992: *Psychosexual medicine: a study of underlying themes.* London: Chapman & Hall.

Skrine, R. 1997: *Blocks and freedoms in sexual life.* Oxford: Radcliffe Medical Press.

Stainer-Smith, A. 1996: Dare we measure patient satisfaction? *Institute of Psychosexual Medicine Journal* 12, 11–14.

Tunnadine, P. 1992: *Insights into troubled sexuality.* London: Chapman & Hall.

Appendix

TRAINING IN PSYCHOSEXUAL MEDICINE

The Institute of Psychosexual Medicine offers training for medical practitioners in brief focused psychosomatic therapy for the treatment of sexual and related difficulties.

Aims of training

At the end of training the doctor should be able to:

- Make a diagnosis in sexually related problems.
- Demonstrate an understanding of the doctor–patient relationship and its use in the diagnosis and treatment of sexual problems.
- Know which problems are suitable for brief psychosexual therapy and which should be referred elsewhere.
- Be competent to receive referrals from other practitioners and agencies.

Objectives of training

The training should increase the skills of the doctor in:

- Basic consultation skills.
  Listening.
  Observation of non-verbal communication.
  Identification of overt and covert problems together with their defences.
- Recognition and use of the doctor–patient interaction.
- Use of the genital examination appropriately as a psychotherapeutic event.
- Negotiation of plans for further work on the problem, including investigations, further appointments or referral, *and*

- The recognition and use of unconscious material (particularly for those wishing to gain the IPM Membership).

Method of training

Training is by the seminar method involving case study. A group of 7–12 doctors meets with an accredited leader for 12 hours per term (6×2 hours or 3×4 hours). Doctors are invited to present clinical encounters for discussion. They must be currently engaged in clinical work with patients so as to have cases to present. Guided by the leader and from the contributions of the group, they learn the skills of psychosexual medicine as described in chapter 6. They learn to listen and observe their patients rather than follow the traditional medical model of history taking. They learn to study what it feels like to be with that patient in the room. The validity of the doctor's approach and the perceptions of the group are tested by follow-up reports. Because of the unique nature of the doctor–patient relationship, each case is studied individually without reference to other cases. Facts, theories and generalizations about human sexual behaviour are not discussed, nor is the doctor's own personal sexual attitude or experience shared. All doctors in training are encouraged to read the Journal of the IPM, which is published several times a year, and to attend meetings of the IPM held in various parts of the country.

Training seminars are available throughout the UK.

Accreditation

Diploma

After a minimum of five terms in a Training seminar, doctors are eligible to sit the Diploma examination.

Membership

The Membership examination is for those doctors who have already obtained the Diploma and wish to make psychosexual medicine a specialist area of interest. Attendance for at least another year in a Further Training seminar is required.

Cost of training (as at January 2001)

Subscription to the IPM (obligatory for those in training): £50 per year.
Training seminars: £180 per term.
Diploma examination: £150.
Membership examination: £200.

Application for training

Information about the IPM and application for training is obtainable from:

The Administrative Secretary
The Institute of Psychosexual Medicine
12 Chandos Street
Cavendish Square
London W1G 9DP
Telephone/Fax: 020 7580 0631
Website: www.ipm.org.uk
Email: ipm@telinco.co.uk

Index

Note: Page numbers in **bold** type indicate figures; *italic* type refers to tables.